Annemarie Mol, Ingunn Moser, Jeannette Pols (eds.)
Care in Practice

Matte*Realities*/Ver*K*örperungen
Perspectives from Empirical Science Studies
Volume 8

Editorial

Since the late 1970s, *empirical science studies* have developed into a key field of research at the intersection of science, technology and society. This field merges a repertoire of theories and methods stemming primarily from cultural anthropology, sociology, linguistics and history. Its main characteristic is the detailed analysis of scientific practices and epistemic cultures and how these become entangled with public discourses and everyday life. This focus tries to reveal specific, local configurations and their epistemological as well as social consequences. Beyond a mere deconstruction, science studies are constantly looking to engage with the fields in which they do their work. The goal of this book series is to offer to scholars a German and English speaking Forum that

- develops inter- and trans-disciplinary bodies of knowledge in the areas of medicine and the life sciences and makes these nationally and internationally available;
- supports young scientists through opening up a new field of work which runs across existing disciplinary structures;
- encourages the formation of *tandems* through co-authorship. In particular, it supports, evaluates and comments on collaborative projects with colleagues from the natural and engineering sciences.

The series is directed towards scholars and students from both the empirical science/social studies and the natural sciences and medicine.

The series is edited by Martin Döring and Jörg Niewöhner.
Scientific Advisors: Regine Kollek (University of Hamburg, GER), Brigitte Nerlich (University of Nottingham, GBR), Stefan Beck (Humboldt University, GER), John Law (University of Lancaster, GBR), Thomas Lemke (University of Frankfurt, GER), Paul Martin (University of Nottingham, GBR), and Allan Young (McGill University Montreal, CAN).

ANNEMARIE MOL, INGUNN MOSER, JEANNETTE POLS (EDS.)

Care in Practice

On Tinkering in Clinics, Homes and Farms

[transcript]

The financing of this book was supported by the Norwegian Research Council and the Section of Medical Ethics, Academic Medical Centre, University of Amsterdam.

**Bibliographic information published by
the Deutsche Nationalbibliothek**
The Deutsche Nationalbibliothek lists this publication in the Deutsche Nationalbibliografie; detailed bibliographic data are available in the Internet at http://dnb.d-nb.de

© 2010 transcript Verlag, Bielefeld

transcript Verlag | Hermannstraße 26 | D-33602 Bielefeld | live@transcript-verlag.de

All rights reserved. No part of this book may be reprinted or reproduced or utilized in any form or by any electronic, mechanical, or other means, now known or hereafter invented, including photocopying and recording, or in any information storage or retrieval system, without permission in writing from the publisher.

Cover layout: Kordula Röckenhaus, Bielefeld
Layout by Rob Kreuger
Typeset by Rob Kreuger
Printed by Majuskel Medienproduktion GmbH, Wetzlar
ISBN 978-3-8376-1447-3

Contents

	page
Care: putting practice into theory Annemarie Mol, Ingunn Moser & Jeannette Pols	7
On recognition, caring, and dementia Janelle Taylor	27
Care and killing *Tensions in Veterinary Practice* John Law	57
How to become a guardian angel *Providing safety in a home telecare service* Daniel López, Blanca Callén, Francisco Tirado & Miquel Domènech	73
Care and disability *Practices of experimenting, tinkering with, and arranging people and technical aids* Myriam Winance	93
Now or later? *Individual disease and care collectives in the memory clinic* Tiago Moreira	119
Animal farm love stories *About care and economy* Hans Harbers	141
Telecare *What patients care about* Jeannette Pols	171
When patients care (too much) for information Brit Ross Winthereik & Henriette Langstrup	195
Care and its values *Good food in the nursing home* Annemarie Mol	215
Good farming *Control or care?* Vicky Singleton	235
Varities of goodness in high-tech home care Dick Willems	257
Perhaps tears should not be counted but wiped away *On quality and improvement in dementia care* Ingunn Moser	277
The syndrome we care for XPERIMENT! Bernd Kraeftner, Judith Kroell, Isabel Warner	301
List of authors	323

Care: putting practice into theory

Annemarie Mol, Ingunn Moser & Jeannette Pols

Whether we like it or not, human beings need food and shelter, and so do the animals that live with them/us.[1] Someone has to harvest or slaughter; someone has to milk; someone has to cook; someone has to build and do the carpentry. Washing is wise as well, since if they are not being washed pots, pans and bodies start to smell. Failing to dress wounds may lead to infection. And as diseases and impairments also come in other forms, there tend to be sick to look after one way or another – while everyone also needs to look after herself. All in all, care is central to daily life. However, the importance of care has not been reflected in the scholarly attention it receives. The Enlightenment tradition celebrated the mind and its alleged rationality, not the body and its pains and pleasures. To the sciences, bodies were interesting in as far as they could be objectified and explained in the laboratory, but not as they shuffled about, gasped for breath, gobbled up or lingered over food, talked, screamed, or needed to be soothed.[2] Thus, for a long time care figured in academia as a more or less tedious practical necessity, rather than as an intellectually interesting topic. Or worse: care hardly figured at all. It was relegated to the private realm: there was no need to study it, or talk about it in public settings. Someone or other just needed to get on with it.

Recently this has begun to change. First nursing theory started to talk about care. And then sociology, anthropology, geography, philosophy and ethics followed suit.[3] This book is a consequence of that process and seeks in turn to strengthen it. For this is our concern: if care practices are not carefully attended to, there is a risk that they will be eroded. If they are only talked about in terms that are not appropriate to their specificities, they will be submitted to rules and regulations that are alien to them. This threatens to take the heart out of care – and along with this not just its kindness but also its effectiveness, its tenacity and its strength. This is our concern. There is not only a domain to salvage but also, and more importantly, a mode, a style, a way of working. And thus, by describing practices to do with care, all the while wondering what care *is*, we here seek to contribute to the vitality of the *logic* of care.[4]

The chapters of this book emerge from different sites and situations. You will read about phone calls taken by operators in a telecare service for the elderly in Barcelona and about yellow tags inserted in the ears of cows in the north of England. You will be presented with stories that analyse public documents and with treatises drawing upon private experiences. Just at the moment when you have started to sympathise with the users (and the non-users!) of an online record system for pregnant women in Denmark, you will be called upon to care for a syndrome of people in a vegetative state in Austria. Diversity unfolds, even though, globally speaking, what we have gathered here is quite provincial, as all our 'materials' come from rich and Northern countries: one chapter is based in Seattle, while the others originate in villages and towns spread around Western Europe. The kinds of care we talk about are not endlessly varied either: you will find nothing here about the care of craftsmen for their creations, gardeners for their plants, wage earners for their families, dressmakers for their sewing, or parents for their children. We restrict our scope to farming, health care and care for people who are old or who cope with disabilities. At the same time, we do not so much share a set of materials as an array of theoretical resources and ambitions.[5] As a consequence a few themes recur through the book. These themes will be highlighted in this introduction. Thus, even if we obviously draw on the past, this introduction does not seek to present an overview of 'the field so far'. Rather, we introduce in the chapters that follow thematically. The themes we highlight are not of equal importance to every chapter. What is crucial to one chapter may be mentioned only in passing in the next. But jointly issues to do with 'public and private', 'the good, the bad and the ambivalent' and 'technology and humanness', constitute what as editors we take to be the originality and the force of this collection.

Public and private: about words

Writing about practices to do with caring started as a way of making public what had previously been hidden in or delegated to the private sphere. As a part of this, words designating other (more obviously public) activities were mobilised to talk about care practices. Rather than representing parental (and specifically motherly) care as a matter of love, beyond all calculation, studies seeking to stress its public importance recast such care as work. The term 'domestic labour' got coined.[6] Rather than exploring the devotion or the generosity with which doctors engage in caring, medical sociologists wrote about the social power, the status and the salary that accompanied the rise of the medical profession. Interestingly, calling motherly care 'work' was a way of adding value to it, while stressing that medical care is a professional endeavour, was done in a critical tone, as if something bad was being unmasked here.[7] There was no dialogue between (celebrating) studies of motherly care and (devastating) studies of paternalist doctors. To make things yet more complex, analysts of nursing care, while exploring how this was organised as 'women's work', argued that, for all that, nursing needed to be understood as a real profession. Rather than a criticism, this was a claim – in pursuit of power.[8] Finally, to complete our short list, the daily activities of farmers were rarely topicalised as 'care' at all. If we do so here, it is because we are struck by the similarities between farming and other caring practices. We wonder about the lessons that emerge in moving from one site to the other.

What about those who 'receive' care? Academic literatures take them to be in a precarious position. Not enough care, care in excess, the wrong kind of care: time and again the question is how to put right something that is failing. This goes for children receiving parental care, but it also applies to the elderly and people with a handicap or a disease in the context of professional care.[9] The core point became the lack of power of care-receivers, their alleged passivity, so tellingly condensed in the term 'patient' As a result other terms were introduced. Public terms. Instead of 'patient', the person who receives care was to be called a 'customer'. Customers, after all, have purchasing power: on the market they make their own choices. The term 'citizen' was introduced as a possibility as well. Addressing people in consultation rooms and care institutions as citizens was meant to emancipate them. As citizens, after all, we are not subjected to decisions, but subjects who can choose. Citizens have no overlords: they are their own rulers.

Using words coined in the public sphere while talking about care practices, drew the latter out of hiding. It sought to make them public, too. However, along the way the *specificities* of care got lost.[10] Framing care as a product for sale on a market makes it difficult to see that a lot of care work is not *bought*, but actually *done* by patients. Far from just 'receiving' care, patients actively attend to their symptoms, swallow their pills, follow their diets, and so on. Even when they are being anaesthetised they engage in the job of counting down. Patients also actively visit their doctor – usually not because they freely 'choose' to shop for care, but rather because they 'have no option'. The term 'citizen' likewise has its limits. When it comes to it, citizenship depends on faculties that people who are in need of care may (temporarily) lack. The term skips over and denies what it is that makes people look for care in the first place: their bodies happen to not submit to their wishes, let alone their commands. They are unruly.

Thus, words coined for the public sphere are ill suited for talking about care practices. What to do? There is no easy solution. Words without problematic histories just don't exist. Therefore, the contributors to this book never just take language for granted. Instead they move their words around, play with them, adapt them to what seems to best accord with what is specific to care in the practices they are describing. For example, rather than talking about *collections* of separate individuals added together, the authors tend to talk about *collectives*, variously connected and divided, from which individuals may emerge.[11] And if *bodies* are being mentioned, they do not figure as a precondition to the life of the mind, but as themselves actively (eagerly, painfully) alive and living. In the chapters about farms, humans are not necessarily in the centre: animals may care for their farmers just as much as farmers care for their animals.[12] Between humans, too, care may move in complex ways. Finally, while trying to put care practices into words, we do not bracket *failure* and *fragility*, but face up to them. For a long time, attending to public affairs has been a matter of exploring modes of control. But even if it is rendered public, care offers no control. It involves living with the erratic.[13]

Writing about care, then, means that we need to juggle with our language and adapt it. However, the most difficult aspect of writing about care is not finding *which* words to use, but dealing with the limits of using *words* at all. Care, after all, is not necessarily verbal. It may involve putting a hand on an arm at just the right moment, or jointly drinking hot chocolate while chatting about nothing in particular. A noisy machine in the corner of the room may give care, and a computer can be good at it, too. And while your cows may respond to the tone of your voice when you talk, they don't much mind what it is that you are saying. Social scientists have often insisted that professionals should listen to their patients and talk with them, rather than just silently using diagnostic techniques and handing over prescriptions. And who would disagree? But stressing the verbal too much misses out on the large non-verbal component of what is specific to care practices.

As authors of this book, we seek to give words to things (events, habits, frictions) that have previously been unspoken. Such articulation work may help to make the specificities of care practices travel. Perhaps, when articulated, when put *in so many words*, care will be easier to defend in the public spaces where it is currently at risk of being squeezed. Perhaps care practices can be strengthened if we find the right terms for talking about them. A language suitable for (self) reflection may also help those involved in care to improve their practices. However, at the same time one can only say so much. Not everything fits into language. What, then, is it to write, to make a book even? Words may carry information or, like tools, help to get something done. They may be evocative, a move in a game, a request for help, a modality of tinkering. But words only go so far. The question, then, a question that recurs throughout this book, is which words to use, and how, at the same time, to best respect the limits of the verbal. Beyond those limits, for sure, come photos and drawings. These may forcefully convey reality in a different way. But when it comes to it, 'conveying' is not the only thing reality calls for.

The good, the bad and the ambivalent

Why did care become an *object of concern* and what is it about care that warrants being studied and attended to in social science writing?[14] This question cannot be answered by pointing to bare facts, but has to do with values. It evokes the *goods* and *bads* that are at stake in care practices. The oppression of women was linked to the (public) invisibility of their (private) care work. Care-givers deserved more credit for their good work, that should also be better organised and more widely shared. Doctors, in their turn, were never taken to be disempowered by the fact that medical care remains largely hidden in consulting rooms. Rather than being too weak, doctors were (for a long time) deemed to be too strong. Their care was not accepted as self evidently good, but taken to imply their domination over others, their patients. Nursing care, again, escaped both generalities. The nursing literature, seeking to strengthen nursing as a profession, delved into the details of what goes on in care practices. In this book we build on that tradition: we unravel and articulate details to do with care. However, our particular aim is not to strengthen *nurses*, but, slightly more widely, to strengthen *care practices* – and whoever is involved in them. Thus, we talk about nursing homes, wheelchairs and webcams – and explore the feeding and slaughtering of farm animals. Rather than using large brushstrokes to cast the care we come across as either good or bad, we give detailed descriptions in the hope of opening up questions to do with qualities and values in new ways.

That this is needed has to do with developments in the care sector. While social scientists were concerned with the broader social effects of care, inside the care sector questions to do with the quality of care were asked in an entirely different way.[15] There, the great variety of activities and interactions typical to care settings, was divided up into separate 'interventions' plus the 'relational work' that facilitates their delivery. This made it possible to use the methods of epidemiology to explore which interventions were 'effective' and which were not. To give a simplified (but instructive) example: a patient and a doctor talk in a consulting room, but this is taken for granted; the drug that is finally prescribed is called *the intervention*; the patient may then take the drug (or not, nobody knows) and after a given time, one or two *parameters* are measured (that may range from blood pressure to scores on a depression test) to see if these have *improved*. One hundred people are prescribed the drug under scrutiny, and a hundred others are given a placebo. If there is more improvement among those who received the drug than among those who received the placebo, the inter- vention is called *effective*. In this way, the *clinical trial* establishes whether or not an intervention equals 'good care'. Alongside this evaluation technique, and in contrast with it, an entirely different way of investing in *the good* was institutionalised: that of medical ethics. At first, medicine was an attractive field for ethics because (unlike most other people) doctors were supposed to have power over life and death. A great normative moment. However, within a few years medical ethics no longer saw decisive doctors as interesting but as paternalistic. Thus, there was a massive shift in medical ethics to arguing in favour of *patient autonomy* and the right of patients to make their own decisions. It evaluated care practices as either respectful (good) or undermining (bad) of patient autonomy.[16]

They form a fascinating pair, clinical trials and medical ethics. In the one, the qualification of care is reduced to measuring a few relatively simple parameters and squeezing these into schemes of accountancy. In the other where patient autonomy is celebrated, what might actually be good to do does not follow from research, but becomes a matter for everyone (given 'the facts') to decide about individually. The contributions to this book venture into the enormous space left open between these two alternatives. Mostly, we go there ethnographically. Thus, while observing care practices we ask what is sought, fostered, or hoped for, then and there: what is performed as good. Likewise, we are curious about what, by contrast, is avoided, resolved, or excluded: what is performed as bad. Working in this way, we hope to learn more about 'good care' and 'bad care'. However, while sometimes the locally relevant 'good' and 'bad' are surprisingly obvious, often they are not. A lot of our stories have to do with complexities and ambivalence.[17] Good and bad may be intertwined; good intentions may have bad effects; if one looks hard enough any particular 'good' practice may hold something 'bad' inside it (and vice versa); 'good enough' care may be a wiser goal than care that is 'ever better'; while sometimes it is simply unclear whether (for whom, to what extent, in which way) some form of care deserves to be praised or to be criticised.

That our stories carry ambivalence is, or so we take it, not a failure of our analyses. Rather, it is in line with earlier contributions to the *ethics of care*. Unlike *medical ethics*, the *ethics of care* never sought to answer what is good, let alone to do so from the outside. Instead, it suggested that 'caring practices' entail a specific *modality* of handling questions to do with the good. The opposition was to other traditions in ethics, and especially to the ethics of justice. In the ethics of justice, 'ethics' is taken to be a matter of sorting out *principles* by means of argumentation. Suitable ethical principles are general, or, better still, universal. In the ethics of care it was stressed that in practice, principles are rarely productive. Instead, local solutions to specific problems need to be worked out. They may involve 'justice' but other norms (fairness, kindness, compassion, generosity) may be equally or more, important – and not in a foundational way, but as orientations among others.[18] We build on this and seek to develop it. In doing so, we do not separate out ethical from other norms (be they professional, technical, economical or practical). In care practices, after all, it is taken as inevitable that different 'goods', reflecting not only different values but also involving different ways of ordering reality, have to be dealt with together. Raising an argument about which good is best 'in general', makes little sense. Instead, care implies a negotiation about how different goods might coexist in a given, specific, local practice. Though 'negotiation' is not quite the right term, as it calls up verbal argumentation. In practice, however, seeking a compromise between different 'goods' does not necessarily depend on talk, but can also be a matter of practical tinkering, of attentive experimentation. In care, then, 'qualification' does not precede practices, but forms a part of them. The good is not something to pass a judgement on, in general terms and from the outside, but something to *do*, in practice, as care goes on.[19]

And what if the doing fails? In traditional ethical repertoires, a failure to do good is a reason for moral blame, a negative verdict. In the ethics of care this is not so obvious. What follows from a failure, remains to be seen. The crucial difference is that in rationalist versions of the world, as in fairy tales, there tend to be happy endings. Order, effectivity, efficiency, health or justice: in one way or another these may be achieved and if they are not, then someone is to blame. But in care versions of the world, the hope that one might live happily ever after is not endlessly fuelled. You do your best, but you are not going to live 'ever after'. Instead, at some point, sooner or later, you are bound to die. Along the way, there will be unfolding tensions and shifting problems. Care is attentive to such suffering and pain, but it does not dream up a world without lack. Not that it calls for cynicism either: care seeks to lighten what is heavy, and even if it fails it keeps on trying. Such, then, is what failure calls for in an ethics, or should we say an ethos, of care: try again, try something a bit different, be attentive. Thus if we had to summarise how the chapters of this book cast *good care* we would put it like this: persistent tinkering in a world full of complex ambivalence and shifting tensions.

Technology and what it is to be human

During the twentieth century it was commonly argued that *care* was other to *technology*. Care had to do with warmth and love while technology, by contrast, was cold and rational. Care was nourishing, technology was instrumental. Care overflowed and was impossible to calculate, technology was effective and efficient. Care was a gift, technology made interventions. Much of the resistance to squeezing care into technological frameworks is informed by this line of thought. It wants to keep care pure: each pole of the dichotomy should be allowed its own domain. Care (and caring relations) at home, technology (and instrumental relations) in the workplace. A life world here, and a system over there. This book sings another song. If we insist on the specificities of caring practices it is on different terms. Rather than furthering purifications, the authors of this book insist on the irreducibility of mixtures. Caring practices, to start there, include technologies: from thermometers and oxygen masks to laboratory tests and video cameras. If they happen to be helpful then they are all welcome. At the same time, engaging in care is not an innate human capacity or something everyone learns early on by imitating their mother. It is infused with experience and expertise and depends on subtle skills that may be adapted and improved along the way when they are attended to and when there is room for experimentation. Technologies, in their turn, are not as shiny, smooth and instrumental as they may be designed to look. Neither are they either straightforwardly effective on the one hand, or abject failures on the other. Instead they tend to have a variety of effects. Some of these are predictable, while others are surprising. Technologies, what is more, do not work or fail in and of themselves. Rather, they depend on care work.

On people willing to adapt their tools to a specific situation while adapting the situation to the tools, on and on, endlessly tinkering.[20]

In one way or another, then, the chapters in this book talk about both care and technology at the same time. Instead of casting care and technology in contrast with each other, we seek to rethink and reframe them together. This is our concern: to contribute to disturbing and complicating the care-technology distinction. And we interfere with other, similar distinctions, too. Care and control; care and economics; care and killing.

What changes along the way? One answer is: what it is to be human. Care practices move us away from rationalist versions of the human being. For rather than insisting on cognitive operations, they involve embodied practices.[21] Rather than requiring impartial judgements and firm decisions, they demand attuned attentiveness and adaptive tinkering. Crucially, in care practices what it is to be human has more to do with being fragile than with mastering the world. This does not imply a docile acceptance of fate: care is active, it seeks to improve life. But what it does imply is that in a care context, the 'human' is not in opposition to the 'mere beast'. Instead, the fact that human beings are animals too is calmly taken on board. No need to silence the 'beast inside us' – it is likely to call for care. No need either to silence real beasts: they deserve to be attended to on their own – nonverbal – terms. The point is not to preach equality, but to attend to everybody's specificities and to the relations in which we make each other be. Like other animals, human beings live with pain and enjoy pleasure. But unlike other animals, human beings have farms where they raise other animals and they have slaughterhouses, too. Thus, they mix care for their animals with killing them. Does killing oppose care, or may it be done in caring ways? Such questions keep presenting themselves while the webs of resonance and interdependence are extensive and complex. What in all our daily life dealings (and dealings with daily life) to call 'care' and where does the term no longer make good sense?

What follows

So these are some of the moves in which this book is caught up. At the same time, each chapter has its own specific argument to make, its own story to tell. Here's a short overview of what you may expect. We start with a chapter by Janelle Taylor who talks about recognition. 'Does she recognise you?' friends and acquaintances almost invariably ask her when they learn that her mother has dementia. The question presumes a narrowly cognitive take on what it is to be human. Mobilising auto-ethnographic stories of daily life in Seattle, Taylor turns this question round to ask instead 'Do we recognise her? How might we grant her recognition?' The recognition that a person like her mother calls for is tied up with care. Care of the mother for her children, whom she cared about. And care as a present practice, making human life worthwhile.

With a large jump we then move to a farm in the south of England in 2001. At that time, an epidemic of foot and mouth disease raged through the country and according to policies intended to halt its spread, veterinarians found themselves killing animals that they would under other circumstances have tried to keep alive. John Law tells stories about ways in which, then and there, tenderness and clinical coolness went together, and in doing so suggests what we may learn about 'care' from this particular setting. One thing is sure: veterinary care has little to do with being soft.

In the setting researched by Daniel López, Blanca Callén, Francisco Tirado and Miquel Domènech, safety is the goal of the care provided. The authors talk about a 'guardian angel': a home telecare service in Catalonia that keeps an eye – or rather a telephone-mediated ear – on elderly people living independently in their own homes. The safety granted to people, or so the authors show, does not follow from total control, but neither from trust in fate. It rather depends on a mixture of faithfully working with procedures and creatively adapting to local circumstances and specific situations.

Myriam Winance explores, in France, the tinkering character of care in a different setting, that of testing out a wheelchair and seeking how to adapt it to the specific needs of the collective in which it is to be used. Caring, she argues, is not a matter of giving something to others who may then passively receive it. To care, in this setting, is rather to meticulously explore, test, touch, adapt, adjust, pay attention to details and change them, until a suitable arrangement (material, emotional, relational) is achieved. Along the way, not only the wheelchair is adapted, but so, too, are the different people involved in using it.

Even in a clinic that was never meant to provide care, but that sought to contribute to finding a cure – a cure for Alzheimer's Disease to be precise – it is possible to catch care at work between the other regimes that order practices. Tiago Moreira shows this by telling us about an anonymised memory clinic somewhere in Britain. What is specific about care in this context, he argues, is that it is not staged as a fight against inevitable cognitive decline and does not promise the relief of a therapeutic solution. Instead it is a matter of handling daily life, of making things work from one day to the next, of tinkering. And the problems such care deals with are not localised in an individual's brain, but in the life of a collective.

With Hans Harbers we move back in time, to a Dutch farm in the nineteen fifties and sixties, the farm where he grew up. The animals on the farm got different forms of care – some were individualised and given a name, others not; some were slaughtered, others not; some were invited into the house, others not. But no universal declarations of animal rights were needed for the human-animal relations to be richer, more complex and layered, than a functionalist gloss on farming might have it. Yes, the family depended economically on their animals. But this (at that historical time?) did not exclude care, but called for it.

Still in the Netherlands, Jeannette Pols tells about present day telecare devices for people with heart failure or lung disease. Different telecare devices, or so we learn, each tackle a different problem: one a disease hidden inside a body; the next an unhealthy life style; and the third isolation and loneliness. Accordingly, the devices provide different care. The first device informs professionals about the disease so that they may tell patients what to do; the next helps patients to hold on to daily life routines that professionals have designed for them; while the third encourages patients to talk to each other so as to learn about more interesting ways of handling their daily lives with a disease. But what is it to unravel such differences, Pols asks, and where to go from here?

In Denmark Brit Ross Winthereik and Henriette Langstrup followed a project that sought to introduce a web-based record for maternity care. It came with the idea of turning the pregnant women involved into 'active patients'. However, rather than taking better care of themselves at home, the women involved were inclined to take on responsibility for the way their health care professionals used their electronic record. Thus the record helped to reconfigure the relations between pregnant women and health care professionals, but in quite unexpected ways. This, or so the authors argue, may well have to do with the inappropriate understanding of 'care' that was built into the record to begin with.

Annemarie Mol then wonders about 'good' care and she does so by telling stories to do with food and eating in Dutch nursing homes. The different *goods* at stake in this context have complex relations between them. Nutritional value and the cosiness of a pleasant meal, for instance, sometimes appear to reinforce each other whilst at other moments they clash. Taste, yet another good to do with food, shifts between food itself and the person tasting it. And seeking to assess the quality of care by measuring individual parameters, frustrates compromises between different locally relevant goods. It thus risks undermining the quality of care rather than improving it.

Seeking to assure quality by introducing systems of control, does not prove to be an unequivocal blessing either. Not in farming practice at least. Vicky Singleton lays this out with the example of the yellow tags that have to be inserted in the ears of every cow in Europe. In daily practice these tags and the bookkeeping linked up with them, are a lot more messy and bothersome than they appear from the outside. Farming practice, after all, is not a matter of individualised control, but involves living together adaptively. Singleton shows that even the relation between inspectors and farmers is put under pressure. As a disappointed informant put it: the care is going out of it.

Dick Willems writes about caring machines. With material from home care in the Netherlands, he unravels how ventilators and oxygen tanks help to constitute the lives of people with severe lung disease. What it is to breath is not a simple given in these stories, but something that changes along the way. What a body is and where it begins and ends also appears to be fluidly adaptable. And finally there is, inevitably, death. But this is not staged as the ultimate bad. Instead, the question is raised as to how the various machines involved may (or may not) help to frame a good death.

The question as to how care may be good is also central to Ingunn Moser's chapter. Seeking to assess the quality of care from the outside by counting, says Moser, does not work. Rather than spending a lot of energy on trying to do this, we would do better to invest in improving care. Detailed stories from a nursing home in Norway where the *Marte Meo* method is deployed provide an example of how this may be done. In this nursing home, videos of care practices are analysed in supervision settings so as to jointly establish what it might be good to do, and to avoid, in specific situations. The knowledge generated is not necessarily easily transportable, but it made immediate improvements to care locally.

The final word is for the research-artists of XPERIMENT! They have been involved in representing a syndrome that textbooks call 'persistent vegetative state'. While observing the intricate details of the care for the comatose patients concerned, the XPERIMENT! participants sought to describe, but especially to draw, what might, in this context, be good care. But along the way they began to wonder what it is to do such work. How to align the versions of the syndrome *represented* to the versions of the syndrome *in the field*? And is it possible for practices of research to be 'care practices' too, in their own, specific ways? Seeking to put these issues into words, the authors are at the same time caringly apprehensive of what it is to use words.

As may be clear from these short introductions, there is no iron logic in the order of our chapters. We have reasons for this particular order so we suggest that you follow it, but if you prefer to take another route then you are unlikely to encounter problems. One way or another, we hope that the texts assembled here inspire you. That you are moved by them, encouraged, sharpened. And that you feel, as you read, that you, as *the reader*, are being cared for.

Notes

1 This text has footnotes, that, beware, do not give an overview of 'the literature'. There is a lot more that is interesting to read! The main aim of these notes is to point the reader to literature that is directly relevant background of this volume. Accordingly, the proportion of titles written by 'our' authors, is very high. We seek to thus bring out how the lines of thought that we follow here, stem from a network-collective. The first 'thank you', too, is to the authors of this volume, for their generous collaborative efforts. Next, we would like to warmly thank Martin Döring and Jörg Niewöhner for being such skillfull and caring series-editors!

2 For the complexities involved in the disentangling of bodily felt passions and publically organised politics, see the contributions to: Kahn, Saccamo & Coli 2006. For a great history of the way that scientists *in practice* were far more concerned with their bodies than they theories acknowledged, see Lawrence & Shapin 1998.

3 For philosophy see Foucault 1990; for the social sciences Robinson 1998.

4 We have been trying to do this for a while. For an elaboration of the term *logic of care*, see Mol 2008; for the argument that 'care' is as creative and generative as 'science' Moser 2008; and for the contrast between 'rights' and 'care', Pols 2003.

5 Most of us have a background in the *Social Studies of Science and Technologies* and from there have moved out to the study of other practices, all the while keeping an open eye for the ways science and technology inform and interfere with these practices. For this background see e.g. Callon & Law 1997; M'charek 2005; Latour 2002; Thompson 2005; Barry 2001.

6 This gave raise to heated debates in the seventies; and the topic is still important, not only because the domestic labour still is far from equally shared, but also because currently it is substantially shifted round the globe by being 'outsourced' to poor regions, see e.g. Anderson 2000.

7 The classic author to quote here is Freidson. More recently, however, Freidson has shifted his way of writing about the medical profession from generalised criticism to a more layered approach, open to internal differentiation. See therefore now: Freidson 2001.

8 This is still going on- for nurses professionalism continues to be a promise at the horizon. See for a recent example Cohen 2008.

9 For literatures that take up the question of the person potentially 'receiving' care (and/or engaging in self-care), see: Epstein 1996; Shakespeare 2006; Moser 2000 & 2005; Callon & Rabeharisoa 2003; Barbot & Dodier 2002; Barbot 2006.

10 For various aspects of the argument that 'customer' and/or 'citizen' might not be suitable terms in this context, see: Mol 2008; Callon & Rabeharisoa 2004; Winance 2007; Pols 2005; Pols 2006b; Moser 2006; Singleton 2007; Langstrup & Ross Winthereik 2008; López & Domènech 2009.

11 The typical reference point here is the work of Callon & Rabeharisoa, but for a good example see also Moreira 2004.

12 Here a crucial reference is the recent work on animal as it revises earlier thoughts on human-animal relations. See for instance Despret 2004.

13 For earlier work on the issue of fragility, see: Struhkamp 2005; Varela 2001; Diedrich 2005.

14 For the notion of 'concern' and its contrast with 'critique', see Latour 2004.

15 For some of the analyses of such (self) surveilance, see: Ashmore, Mulkay & Pinch 1989; Pols 2006a; May, Rapley, Moreira, Finch & Heaven 2006; Struhkamp, Mol & Swierstra 2009.

16 Obviously there is a lot more to say about this that complicates these catchy phrases. See for the approaches of ethics and ethnography: Parker 2007; Pols 2008.

17 For the issue of ambivalence *within* technoscience see: Singleton & Michael 1993; and Singleton 1998.

18 The classic reference is: Tronto 1993; for a more recent publication in this line of work, see: Hamilton & Miller 2006. For a sociological approach, concentrating on the value generosity, see Frank 2004; and for the value dignity, see Nordenfelt 2009.

19 For an example of this, see Winance 2006.

20 For the argument that *technology* is far more messy than most analists have it, and depends on care, see: Law and Singleton 2000; Law 2002; Latour 2002; Oudshoorn & Pinch 2005; Harbers 2005. For the argument that *care* always already includes technology, see: Hendriks 1998; Akrich & Pasveer 2000; Willems 2002; Harbers, Mol & Stolmeijer, 2002; Moser & Law 2003; López & Domènech 2008. For an explicit discussion of the 'warmth' involved, see Pols & Moser 2009.

21 This comes with a re-thought 'body', too – the body is no longer taken to be given and waiting for the medical gaze to discover it, but is studied as it interacts with medical technologies, while thus being performed in quite particular, varying ways. See for this: Mol 2002; Taylor 2005; Mol & Law 2004; Pickstone 2000; Moreira 2006; Taylor 2008. An imaginative exploration of the body in care practice was presented by Xperiment! in the exposition *Making Things Public* in 2005. For a trace of that, see XPERIMENT! 2005.

References

Akrich, M. & Pasveer, B. (2000) Multiplying Obstetrics: Techniques of Surveillance and Forms of Coordination, in: *Theoretical Medicine and Bioethics*, 21, 63-83.

Akrich, M. and Pasveer, B. (2004) Embodiment and disembodiment in childbirth narratives, *Body & Society* 10 (2-3), 63-84.

Anderson, B. (2000) *Doing the dirty work: the global politics of domestic labour*, Zen Books.

Armstrong, D. (2002) A New History of Identity. *A Sociology of Medical Knowledge*, Basingstoke: Palgrave Macmillan.

Ashmore, M., M. Mulkay & T. Pinch, (1989) *Health and Efficiency. A sociology of health economics*, Open University Press.

Barbot J. (2006) How to build an 'active' patient' The work of AIDS associations in France, Social Science & Medicine, 3, 538-551.

Barbot, J. and Dodier, N. (2002) Multiplicity in Scientific Medicine: The Experience of HIV-Positive Patients, in Science, *Technology and Human Values*, 27, 3, 404-440.

Barry, A. (2001) *Political Machines. Governing a Technological Society*, London: Athlone Press.

Callén, B.; López, D.; Domènech, M. y Tirado, F. (2009) Telecare Research: Cosmopolitizing Methodology, in: *European Journal of Disability Research*, 3, 2, 110-122.

Callon, M. and Rabeharisoa, V. (2003) Research in 'the wild' and the shaping of new social identities, in *Technology and Society*, 25, 2, 193-204.

Callon, M. and Rabeharisoa, V. (2004) Gino's lesson on humanity: genetics, mutual entanglements and the sociologist's role, in *Economy and Society*, 33, 1, 1-27.

Cohen, S. (2008) Our image, our choice. *Perspectives on sharing, empowering and elevating the nursing profession*, Marblehead: Hcpro Inc.

Despret, V. (2004) The Body we Care for: figures of anthropo-zoo-genesis, *Body and Society*, 10 (2-3), 111-134.

Diedrich, L. (2005) A bioethics of failure. Anti-heroic cancer narratives in: Shildrick, M. & Mykitiuk, R. Ethics of the body. *Postconventional challenges*, Cambridge, Mass: MIT-Press.

Epstein, S. (1996) *Impure Science. AIDS, Activism and the Politics of Knowledge*, Berkeley, Univ. of California Press.

Foucault, M. (1990) *Care of the self, The history of sexuality 3* (translation: R. Hurley) Penguin Books.

Frank, A. (2004) *The Renewal of Generosity. Illness*, Medicine and How to Live, Chicago: The University of Chicago Press.

Freidson, E. (2001) *Professionalism, the third logic*, Polity Press.

Hamington, M. & D. Miller, eds. (2006) *Socializing Care*, Oxford: Rowman & Littlefield.

Harbers, H. (ed) (2005) *Inside the politics of technology. Agency and normativity in the co-production of technology and society*. Amsterdam: Amsterdam University Press.

Harbers, H. Mol, A. & Stollmeijer, A. (2002) Food Matters. Arguments for an Ethnography of Daily Care, in: *Theory, Culture and Society*, 19 (5/6), 207-226.

Hendriks, R. (1998). Egg timers, human values and the care of autistic youths. *Science, Technology & human values*, 23 (4), 399-424.

Kahn, V. Saccamano, N. and Coli, D. eds. (2006) *Politics and the Passions* 1500-1850, Princeton: Princeton University Press.

Langstrup, H. and Ross Winthereik, B. (2008) The Making of Self-Monitoring Asthma Patients: Mending a Split Reality with Comparative Ethnography, in *Comparative Sociology*, 7, 3,362-386.

Latour, B. (2002) Morality and Technology: The End of the Means, in: *Theory, Culture & Society*, 19, 5/6, 247-260.

Latour, B. (2004) Why has critique run out of steam? From matters of fact to matters of concern, *Critical Inquiry* 30, 225-248.

Law, J. (2002) *Aircraft stories. Decentering the object in technoscience*, Durham: Duke University Press.

Law, J. (2004) *After method. Mess in social science research*, London: Routledge.

Law, J. and Singleton, V. (2000) Performing technology's stories: On social constructivism, performance, and performativity, in: *Technology and Culture*, 41, 4, 765-775.

C. Lawrence & Shapin, S. (1998) *Science incarnate. Historical embodiments of natural knowledge*, Chicago: University of Chicago Press.

López, D. and Domènech, M. (2008) On inscriptions and ex-inscriptions: the production of immediacy in a home telecare service. in: Environment and Planning D: *Society and Space*, 26, 663-675.

López, D. and Domènech, M. (2009). Embodying autonomy in a Home Telecare Service. *Sociological Review*, 56, 2, 181-195.

May, C., T. Rapley, T. Moreira, T. Finch & B. Heaven (2006) Technogovernance: Evidence, subjectivity, and the clinical encounter in primary care medicine, in: *Social Science & Medicine*, 62, 4, 1022-1030.

M'charek, A. (2005) *The Human Genome Diversity Project. An Ethnography of Scientific Practice*, Cambridge: Cambridge University Press.

Mol, A. (2002) *The Body Multiple: Ontology in Medical Practice*. Durham, Duke University Press.

Mol, A. (2008) *The Logic of Care. Health and the Problem of Patient Choice*, London: Routledge.

Mol A. & Law J. (2004) Embodied action, enacted bodies. The example hypoglycaemia. *Body and Society*, 10, 43-62.

Moreira, T. (2004) Self, agency and the surgical collective: detachment, in; *Sociology of Health & Illness* 26, 1, 32-49.

Moreira, T. (2006) Heterogeneity and Coordination of Blood Pressure in Neurosurgery, in: *Social Studies of Science*, 36, 1, 69-97.

Moser, I. (2000) Against normalisation: Subverting norms of ability and disability, *Science as Culture*, 9, 2, 201-240.

Moser, I. (2005) On becoming disabled and articulating alternatives: the multiple modes of ordering disability and their interferences, in *Cultural Studies*, 19, 6, 667-700.

Moser, I. (2006) Disability and the promise of technology: Technology, subjectivity and embodiment within an order of the normal, in: *Information, Communication and Society*, 9, 3, 373-395.

Moser, I. (2008) Making Alzheimer's Disease matter: Enacting, interfering, doing politics of nature, *Geoforum*, 39, 1, 98-110.

Moser, I. & Law, J. (2003). 'Making Voices': New Media Technologies, Disabilities and Articulation. In: Liestöl, G., Morrison, A. and Rasmussen, T. (eds) *Digital Media Revisited. Theoretical and Conceptual Innovation in Digital Domains*. Cambridge: MIT-Press, 491-520.

Nordenfelt, L. (ed.) (2009) *Dignity in care for older people*, Chichester: Wiley-Blackwell.

Oudshoorn, N. & Pinch, T. (eds) (2005) *How Users Matter: The Co-Construction of Users and Technology*, The MIT-Press.

M. Parker (2007) Ethnography/ethics, in: *Social Science & Medicine*, 65, 11, 2248-2259.

Pickstone, J. (2000) *Ways of knowing. A new history of science, technology and medicine*, Manchester: Manchester University Press.

Pols, J. (2003) Enforcing patient rights or improving care? The interference of two modes of doing good in mental health care, in: *Sociology of Health & Illness*, 25, 3, 320-347.

Pols, J. (2005) Enacting appreciations: beyond the patient perspective. *Health Care Analysis*, 13, 3, 203-221.

Pols, J. (2006a) Accounting and Washing, in: *Science, Technology & Human Values*, 31, 4, 409-430.

Pols, J. (2006b) Washing the citizen: washing, cleanliness and citizenship in mental health care, *Culture, Medicine & Psychiatry* 30, 1, 2006, p.77-104.

Pols, J. (2008) Which empirical research, whose ethics? Articulating ideals in long-term mental health care. In: Widdershoven, G., Hope, T., Van der Scheer, L. & McMillan, J. (eds) *Empirical Ethics in Psychiatry*. Oxford University Press, 51-68.

Pols, J. & Moser, I. (2009) Cold technologies versus warm care? On affective and social relations with and through care technologies, ALTER, *European Journal of Disability Research*, 3, 159-178.

Robinson, F. (1998) *Globalising Care: Feminist Theory, Ethics and International Relations*, Boulder CO: Westview Press Inc.

Shakespeare, T. (2006) *Disability rights and wrongs*, London: Routledge.

Singleton, V. & Michael, M. (1993) Actor networks and ambivalence. General practitioners in the UK Cervical Screening Program. *Social Studies of Science* 23, 227-64.

Singleton, V. (1998) Stabilizing instabilities: The role of the laboratory in the United Kingdom Cervical Screening Programme, in Berg, M. & Mol, A. eds. (1998) *Differences in Medicine. Unravelling practices, techniques and bodies*, Durham: Duke University Press.

Singleton, V. (2007) Training and resuscitating healthy citizens in the English New Public Health – normativities in process, in: K. Asdal, B. Brenna and I. Moser (eds.) (2007) *Technoscience: The politics of interventions*, Oslo: Oslo Academic Press, unipub Norway.

Struhkamp, R. (2005) Wordless pain. Dealing with suffering in physical rehabilitation, Cultural Studies, 19, 6, 701-718.

Struhkamp, R. A. Mol & T. Swierstra (2009) Dealing with Independence: Doctoring in Physical Rehabilitation Practice, in: Science, *Technology and Human values*, 34: 55-76.

Taylor, J. (2005) Surfacing the Body Interior, in: *Annual Review of Anthropology*, 34, 741-756.

Taylor, J. (2008) *The Public Life of the Fetal Sonogram. Technology, Consumption and the Politics of Reproduction*, Rutgers University Press.

Tronto, J. (1993) *Moral Boundaries: a political argument for an ethic of care*, London: Routledge.

Varela, F. (2001) Intimate distances: fragments for a phenomenology of organ transplantation, *Journal of Consciousness Studies*, 8, 5-7.

Willems, D. (2002) Managing one's body using self-management techniques: practicing autonomy, in: *Theoretical Medicine and Bioethics*, 31, 1, 23-38.

Winance, M. (2006) Trying Out the Wheelchair. The Mutual Shaping of People and Devices through Adjustment, in: *Science, Technology & Human Values*, 31, 1, 52-72.

Winance M. (2007), Being normally different? Changes to normalisation processes : from alignment to work on the norm, in: *Disability and Society*, 22, 6, 625-638.

XPERIMENT! (2005) What is a Body / a Person? Topography of the possible, in: Latour, B. & P. Weibel eds., *Making Things Public*, Cambridge, Mass.: MIT Press, p 906-909.

On recognition, caring, and dementia

Janelle S. Taylor

My mother is living with progressive dementia. Since my father died, about three and a half years ago now, I have been very involved in her care.

I am listening for it. Because I am writing these words rather than speaking them, I cannot hear your response, but I am listening for the question that, as I have learned, always comes.

I speak about my mother and her condition to friends, coworkers, and others around me, as openly as I would about any other important aspect of my family life. Over time, I have noticed that at the mention of dementia, memory loss, or Alzheimer's, *everyone*, almost without exception, responds with some version of the same question:

> 'Does she recognize you?'

There are variants, of course:

> 'Does she still know who you are?'
> 'She's aware of you, though?'
> 'But at least she still knows your name, right?'

However it may be phrased, the question is always whether my mother *recognizes* me, meaning: can she recite 'the facts' of who I am, what my name is, and how I am related to her?

Frequent repetition has made this question sound strange to me. As a daughter, I have learned that when someone you love asks you the same question over and over again, it is probably a symptom of dementia. As an anthropologist, however, I am convinced that when *many* people ask the same question over and over again, it is probably a symptom of something important and unresolved about social life. If the mere mention of dementia very regularly calls forth particular kinds of questions about 'recognition', this seems to me a social fact worthy of reflection.

In this essay, I take such questions as the entry point for an inquiry into recognition, its linkages to care, and what these linkages imply –

for people living with dementia, and for the rest of us, the 'Temporarily Able-Brained' (Friedell 2003) who share a world with them today, and who may ourselves join their ranks in the future.

The research on which I report here is of the decidedly unchosen variety, thrust on me by life-changing losses that I would have avoided if I could, but from which I have learned a great deal nonetheless. My training as a medical anthropologist has moved me, through all that has happened, to keep notes and record observations about conversations, events, and experiences that seemed important, to collect materials and documents that seemed relevant, and to search out and read scholarly analyses as well as personal accounts of dementia. The account that follows is thus 'autoethnographic', in the sense that it addresses certain aspects of the social world that have become visible and interesting to me by virtue of my particular position as daughter of a lovely and beloved mother with advanced dementia. It is an attempt to tell the truth as I see it, from where I now stand.

'Does she recognize you?'

It is tempting to look beyond and behind this question for the intentions that motivate any particular person to ask it. I believe it is worth resisting the impulse to jump to explanations pitched at the level of individuals, however, at least long enough to ponder the very specific and widely-shared form that this question takes, as a query about 'recognition'.

The philosopher Paul Ricoeur, in *The Course of Recognition* (Ricoeur 2005) seeks to develop a philosophical approach to 'recognition' that could embrace the full range of the term's many meanings. Beginning from the definitions listed in dictionaries, Ricoeur considers the points of etymological and semantic overlap that link one sense of 'recognition' to another. Underlying this proliferation of meanings, he identifies three significant semantic clusters, which he construes as moments in a dialectic that begins from recognition as identification (of things), moves through self-recognition, and finally concludes with recognition by an Other. As he shows, critical transformations take place in the course of the movement from the first of these moments to the last: 'recognition' changes from the active to the passive voice, as it moves from a cognitive and intellectual matter to an ethical and political one. What begins in the sovereign self's active intellectual 'recognition' of external objects ends in the socially and politically embedded subject's passive receipt of 'recognition' granted by others.

It is the broad scope of Ricoeur's framing of 'recognition' that I find so helpful. When a friend or acquaintance or coworker asks me, 'Does she recognize you?' he or she is, in Ricoeur's terms, giving voice to the first of the three distinct 'moments' in the 'course of recognition': the question concerns my mother's ability, as a sovereign self, to actively draw intellectual distinctions among the objects and people around her. I have come to think, however, that also at stake here is Ricoeur's third and final 'moment', when the subject is granted social and political recognition by others.

Ordinarily in my life, when someone asks me a question that I find baffling or rude, I respond with a query of my own: 'Why do you ask?' Riceour's analysis helps me to similarly turn around the question that people are always asking me about my mother, and respond with a query of my own. How are claims to social and political 'recognition' linked to, or premised on, the demonstrated capacity to 'recognize' people and things? When elderly people with dementia suffer cognitive changes, how do these get invested with decisive importance in determining whether and how they are (or are not) granted "recognition" as fully social persons and members of a community?

When everyone keeps asking me 'Does she recognize you?' I believe the question really is – or should be – 'Do you, do we, recognize *her*? Do we *grant her recognition*?'

'Does she recognize you?'

I was first led to ponder at length the meanings of the term 'recognition', by the simple fact that I found this question both ubiquitous and quite difficult to answer.

My Mom is always glad to see me. Does she still know my name? It has been years since I've heard her say it. Not long ago, she pointed to a painting of her father that hangs in her room, and said, 'That's my Dad'. And at least up until a year or so ago, she referred by name to Chuck, my father, to whom she was married for forty-nine years until his death. But I have heard her speak no other names for a very long time. At this point, my mother has considerable difficulty finding all kinds of words, let alone names. When words do come, they disperse too quickly, and rarely hang together long enough to form a full sentence. I do not expect that I will ever again hear my name spoken in my mother's voice.

Even before she became impaired, however, my mother rarely ever called me Janelle. That was the name she gave me at birth, and it has always been the name I use outside my family, but over the years my Mom gave me many other names as well. At home I was Nellie, or sometimes Nelle-Belle. But usually, I was Sweetie, Honey, Kid, Pumpkin, Friend, Pest or any one of many other silly nicknames.

And now, I am Stranger. One day some months ago, I walked into the activity-room of the secure dementia unit where my mother now lives, and found her sitting at a table with three other white-haired ladies and two pretty young aides, playing some version of poker with a set of enormous playing-cards. Mom saw me, and a smile slowly spread over her face, as she raised her hand to point at me, and said: 'Well, hello there, Stranger!' It's a name that one would use, of course, only for someone who is very familiar. When she calls me Stranger, I know that I am no stranger to her.

Not only is it hard to know whether my mother 'recognizes' me, in the narrow sense of remembering my name, but the question itself also seems to me more and more irrelevant. I know that it is out of concern for me, as well as for my mother, that well-meaning friends and acquaintances ask me this question. They are seeking a landmark by which to gauge the stage of my mother's progress along what everyone understands to be a one-way journey downhill. Those who have little firsthand experience with dementia tend, I think, to imagine it as a more or less purely cognitive loss of a store of remembered facts, manifested in a loss of the ability to recite names and dates and other bits of information. Knowing the names of one's own children presents itself, in this view, as the most obvious and dramatic of what Elinor Fuchs calls the 'stills'. Fuchs writes:

> One can measure the advance of dementia by the 'stills'. The social worker will ask the *still* questions: Does she *still* feed herself? *Good!* Still chew? *Good!* Still toilet? Well, that's to be expected. And we have ours: Still like to dress up? Get her hair done? Her nails? Still hang on to her French and German? Yes, a few words, pretty good accent. Still play the piano? Oh yes, the 'Anniversary Waltz', over and over. Still like parties? Oh-ho, *does she ever*! (Fuchs 2005:4).

Yet it is worth noting that the ability to remember names does not even merit a place in Fuchs's own list of 'stills'. Set in the context of questions about the degree to which a person is able to eat, bathe, dress, or speak, and so on, whether he or she remembers names may not seem so important.

For those who have some personal experience with dementia, the 'stills' are paralleled by the 'firsts'. The first time my mother repeated the same question several times in the course of a short telephone conversation, almost nine years ago now, I wept inconsolably at the prospect of, as I then feared, 'losing her'. In retrospect, that first 'first' seems to me quite innocuous, and my response to it rather overwrought. I marvel that such a minor impairment once seemed to me so terrifying. Other 'firsts' that have come since have been harder. The first time after my father's death that Mom asked where he was. The first time I had to make a decision about her medications. The first time she tried to sign her own name and could not. The first time she needed my help in the shower.

Yet it bears saying that not all of the 'stills' and the 'firsts' necessarily tell a grim story of unremitting decline, loss, humiliation and disappearance. Despite all the changes she has been through, my mother 'still' is in many ways the cheerful, affectionate person I have always known her to be. Mom still enjoys gentle joking and teasing, as she always has. She still enjoys being around people, still beams radiantly at small children when she sees them, still enjoys the give-and-take of conversation. And for my part, I must say that some of the 'firsts' have been tender moments that I cherish. The 'first' time since my early childhood that my Mom and I walked down the street holding hands. The first time I tucked her into bed at night with her stuffed animals all around her. The first time (in at least forty years) that we sang together a loud and unabashed, if slightly out-of-tune, chorus of 'She'll Be Coming Round the Mountain'.

Amid so many 'stills' and 'firsts', many sad and painful, some sweet and funny, the more I become involved with the practicalities of caring for my mother, the weirder it seems to me that everyone else seems to care only about the one very narrow question of whether she still 'recognizes' me in the very specific sense of being able to identify me by name.

'Does she recognize you?'

The weirdness of the question becomes more obvious when one pauses to consider the procedure that would be required to answer it.

Imagine that you come upon two people, and one of them is urgently questioning the other: *'What is my name? Who am I? How old am I? How do we know each other?'* Would you not assume that it is the *questioner*, rather than the one being questioned, who suffers from a loss of memory?

I don't *need* my mother to tell me my name, or how I am related to her. I already *know* these things. And I *know*, furthermore, that she suffers cognitive losses – that's just what it means to have dementia. So why, then, would I make a point of asking her these questions that I *know* she cannot possibly answer? To do so seems to me rude by all normal standards of social intercourse, if not downright mean. I can't bring myself to do it. I guess you could say that my mother raised me better than that.

But of course, by the time one embarks on such interrogations, one is already acting on the judgment that 'normal standards of social intercourse' do not apply. And in many ways they really *cannot* apply to people with dementia, who often speak or behave weirdly, and in that sense are rude, simply because their impairment prevents them keeping straight the rules of social intercourse and the sense of how to act within them. Still, I find it remarkable that for many people whose cognitive functioning is *not* impaired, who *can* still observe social niceties, the mere suspicion that someone else *might* suffer dementia seems to justify, or even require, that they suspend all the rules and habits learned over a lifetime, about how to treat another person politely and with kindness. Lauren Kessler recalls:

> I always corrected her when she called me Judy (her sister). Every time I visited, I took down the framed photographs from her dresser – the ones I had brought in to remind her of her family – pointed to each, and quizzed her. 'You know who this is, don't you, Mom?' Of course, she didn't. So I told her, again and again, each visit, who was who. And then quizzed again… Thinking back on this now, I am appalled at my insensitivity. What did I think I was doing? After months of reality orientation, I managed to accomplish only two things: I made myself miserable, and I made my mother irritable. (Kessler 2007:88).

Kessler is unusual only in the degree of critical reflection with which she now recalls these matters. The kind of grilling to which she once subjected her mother is common – common enough that one very nice little book offering practical tips on how to talk to a family member or friend with Alzheimer's specifically advises: 'Don't ask them to tell you what your name is, or how you are related to them' (Strauss 2001:95)

'Does she recognize you?'

When my friends inquire whether my mother still recognizes me, they speak out of sympathetic concern for me, and the emotional suffering they assume I must experience, from what is regularly described as 'the horror of Alzheimer's'. One component of this horror is an ethical judgment.

Not only is it tragic, but it is *wrong* for a person to forget their close relations, especially family relations. Philosopher Avishai Margalit, in a book entitled *The Ethics of Memory*, asks:

> Is there an ethics of memory?... Are we obligated to remember people and events from the past? If we are, what is the nature of this obligation? Are remembering and forgetting proper subjects of moral praise or blame? (Margalit 2002:7).

Margalit concludes that there is an *ethics* of memory, but very little *morality* of memory. In his argument, ethics pertains to 'thick' social relations with those nearest and dearest to us in our lives, whereas morality concerns 'thin' social relations with people to whom we are not bound by any special ties, 'the stranger and the remote'. Shared memory is, he contends, 'the cement that holds thick relations together'.

Memory of names is an especially important ingredient of that cement. *The Ethics of Memory* begins with the story of an Israeli army commander who publicly admitted that he had forgotten the name of a soldier in his unit who was killed under his command. His comment drew responses of angry outrage because, Margalit explains, remembering the name of the soldier is just a metonym for remembering the young soldier himself – it is remembering the person that is important. Remembering the person is important because without it, caring is not possible:

> What is at stake here is the officer's *caring*... The relation between memory and caring... is, I maintain, an internal relation – a relation that could not fail to obtain between these two concepts since memory is partly constitutive of the notion of care. If I care for someone or for something, and then I forget that person or that thing, this means that I have stopped caring for him or it (Margalit 2002:27-28).

For Margalit, 'caring' is primarily an attitude toward others. He works to specify just what kind of attitude it is, and how it differs from others: caring 'suggests regard for other people' (p. 31), it 'is concerned with their wants and needs' (p. 34), it 'is a selfless attitude' (p. 35), and it is 'a demanding attitude toward others' because 'what we find hard is the *attention* that is implied by caring' (p. 33). However we may specify it, though, 'caring' remains a subjective and internal state of mind and feeling of a discrete individual, and one that is premised upon a capacity for 'recognition' in its narrowly cognitive sense.

On Margalit's account, if my mother has forgotten my name, and does not 'recognize' me, then she has surely stopped 'caring' about me.

'Does she recognize you?'
I am not so convinced that the inability to remember names necessarily means that a person with dementia cannot 'recognize' or 'care' about other people, for reasons I will explore below. But very often, it does mean that other people stop 'recognizing' and 'caring' about *them*.

When my father died, five hundred people attended his memorial service. Many of them were people I did not know, part of the large circle of friends, acquaintances, colleagues, and former students he had come to know over the decades that he worked at a Seattle-area public high school as a principal with a very hands-on administrative style and an outgoing, friendly demeanor. Many of these people knew my mother, however, and some were longtime friends of my parents whom I recognized, by face or at least by name, from my earliest childhood. Others were people they knew through the various groups in which they had taken part: the investment club, the monthly discussion 'salon', the group of people who walked with them every morning at the local mall, and others. Some were primarily my mother's friends: neighbors, women she had worked with at her various office jobs over the years, mothers of the friends of some of her children with whom she had become close, old friends from her college days. On that day, united with her in grief, all of these people greeted Mom with hugs, and tears, and condolences.

And then they disappeared. A few did come to see Mom at least once or twice, in the first months after Dad died. But those few visits aside, whenever I scanned the 'guest sign-in' sheet at the facility where Mom lived, I saw – no one. Two and a half years later, when it came time to move Mom into a specialized dementia unit located in a different assisted-living facility, I wrote to all of my parents' friends for whom I had any contact information, updating them on her situation, letting them know her new address, telling them that she would doubtless enjoy receiving visits, asking them to please forward my note to anyone else I may have missed, and to please contact me with any questions they might have. No one replied.

Only one friend remains present in my mother's life. Every month or two, Eli Davis drives an hour and a half from her home to Seattle to visit Mom, bringing treats, and hugs, and her perennially cheerful self, even pre-arranging with the staff to lead a storytelling session for all the dementia-ward residents. I love her dearly for it – and I wonder: where are the others? Where are the couples with whom my parents socialized, the women with whom Mom spent hours and hours on the phone all through my childhood? What has become of all their friends? I think about the individual friends of my parents whom I know; each one is a warm, funny, kind person. The sad fact is, however, that as a group, they have abandoned her.

This should not surprise me as much as it has. It is, perhaps, hardly fair to expect friends to step up to challenges from which even close kin often shrink. The same may not be true everywhere (and I venture to hope that further life experience may prove it untrue here too) but it seems to me that middle-class American friendships are not generally expected to bear the weight of deep and diffuse obligations to care. More like pleasure crafts than life rafts, they are not built to brave the really rough waters – and these are rough, corrosive, bitter waters indeed. Dementia seems to act as a very powerful solvent on many kinds of social ties. I doubt that many friendships survive the onset of dementia (and, perhaps tellingly, I have been unable to locate any published research about friendships and dementia).

Often, in the social world that my parents (and I) inhabit, friendships are grounded in shared experiences of dealing with the practicalities of life, as 'consociates' who work in the same office, are enrolled in the same institution, pick up kids at the same daycare, and so forth, and tend to fade away once those realities are no longer shared (Plath 1980). Once my mother was retired from work, her children grown up and gone, many such connections atrophied, and she formed few new ones. As her capacities diminished, her social world contracted severely, until it centered almost exclusively (and rather oppressively) on my father.

Friendships in this social world are also built up and sustained through ongoing exchanges of invitations, confidences, favors, gifts, cards, and the like. As Ricoeur discusses, 'the logic of giving gifts usually entails reciprocity, which is minimally evident in gratitude and more often demands a return in kind' (Connolly 142). When friendship is grounded in reciprocity, then a person who no longer can engage in the usual social exchanges, is difficult to 'recognize' any longer as a friend. At my father's memorial, I saw one of my parents' old friends for the first time in many years, and explained to her briefly that Mom has what seems to be Alzheimer's. She exclaimed, 'Yes, well, I haven't gotten a *Christmas* card from her in *years!*' She still sounded quite indignant.

The fact of my mother's having moved into an institution may also go far toward explaining her social abandonment. The facility where my siblings and I placed her after our father's death was not a nursing home, but a 'retirement community' catering to the wealthy and the well-insured, where only a few residents were impaired, and Mom had her own pleasant little apartment furnished with her own belongings. The place had more the feel of a college dormitory than of a scary medical institution. Still, any medical institutionalization arguably entails a form of 'social death'. Writing about Alzheimer's units in nursing homes, J. Neil Henderson describes this view:

> ...When a person is institutionalized, he or she experiences a process of mortification (Goffman 1961). The root *mort*, as in *death*, is not accidental in Goffman's use of *mortification* to characterize the effect of placement... When a person is extracted from home because of dependencies that interrupt his or her ability, or his or her family's ability, to cope with the exigencies of life, the nursing home placement process becomes step one in a double burial ritual... The now-institutionalized person's psychosocial self is slain at the nursing home door. At this point, the sometimes lengthy step two of the double burial ritual begins. Rather than lie supine on the burial scaffold, as in some cultures, the patient languishes in long-term patienthood until biological functions cease, at which time the second, and final, burial occurs... (Henderson 2003:155).

Not only friends, but even their close family members often virtually abandon elderly people who are institutionalized with dementia. The vast majority visit them only briefly and occasionally (Yamamoto-Mitani 2002). And even among family who serve as primary caregivers of people with dementia, 'in practice, the ability to recognise others appears to be the most important determinant of whether or not social death occurs' (Sweeting and Gilhooly 98).

'Does she recognize you?'

After the inevitable question comes, very often, the anecdote. It takes the form of a story about an encounter with someone who does not remember the speaker. Failure to remember a name almost always serves as the punchline:

> '...but I don't really think she even knew the children's names.'
> '...and then I realized that she didn't even remember me at all.'

I know that the people who tell me these stories do so out of a sympathetic impulse, but I am always left somewhat at a loss. What am I supposed to say? Usually I mumble some sort of awkward defense of the person, 'Well, yeah, she probably has some memory loss... I'm sure she can't help it'.

Over time, I have come to think that what is important about these stories is the way that evidence of dementia always serves to *end* them. It is as if someone with dementia never *could* any longer be part of any story that might continue – and if the life *story* is over, then the life must be over too. More than once, some compassionate interlocutor has remarked to me how difficult it must be to have lost both my father and my mother. I find myself having to insist: 'But I have not lost my mother, she is not dead'.

It is not insignificant, I think, that the term *Alzheimer's* (with which all forms of dementia are commonly equated) is so frequently conjoined with the word 'horror'. When it comes to speaking or writing about dementia, horror seems to be the default genre. A person you love, and to whom you are bound by unbreakable ties, turns out to be someone you do not know at all, who does not 'care' about you and may even seek to harm you: this is the classic gothic plot. It surfaces everywhere. To take just one example, consider this passage from Stephen Holden's *New York Times* review of Bille August's 2002 film, 'A Song for Martin':

> Like 'Iris', 'A Song for Martin' unblinkingly focuses on the special horror of Alzheimer's as Barbara helplessly watches her husband turn into a stranger and disappear before her eyes... (Holden 2002: E13).

Or, alternatively, a person dies but their body lives on: this is the basic zombie story. In an article titled 'Death in Slow Motion: A Descent Into Alzheimer's', which I read in *Harper's* magazine around the time I first began to use the term *Alzheimer's* in connection with my own mother, Eleanor Cooney described her mother in terms strongly reminiscent of the zombie story:

> I grieve for her exactly as if she'd died. She's gone, I've lost her, but I'm still responsible for her living, breathing body and the ghosts in her head... (Cooney 2001: 57).

Even organizations that advocate for people with Alzheimer's fall into horror stories. The Dallas chapter of the Alzheimer's Association, on its webpage, seeks to spur potential donors into action by evoking images of fearsome body-snatchers coming to get you:

> *It's a nightmare. And you can't wake up...* Alzheimer's will strike 986 more Americans today. And tomorrow. We don't know who will be in that group of victims. It could be someone you know. Someone in your family. Your closest friend. It could be you. We just don't know. *We know this: 986 more will be taken today, and every day, until we stop it!* (Greater Dallas Chapter 2007; emphasis in original).

Both the gothic and the zombie variants of the Alzheimer's narrative depart from the same basic premise: the body may continue to live, but the person with Alzheimer's is dead, gone, no longer there, no longer a person. He or she does not know your name, does not 'recognize' you, therefore cannot 'care' about you, but you must 'care' for him or her – and such 'care' is conceived as an unending toil of unrelieved grimness.

Such narratives are not 'mere' stories. A caregiver's judgment that a person with dementia is 'socially dead' does very real harm, when it leads them to ignore the person with dementia, or to treat him or her in dehumanizing ways. One of the caregivers interviewed by Helen Sweeting and Mary Gilhooly, in their interview-based study of 'dementia and the phenomenon of social death', described to them his wife and how he treats her:

> I suppose people would say it's like living with the living dead... She doesn't speak, she does nothing, she just sits there... it's very easy, really, she's just a big baby... I mean you're sitting there ignoring her basically... you know you've got to toilet her and things like that... but it's not as if you

can sit beside her and talk and try to get her to smile – I've got beyond that (Sweeting and Gilhooly 1997:105).

Indeed, just how far 'beyond that' this man has gotten becomes all too clear in his description of how he leaves his wife tied to the toilet, when he wants to go out of the house for a while. (Sweeting and Gilhooly 1997:105)

In the case of hospitalized people who are attached to various kinds of life-sustaining technologies, the judgment that a person with dementia is 'as good as dead' may become a self-fulfilling prophecy, when it serves as 'a rationale for facilitating death' (Kaufman 23) and leads to decisions that allow death to happen. As Sharon Kaufman notes, the construction of dementia as 'a condition both of death-in-life and of life-in-death' (23) finds expression in the clinical context, in the contradictory statements and stances of medical professionals toward dementia-near-death in hospital settings.

> Physicians sometimes unwittingly offer contradictory directives to families, and a kind of doublespeak... revolves around the mystery of life... It emerges in the language that physicians use to explain physiological decline, the absence of beneficial treatments, and the role dementia plays in the nearness to death. It takes the following shape: 'Your mother is not actually (or completely) dead, or dead yet, but neither is she alive.' Or, 'She's not really alive, but we can keep her alive a bit longer'. Or, 'He has no meaningful life, but we can continue to take care of him'. Practically, *life* and *death* merge in this language... (Kaufman 40).

The single term *dementia*, it is worth noting, embraces a very wide range of different conditions and degrees of impairment. The hospitalized people on life-support whose predicament Kaufman discusses are far more severely limited in their capacities than someone such as my mother, and in their situation the line between 'life' and 'death' is indeed very ambiguous. By collapsing all such differences, however, and equating all forms of dementia with death, 'horror stories' effectively pronounce a sentence of social death on anyone, whatever their degree of impairment, to whom that label has become affixed.

'Does she recognize you?'

When a person with dementia is narratively construed as 'dead', the main drama centers not on him or her but on the suffering of the spouse and family members. As Lawrence Cohen has noted, public discussions of Alzheimer's describe it

> as 'a marathon', an 'exhausting vigil' given bodies 'who need to be constantly watched or restrained', an 'ordeal'... and most tellingly, an 'endless funeral'...The suffering conveyed... by such temporal language is not that of the old person [but that of] 'the other victims'... The continually reiterated discovery of Alzheimer's journalism is that it is the caretaker who is the *real* victim (Cohen 1998:54).

Caring for someone as dementia progresses and capacities recede is indeed an enormous job. I will be the first to point out that I am not the one who does most of the hard work of meeting my mother's practical needs. Up until his death, my father was the one who took over all of the many tasks my mother used to do as, one by one and year by year, she lost the ability to manage them. By the time he died, he was doing all of the bills, all of the shopping, all of the cooking, all of the housework, as well as the yardwork, the laundry, the correspondence, and everything else that he had for most of a lifetime happily left to my mother (and before that, his mother). It's possible, I think, that the strain of caring for her – or perhaps more accurately, the strain of caring for her while refusing all help and striving to 'protect' her by concealing from others the extent of her impairment – may have been a factor contributing to the heart attack that killed him.

Today, three and a half years later, my Mom also needs help with toileting, showering, dressing, brushing teeth, going to bed, and must sometimes be reminded to eat. The vast bulk of this work is done by the kind, attentive, overburdened and seriously underpaid workers – many of them first-generation immigrants from Somalia, Vietnam, the Philippines, and elsewhere – who staff the secure dementia ward of the upscale assisted-living facility where, thanks to a generous long-term-care insurance policy, my mother can afford to live. Even so, there remains plenty for my brothers and sister and me to do. My brothers and I take turns accompanying our Mom to checkups with doctors, dentists, ophthalmologists, and (more frequently than seems to me reasonable) nurses hired by the insurance company to conduct 'assessments' of her cognitive capacities. I shop for clothes or other items when Mom needs them, and talk with the staff at her facility about many small issues that arise from day to day. My sister manages our mother's finances. The four of us e-mail each other regularly about this or that small issue that comes up. And of course, we visit her. When people ask me whether my mother still 'recognizes' me, they are expressing concern for me, asking me how I am bearing up under the burden of suffering that her dementia must place on me. When friends who have little experience of dementia sympathetically imagine what I must be going through, I suspect that they probably picture such day-to-day practicalities merging seamlessly with extreme emotional suffering, as part of 'the horror of Alzheimer's'. And they are quite ready to hear about my burdens and my suffering.

What they find much harder to hear, I think, is that I am *not* a victim, and being around my mother is *not* a nightmare or a horror. She is not 'dead', she is not 'gone', and she is not just a 'body'. It is true that we have been very lucky: my mother's decline has been very slow and gentle, and she has remained good-tempered and affectionate throughout. I have never (yet) seen her become angry, suspicious, or violently agitated. She does not seem depressed. Aside from her dementia, my Mom is generally very healthy, remains physically mobile, suffers no chronic pain, and takes very little medication. Even though my Mom is seriously impaired she is still sweet, cheerful and sociable. I enjoy her company. Many other families are far less fortunate in their experience of dementia, and for them perhaps the gothic and zombie stories do resonate. But my experience with my mother's dementia is no 'horror story' – and this, too, lies within the domain of the possible.

'Does she recognize you?'

'Recognition', write the philosophers Nancy Fraser and Axel Honneth,

> has become a keyword of our time. A venerable category of Hegelian philosophy, recently resuscitated by political theorists, this notion is proving central to efforts to conceptualize today's struggles over identity and difference. Whether the issue is indigenous land claims or women's carework, homosexual marriage or Muslim headscarves, moral philosophers increasingly use the tem 'recognition' to unpack the normative bases of political claims. They find that a category that conditions subjects' autonomy on intersubjective regard well captures the moral stakes of many contemporary conflicts... (Fraser & Honneth, p. 2003).

It was only after constantly being confronted with questions of 'recognition', that I became aware of philosophical writings on 'the politics of recognition'. I turned to these works hoping to find there theoretical frameworks that would give me some critical purchase on the questions that have been bothering me: What social processes are at work behind this constant question about 'recognition'? Why is it apparently so difficult for people to 'recognize' – as a friend, as a person, as even being *alive* – someone who, because of dementia, can no longer keep names straight? How does the turning-away of friends, at the level of personal networks relate to processes of 'social death', social exclusion, and abandonment of people with dementia on a broader level? In short, how do questions about 'recognition' in its narrowly cognitive sense get implicated in the 'politics of recognition' on a broader scale?

The philosopher Charles Taylor, in a landmark essay on 'the politics of recognition', contends that because a person's sense of self is grounded in his or her membership in a cultural group, when the political system in which they live fails to recognize the cultural identity of the group to which they belong this causes real harm to individuals. As he writes, 'Misrecognition shows not just a lack of due respect. It can inflict a grievous wound, saddling its victims with a crippling self-hatred' (Taylor 1994:26). This framework, developed in the context of engagement with debates concerning multiculturalism and identity politics, especially in North America, does not readily address the situation of people with dementia. Dementia sufferers do not constitute a cultural group in a way comparable to others that Taylor considers. Surely no one *develops* their primary sense of self centered upon identification with dementia-sufferers as a cultural group. Discourses that equate Alzheimer's with death may indeed lead some people with dementia to suffer 'crippling self-hatred', especially now that the disease is often diagnosed early enough on that the affected person may be quite cognizant of the stigma attached to it. Yet political 'misrecognition' such as Taylor describes is far from the only or primary challenge that dementia presents to the sense of self.

Nancy Fraser has developed a conception of 'recognition' centered less upon problems of the development of an individual's sense of self, than upon what she calls 'the intersubjective condition of participatory parity', (Fraser 36), in other words the 'institutionalized patterns of cultural value' (Fraser 37) that either allow or deny people possibility of participating along with others on an equal footing, in a given activity or interaction. Fraser is concerned to develop an account of justice that can address, and distinguish among, the claims and demands made by various self-identified groups. Dementia Advocacy and Support Network International (DASNI), founded in 2001, is to the best of my knowledge the only identity-based group coalescing around the shared fact of having dementia. DASNI claims that roughly one-third of its members are people who have dementia themselves (DASN International 2008). DASNI's leadership includes people with dementia, and one of the group's primary aims is finding 'ways the Alzheimer's movement might become more inclusive of people with dementia' (DASN International 2008). One of the challenges that DASNI faces, however, is that people with dementia generally do not 'identify' with their condition, nor claim common membership in a group of people with whom they share it. And, as Michael Bérubé points out, discussing 'citizenship and disability' with reference to his son Jamie, who has Down's syndrome:

> Fraser writes as if the promise of democracy entails the promise to enhance participatory parity among citizens, which it does, and she writes as if we knew what 'participatory parity' itself means, which we don't (Bérubé 2003).

It is not clear what forms of political participation lie within reach of people such as my mother, who (as documented by the 'mini-mental status exam' that the insurance company demanded) cannot say what day, month, season or year it is, nor what city, state or country we are in. That the question is unclear does not mean that it is unimportant, no need we necessarily jump to the conclusion that people with dementia *cannot* be more fully 'recognized' as citizens, in terms of the 'politics of recognition' as developed by Fraser, Taylor, and others. It does mean, however, that available theoretical frameworks fall short when they encounter dementia.

Developing philosophical arguments about 'the politics of recognition' that might more easily accommodate the predicament of people with dementia will, I suspect, likely require looking for other ways of understanding 'selves'. We may need to stop looking only to individuals as the bearers of 'selfhood', and start looking more at how 'selfhood' is distributed among networks, sustained by supportive environments, emergent within practices of care. The critique that Ingunn Moser (N.d.) levels at a narrowly biomedical understanding of dementia is, I think, relevant also to political theory, to the extent that it too is premised upon a rationalist and individualist understanding of the 'self':

> Locating and fixing subjectivity and humanness in cognitive competencies and making autonomy and independence the gold standards for human subjectivity and agency, the biomedical version of dementia becomes fatal to the subject (Moser N.d.).

In order to address how 'recognition' in its narrowly cognitive sense get implicated in the 'politics of recognition' on a broader scale, arguments about the 'politics of recognition' must be stretched to encompass what Annemarie Mol terms a 'politics of what' (Mol 2003: 177). 'Recognition' is inseparable from 'caring', and both can be understood as not just the interior emotional or intellectual states of individuals, but as *practices*, particular forms of activity, at once social, representational and very concretely material.

'Does she recognize you?'

My mother would certainly fail a pop-quiz about my name, but she lights up when she sees me. She is eager to talk, and tries to speak, but words often elude her, and sentences get distracted and wander off in unanticipated directions. The difficulties of talking don't seem to bother her terribly, though. There is pleasure in it still.

In a café, as we share a scone, Mom and I make what passes for conversation. I've learned to ask only the sort of question that does not require any specific information to answer: 'So, things going okay with you these days?' 'How's my favorite Mom doing, you doing alright?' I tell her funny little stories about my kids. Sometimes we leaf through a magazine, looking at the pictures and commenting on them. Sometimes we look out the window, and I make general observations that require no specific response. 'Looks like spring is coming, look at those leaves coming out on the trees.' 'Sure are a lot of people out walking around today!' 'That guy's hair is really curly.' With each exchange Mom smiles at me, beaming affectionately in that familiar, slightly conspiratorial way, as if we are both in on the same joke.

And I begin to see, too, that Mom has her own experience of the world that is different from mine, and interesting in its own way. The loosening of memory that leaves her stranded in the present moment also allows her to inhabit it more fully than I am able to, caught up as I always am in the rush of my days, so full of schedules, deadlines, plans and arrangements. Morris Friedell, himself affected by Alzheimer's, describes how:

> I find myself more visually sensitive... Everything seems richer: lines, planes, contrast. It is a wonderful compensation... We [who have Alzheimer's disease] can appreciate clouds, leaves, flowers as we never did before (Shenk 2001:193).

Acknowledging this compensation is, in the words of Floyd Skloot (who write beautifully about, and despite, his dementia):

> not so much a matter of making lemonade out of life's lemons, but rather of learning to savor the shock, taste, texture and aftereffects of a mouthful of unadulterated citrus (Skloot 2003:197).

As Mom and I walk slowly, hand-in-hand, around the neighborhood of the facility where she now lives, she responds with interest to so many things around us: the cuteness of a small child, the blueness of a blue house, the puzzling fact of an open car door, the surprise of a dog wearing a sweater, the improbable angle described by a man carrying a bag so heavy that he leans all to one side as he walks. Sometimes, in Mom's company, I am able to slow down enough to gain a new appreciation of the moment. A few days ago we spent a half hour looking out my mother's bedroom window to where a woman sat on the sidewalk outside, next to her baby in its stroller, blowing bubbles. The breeze caught the bubbles and carried them up, whirling and dancing, catching the afternoon light in brief rainbow flashes. It was the kind of thing I would not normally sit and watch – and it was beautiful. A young mother I do not know created a fleeting moment of wonder, and my own aging and impaired mother helped me to see it.

So. Our conversations go nowhere, but it hardly matters what we say, really, or whether we said it before, or whether it is accurate or interesting or even comprehensible. The exchange itself is the point. Mom and I are playing catch with expressions, including touches, smiles and gestures as well as words, lobbing them back and forth to each other in slow easy underhand arcs. That she drops the ball more and more often doesn't stop the game from being enjoyable. It is a way of being together. Reflecting on his own mother's slide into dementia, the novelist Ian McEwan writes of her small comments and observations: 'I understand her to be saying simply that she is very happy for us to be out together seeing the same things. The content is irrelevant. The business is sharing'. (McEwan 2001).

Like many people whose knowledge of dementia comes primarily from the experience of caring for someone who has it, I came upon this perspective as if it were my own original discovery, not realizing until later that many scholars and researchers had already argued compellingly that, as Cohen puts it, 'the senile deformation of meaningful utterance is not necessarily a turn to meaninglessness' (Cohen 2003:125).

> It sounds crazy. It makes no sense if you pay attention to the words. But if you listen instead to the tone and the voice patterns, if you look at the body language, then it seems very much like a conversation. He asks. She answers. He comments. She comments. They take turns. They look at each other. Clearly they are connecting…We are so focused on words… on the act of talking, that we have forgotten how to communicate without them. More than that, we think there is no communication without words – which, of course, means that we believe we can't communicate with those who, in the later throes of Alzheimer's, have lost most of their language. These sentences Hayes and Frances M. say to each other may not make sense as conversation, yet there is meaning here… They are getting something out of this moment (Kessler 2007: 122).
>
> Even when speech is incoherent and void of linguistic meaning, in face-to-face interaction there is a smooth and appropriate alternating pattern of vocalizing, as well as gesticulating, back and forth. With the utterance of only 'Bah', 'Shah', 'Brrrr!' and 'Bupalupah', Abe and Anna were able to communicate without any recourse to intellectual interpretation. There was a fittingness and a meaningful relationship between the rise and fall of their pitch, their pauses, and their postural shifts… What this example illustrates is Merleau-Ponty's argument that communication dwells in corporeality or, more specifically, in the body's capability to gesture (Kontos 2006:207).
>
> In the nursing home, a lot of residents had problems addressing one another or understanding what was being said. Yet the social convention of neighbour-talk about the weather was one they all understood. This enabled them to have conversations even with people suffering from aphasia who did not use words in a conventional way. The intonation was right for a chat about the weather, so the urgency to produce the right content was less. The transcript of such a conversation does not make sense at all, but in the specific situation the conversation can be smooth, pleasant and clear to everyone present (Pols 2005:209).

There is, in short, much more to conversation than speech, and much more to speech than the transmittal of information. It is a commonplace of scientific research into Alzheimer's and other forms of dementia, that procedural memory (knowing *how to do* such-and-such) often persists much longer than propositional memory (knowing *that* such-and-such). People who are no longer able to speak coherently may often still take part in, and enjoy, activities such as walking, dancing, or singing that rely on embodied procedural memory.

Conversation itself is, for my mother, one of these activities. So much of it really is procedural, a knowing *how to* interact with people. When I make a joke, she laughs. When I tell some small story about something that happened, she murmurs sympathetically. When I express an opinion, she agrees. When we sit together she attends to my presence, reaches out to me, pats my hand. These communicative practices are, I believe, also practices of *caring*- my mother *cares about* smoothness of the back-and-forth flow, *takes care* to keep it all going, and in doing so she acts in a *caring* way toward me and other people around her.

'Does she recognize you?'

She may not 'recognize' me in a narrowly cognitive sense, but my Mom does 'recognize' me as someone who is there with her, someone familiar perhaps, and she does not need to have all the details sorted out in order to 'care' for me. The impulse to care, the habit of caring, the embodied knowledge of how to take care – these things run deep in my mother, a good woman according to the norms of her generation who, for most of her life, was very engaged in caring for other people: her children, her husband, her grandchildren, her friends. Not long ago, when I arrived to visit Mom, I found her sitting in the activity room holding in her lap, with practiced ease, a very realistic baby doll dressed in a purple outfit. Seeing me, she smiled, and beamed down at the doll. 'Look at him! So cute!' She shifted him gently in her arm, fussed a little with his outfit, and looked up at me again. 'I don't think he's going to wake up.' The fact that my mother was holding a doll, and that she likely could not clearly distinguish it from a real live baby is, to me, less important than the revelation that this moment offered, of the persistence within her of the procedural knowledge of how to care, and the desire and need to do so. The progress of her dementia makes it difficult for Mom, now, to comprehend the nature of other people's needs or the sources of their suffering, but she still does notice and respond to others, and is still moved to try to alleviate their distress.

Sometimes, this disjunct between a severely diminished capacity to comprehend and an undimmed capacity to care can lead to painfully ironic situations. On the day that my father died, my brothers and sister and I gathered at our parents' house, stunned, trying to comprehend what had happened and what we must do next, drinking the still-warm coffee that Dad had brewed that morning, and weeping. Though we had explained it to her, Mom did not grasp that her husband of forty-nine years was gone. At one point, she looked at my younger brother and noticed that his eyes were all red and swollen. Reaching out to caress his arm, her face drawn into an expression of sympathetic concern, she looked up at him and asked, tenderly, 'What's wrong? Do you have a cold?'

But sometimes, when distress is simpler and its sources less dramatic, such caring alone is a precious gift. One time, a little more than a year ago, I stopped by the assisted-living facility where my Mom was living at the end of a very busy day in an especially hectic week – I had stayed up very late the night before trying to finish grading student papers, then spent the whole day teaching and in meetings. I found her sitting in a common area, and went with her up to her room. I turned on the TV and we sat down together on the couch. Exhausted, I leaned back and yawned. Mom patted my hand, and said to me, 'You're tired! Just go ahead and sleep! You can just lay down right here'. And so I sat there next to my Mom, holding her hand, feeling her warmth against me all along one side of my body, and I leaned my head on her shoulder, and slept. When I awoke twenty minutes or so later, I felt better – a little bit rested, and deeply comforted by the fact that the mother I now take care of can still, in some small but important ways, also take care of me.

Even some of the odd behavioral quirks that my Mom has developed make sense to me in these terms, as expressions of care couched in the idiom of dementia. People with dementia often develop strong impulses to engage in particular forms of repetitive behaviors, and Mom is no exception. When I take her out to a café, I usually get a cup of black coffee for myself, and order a cup of hot chocolate for her (not too hot, and don't forget the whipped cream on top!). As we drink them, she checks constantly to see whether my cup and hers are 'even', whether the liquids have been drunk down to the same level. If not, she will hurry up and drink more to 'catch up', or else stop and wait for me. If we share a cookie, she is concerned to make sure that the halves be the same size, and that we eat them at the same rate. Cookies also leave crumbs, of course, and those disturb her – surfaces should be smooth and clean. She will wipe all the crumbs off the table and onto a napkin, then carefully fold up the napkin with the crumbs inside. Or she will take another napkin and wipe away at the inside of her cup, where the receding hot chocolate has left a little residue of foam and whipped cream. Then she will carefully pile up the hot-chocolate napkin, the cookie-crumb napkin, and any other napkins on the table, along with any other papers within easy reach, into a neat and symmetrical stack. She likes to secure such piles, when she can, by wrapping them up with rubber bands, or clipping them together, or putting them inside a plastic Ziploc bag or envelope or into her pocket. Given the opportunity and the materials, she tends to prefer to wrap, clip *and* enclose. When my siblings and I sorted through our parents' forty years of accumulated stuff, clearing out their house so that it could be sold, we found among Mom's things (with a mixture of hilarity and dismay) many strange little bundles, odds and ends multiply wrapped and rubber banded and clipped together.

Such behaviors are a little weird, to be sure. It is the sort of thing that makes people uncomfortable. Other people in the café give us odd looks when Mom starts in on her wiping and folding. The other residents at the place she used to live, most of whom were not impaired themselves, did not much like it when she began collecting their mail out of their cubbies and 'organizing' it into piles. The nurse there regarded Mom's pile-making as a symptom of 'obsessive-compulsive disorder' and suggested to me that we start her on Prozac. (I refused.)

I think it is also possible, however, to read such behaviors as, at least in part, expressions of *care*. Explaining her use of the term 'logic of care', Annemarie Mol explains that she:

> seeks a local, fragile, and yet pertinent coherence. This coherence is not necessarily obvious to the people involved. It need not even be verbally available to them. It may be implicit: embedded in practices, buildings, habits, and machines. And yet, if we want to talk about it we need to translate a logic into language. This, then, is what I am after. I will make words for, and out of, practices (Mol 2008:8).

Ingunn Moser (N.d.) and Jeannette Pols (2005) have documented how a 'logic of care' is implicit within practices of dementia nursing care. Such a logic may be present also within the practices of people with dementia themselves. Keeping track of whether our drinks and cookies are 'even' comes naturally to a woman who has always had to carefully divide quite limited resources, first with her own brothers, and later among her four children. When she starts in on her work of wiping crumbs and clipping together papers, her hands are well practiced in such motions from the years that she spent cleaning the kitchen counters, picking up after me and my siblings, working to create an orderly home. She has cared about such details all her life – and caring about them, taking care of them, was also a way in which she cared for other people. My Mom has always struggled to impose upon the resistant matter of her world an order, at once aesthetic and moral, of evenness, fairness, smoothness, and security. Dementia has made such efforts far more difficult, but they deserve nonetheless to be 'recognized'.

'Does she recognize you?'

Two and a half years ago now, ten months after my father's death, I arrived at my Mom's apartment one day and found her sitting on her couch, busily going through some papers. 'These are for my Dad', she explained.

I sat down next to her, to join in with her in her task. She was taking pieces of paper out of her purse, which was crammed to bursting with them, looking at each one, and then putting them into a pile next to her. I took this pile onto my lap and looked through it. It contained a very random assortment of things: blank sheets of stationery decorated with a floral design, condolence cards that friends had sent to her, subscription-reply cards from magazines, sections of months-old newspapers, napkins. And on top of these, there was a very old airmail-envelope, yellowing and brittle, with a letter inside.

I took the letter out and opened it up. Dated April 7th, 1968, it was written in my maternal grandfather's spidery handwriting. 'Dear Aunt Pearl', he wrote. 'Now. Please do not faint, but after reading your letter that you sent Ruth last February and she sent on to me, I just had to write and thank you for your kind cooperation. My oldest Boy 'Bill' has the Idea that he wants to know more about the family. Your letter, which I forwarded to him to-day, should be a great help.' He went on to reminisce fondly about visiting with her and her family in 1931, and sent news of his daughter and two sons, including the names and ages of my mother's four small children. 'Thank you again for your cooperation', he ended, 'and now that I realize I can write, I just may drop you another line'.

To come across a letter you have never seen before, written by a person you loved who died many years ago, can be a moving experience

– perhaps especially when the letter is one of very few artifacts left behind at the end of a humble life such as my Grandpa lived. And I was touched to see that my uncle Bill, also dead now, who in 1996 self-published a book-length family history of which he was very proud, had already begun work on this project thirty years earlier, when still a quite young man.

What staggered me, though, was what I saw written in the blank space at the top of the letter, in my mother's handwriting:

> *Licends – Please try to keep cares together!*
> We will try to keep Diana, Janelle, Mike and Pat. Will try to keep the cares together.

I cannot know exactly when my mother wrote this, but it is clear – from the oddness of the spelling and phrasing, as well as the shakiness of her handwriting – that she was already quite far along her path of progressive dementia.

It is tempting to grasp onto these words as representing a coherent and stable, if hidden, 'perspective' on the world, but I know that that would be a mistake (Pols 2005). Mom can no longer write. If I were to show her this note today, she would probably not be able to read it, nor would she recognize the words as her own. This note is nothing more, and nothing less, than a small fragment of wisdom, the material trace of one moment in her mighty effort to resist her losses. At some point – struggling to write, struggling to order her thoughts and her life – my mother named us, her children, as 'the cares', and exhorted herself to 'try to keep the cares together!', and promised to do so. The slip of paper on which she chose to write this note to herself was a letter from her much-loved and long-lost father, to a relative he had not seen for many years, thanking her for helping his son try to document family history. Generation upon generation, writing upon writing, layer upon layer of struggles, across the years, to 'keep the cares together'. With this essay, I suppose, I add yet another layer of my own.

'Does she recognize you?'

For a while, after we first moved my mother into an assisted-living facility, she often said that she wanted to 'go home'. I understood this to mean that she wanted to move back to where she had lived for forty years until my father's death, the house in which I grew up. Usually, I responded with my own mild version of 'reality orientation', explaining, as gently as possible, that that house was all empty and cold now, and nobody was there to keep her company or help her do stuff, so it was probably better to stay here.

One time, though, I asked her a question instead. 'You mean home to the house up in Edmonds?'

'No, on the farm', she answered. 'You go down...' With her raised arm, she traced out the curve of a long-ago road. For the first seven years of her life, my mother had lived on a small farm in southern Idaho, before her father moved the family to Seattle during World War II to seek work on the docks.

'They're inside there', she added.
'Who?' I asked.
'My Mom and my Dad'.

My mother is a woman in her seventies. Her parents are not waiting for her inside an Idaho farmhouse. Taken one way, a moment such as this gives clear evidence of my mother's inability to 'recognize' people and things around her. You could use that evidence to draw a clear line between us: place me here, on the side of reality, competence and personhood, and put her over there, on the side of delusion, incapacity and the not quite (or no longer) fully human.

What I took from that moment, however, was something different. I realized that what she was longing for was not *my* childhood home, but *hers*. She missed her Mom and Dad. She was trying, in her own way, to hold on to them – just as I was trying, against the odds, to hold on to her. Our predicament is exactly the same.

The ravages of time, aging and disease mean that my mother's efforts to 'keep the cares together' are ultimately doomed to fail. In that respect, however, she is hardly alone. Everyone becomes impaired in one way or another, unless we die first. Every human being begins life utterly reliant on kindnesses he can neither remember nor repay, and many of us will end our lives in a similar state. *As individuals*, every one of us is bound to fail to 'keep the cares together'. It is only as members of communities that any of us can hope to transcend forgetfulness and death.

Why then should a person be cast out and abandoned, condemned to social death and denied recognition as a friend, a person, a fellow human being, just because she shows signs of succumbing to the same forces that we know will eventually claim each one of us? Can we not resist this 'erosion of personhood' (Luborsky 1994), and 'overcome the notion that cognition is the decisive carrier of personhood' (Leibing 2006:258)? Rather than make an individual's claim to social and political 'recognition' contingent on the narrowly cognitive ability to 'recognize' people, words and things, we would do well to emulate this humble, ailing individual woman's effort to hold fast to 'the cares' – what she has cared about, who she has cared for and taken care of. Let us strive to hold on to 'care' as something that makes life worthwhile.

'Does she recognize you?'

I wish that just once, someone would ask me a different question. I can picture it very clearly. This is how it will happen. I will run into a friend, or coworker, or acquaintance, or neighbor, or one of my mother's old friends. We will chat about this and that. I will mention my mother, and her dementia. This person will look into my eyes and ask me:

'Janelle, are you keeping the cares together?'
'I'm doing my best', I will answer.
'...And you?'

Postscript

This essay was originally written in May 2008. Fifteen months have passed since then, and my mother's condition has continued to progress. Some of the small forms of shared activity described here (going to a café, walking around the neighborhood, etc), I now regard, with some longing, as the lost joys of a better time. The truth in my mother's words has, however, only become more vitally important to me. I continue to do my best to keep the cares together – as, within her limits, does she. Reader, I hope that you do too.

Acknowledgments

My husband, Michael Rosenthal, helps me live through difficult things, as well as understand them. A philosopher by training, he also provided indispensable guidance for my trespassings into the philosophical literature. For helping this essay come into being by believing in it when it was still a half-formed idea, I thank him, as well as Lorna Rhodes, Lesley Sharp, Tina Stevens, and especially Annemarie Mol, Ingunn Moser and Jeannette Pols. I am grateful to Anne Fadiman, Sara Goering, Mimi Kahn, Sharon Kaufman, Erica Lehrer, Lynn Morgan, Rayna Rapp, Lesley Sharp, Raymond T. Smith, and Kathleen

Woodward, for helpful and encouraging comments on a draft version of this essay. I'm grateful as well to Lawrence Cohen, Mark Luborsky, and Andrea Sankar, for helpful comments on and responses to this essay in its previous incarnation, as an article in *Medical Anthropology Quarterly*. I thank my siblings Diana Taylor-Williams, Mike Taylor, and Pat Taylor for helping me live, and laugh, through it all. Deepest thanks go, of course, to my mother, Charlene Taylor.

References

Bérubé, M. 2003. 'Citizenship and Disability.' Dissent 50(2):52-58.

Cohen, L. 2003. 'Senility and Irony's Age.' In *Illness and Irony: On the Ambiguity of Suffering in Culture*. M. Lambek and P. Antze, eds. New York & Oxford: Berghahn Books.

Connolly, J. 2007. 'Charting a Course for Recognition: A Review Essay.' *History of the Human Sciences* 20: 133-144.

Cooney, E. 2001. 'Death in Slow Motion: A Descent into Alzheimer's.' *Harper's*, Oct. 43-58.

DASN International. *http://www.dasninternational.org/index.php*, accessed April 30, 2008.

Fraser, N. 2003. 'Social Justice in the Age of Identity Politics: Redistribution, Recognition, and Participation.' In *Redistribution or Recognition? A Political-Philosophical Exchange*, N. Fraser and A. Honneth, eds. Pp.7-109 London: Verso.

Fraser, N. and A. Honneth. 2003. 'Introduction: Redistribution or Recognition?' In *Redistribution or Recognition*? A Political-Philosophical Exchange, N. Fraser and A. Honneth, eds. Pp 1-6. London: Verso.

Friedell, M. 2003. 'Tedious No More!' *http://members.aol.com/MorrisFF/Tedious.html* Accessed 4/29/2008.

Fuchs, E. 2005. *Making an Exit: A Mother-Daughter Drama with Alzheimer's, Machine Tools, and Laughter*. New York: Henry Holt and Company.

Goffman, E. 1961. *Asylums: Essays on the Social Situation of Mental Patients and Other Inmates*. New York: Doubleday.

Greater Dallas Chapter. 2007. Home Page. Electronic document, *http://www.alz.org/greaterdallas/*, accessed September 1, 2007.

Henderson, J.N. 2003. 'Alzheimer's Units and Special Care: A Soteriological Fantasy.' In *Gray Areas. Ethnographic Encounters with Nursing Home Culture*. P.B. Stafford, ed. Pp. 153-172. Santa Fe, N.M.: School of American Research Press.

Kaufman, S. 2005. "Dementia-Near-Death and 'Life Itself'" In *Thinking about Dementia: Culture, Loss, and the Anthropology of Senility*. A. Leibing and L. Cohen, eds. Pp. 23-42. New Brunswick, NJ: Rutgers University Press.

Kessler, L. 2007. *Dancing with Rose: Finding Life in the Land of Alzheimer's*. New York: Viking.

Kontos, P. 2006. 'Embodied Selfhood: An Ethnographic Exploration of Alzheimer's Disease.' In *Thinking about Dementia: Culture, Loss, and the Anthropology of Senility*, A. Leibing and L. Cohen, eds. Pp. 195-217. New Brunswick, NJ: Rutgers University Press.

Leibing, A. 2006. 'Divided Gazes: Alzheimer's Disease, the Person within, and Death in Life.' In *Thinking about Dementia: Culture, Loss, and the Anthropology of Senility*, A. Leibing and L. Cohen, eds. Pp. 240-268. New Brunswick, NJ: Rutgers University Press.

Luborsky, M.R. 1994. 'The Cultural Adversity of Physical Disability: Erosion of Full Adult Personhood.' *Journal of Aging Studies* 8(3):239-253.

Margalit, A. 2002. *The Ethics of Memory*. Cambridge, Mass.: Harvard University Press.

McEwan, I. 2001. "Mother Tongue." *http://www.ianmcewan.com/bib/articles/mother-tongue.html*, accessed September 9, 2008.

Mol, A. 2008. *The Logic of Care: Health and the Problem of Patient Choice*. New York and London: Routledge.

Mol, A. 2003. *The Body Multiple: Ontology in Medical Practice*. Durham, N.C.: Duke University Press.

Moser, I. N.d. 'Should We Hope for a World Without Alzheimer's? Re/articulating Subjectivity and Humanness in Biomedicine, Dementia Care, and STS.' Unpublished manuscript.

Plath, D.W. 1980. *Long Engagements: Maturity in Modern Japan*. Palo Alto: Stanford University Press.

Pols, J. 2005. 'Enacting Appreciations: Beyond the Patient Perspective.' *Health Care Analysis* 13(3):203-221.

Ricoeur, P. 2005. *The Course of Recognition*. Cambridge, Mass.: Harvard University Press.

Shenk, D. 2001. *The Forgetting: Alzheimer's, Portrait of an Epidemic*. New York: Random House.

Skloot, F. 2003. *In the Shadow of Memory*. Lincoln: University of Nebraska Press.

Strauss, C.J. 2001. *Talking to Alzheimer's: Simple Ways to Connect When You Visit with a Family Member or Friend*. Oakland, CA.: New Harbinger Press.

Sweeting, H. and M. Gilhooly. 1997. 'Dementia and the Phenomenon of Social Death.' *Sociology of Health & Illness* 19(1):93-117.

Taylor, C. 1994. 'The Politics of Recognition.' In *Multiculturalism: Examining the Politics of Recognition*, Amy Gutman, ed. Pp. 25-73. Princeton, N.J.: Princeton University Press.

Yamamoto-Mitani, N., C.S. Aneshensel, and L. Levy-Storms. 2002. 'Patterns of Family Visiting with Institutionalized Elders: The Case of Dementia.' *Journal of Gerontology: Social Sciences* 57B(4):S234-S246.

Care and killing
Tensions in veterinary practice

John Law

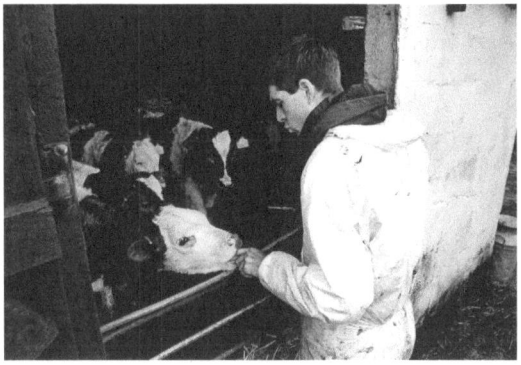

Vet and calves prior to sedation. From: Silence at Ramscliffe, Foot and Mouth in Devon. © Chris Chapman 2001

Slaughter at Ramscliffe

This photograph is one of a series by photographer Chris Chapman which witnesses the culling of animals in Devon during the UK's foot and mouth epidemic in the spring of 2001.[1] The whole series, plus a commentary and poems by James Crowden, are assembled in a remarkable document, *Silence at Ramscliffe*, which witnesses that foot and mouth slaughter at Ramscliffe Farm, Beaford in North Devon. Ramscliffe was a smallish dairy farm, run by Philip Lake with help from his father, Percy, and his mother Roma. 216 cattle and 22 sheep were slaughtered on 6th April 2001.[2] None had the disease themselves, but it had appeared on Lake's cousin's adjacent farm where the stock had been slaughtered. Official policy, clear in theory if not in practice, was that animals on 'contiguous premises' should be culled in order to prevent the spread of the disease.[3] This is why slaughter came to Ramscliffe.

Chris Chapman tells us that there were four people in the team[4]: a slaughterman from Launceston; an AI man from Essex; a young man, just out of training from somewhere 'up country'; and a vet, Robert Kilby, from East Devon. Chapman took Kilby on one side shortly after the latter arrived and explained that he wasn't a hired farmhand but a photographer. Kilby was taken aback:

There was a pause and then without looking up he snapped at me. 'OK, you can stay, but I want you in white overalls and that camera wrapped in a plastic bag.' I felt a flush of relief followed by an awkward feeling of joy.[5]

Chapman describes in words and photographs the killing of the animals at Ramscliffe. First the milking cows. They were driven into the yard in front of the milking parlour, and then inside and into the stalls. He notes that they were confused, not used to this break in routine. Then they were sedated and 'gently ushered out' one by one and guided to the empty silage clamp. The floor was wet with a mixture of rainwater and slurry, and Lake brought straw for them to lie on. Once they were gathered together the slaughter man killed each animal with a captive bolt gun. Then the vet and the AI man used the pithing rod to be sure that each animal was dead, pushing it through the hole in the skull and stirring its brains around. The vet confirmed each death, and the carcasses were marked with blue spray paint. Later it was the turn of the store cattle, and the heifers in-calf. And then, finally, the calves. Chapman's photos of the latter first show Kilby preparing the sedative for the calves. Then we see three or four calves peering through the barrier in the calf shed. They look alert, well. Then comes the photo above. Robert Kilby is at the same gate. One of the calves is suckling on his finger.

> How do I tell a new born calf
> That it is about to be shot and burned?[6]

asks poet James Crowden on the page facing the photograph. Then the sequence of photos shows us a distant view of the vet and two other members of the team sedating the calves, and the four members of the team moving the calves to be slaughtered. And in the final picture in the sequence, Kilby and the AI man are shown carrying the last calf to be slaughtered.

'I watched', writes Chapman, 'as… [the calves] were led across the yard, the last one having to be carried. I had seen enough. I couldn't photograph them being shot. I wandered about the farm in a daze'.[7]

I experience the photographs as an extraordinarily powerful document. They witness an important component in the devastation wreaked by foot and mouth as it visited 2000-plus premises in 2001. There is the slaughter itself: dairy cows turned into carcasses. And then there are the people. So in one photograph we see the farmer, Lake, slipping away into the farmhouse. We've already learned 'that he would help move the cattle but he didn't want to watch anything being killed'.[8] We sense, possibly wrongly, that Kilby, the vet is also protecting himself. Chapman:

> I tried to strike up a conversation [with him] about the merits of the contiguous cull but his brow furrowed. 'You have to look at the bigger picture' was all he could offer. He was in work mode now and the job in hand required all his concentration.[9]

How to handle a document of the kind created by Chapman? The issues and the emotions that it raises were clearly problematic. There is a risk of voyeurism. Crowden catches this in another poem:

> Vietnam in North Devon and Cumbria,
> Hedgerows rank with inquisitive film crews
> Relaying the drama as if it was Beirut,
> Jerusalem, the West Bank.
>
> In England's green and pleasant land,
> Digital images broadcast every night
> into the sofa-safe soft plush depths
> Of countless suburban sitting rooms.[10]

Earlier Chapman finds himself next to a national press photographer and decides that peering through hedges with telephoto lenses is not what he wants to be doing. He ought, he thinks, to work in a way that records the horrors much more intimately. Ian Mercer, the author of the Devon County Council report on the outbreak, observes that emotions are difficult to write down but nonetheless real.[11] However, in this piece I will sidestep the politics and normativities of voyeurism and emotion by attending to the materialised and embodied complexities of veterinary care in the slaughter of 2001. I return, then, to the photograph of Robert Kilby and the calf because I think that it condenses many of those embodied complexities.

The Commentary of a Vet

I ask one vet I'm interviewing, I'll call him Peter, what he thinks or sees when he looks at this photo. He knows it well, the photo. He takes the book, *Silence at Ramscliffe* down from his shelf and we look at it together. Here are my notes. They aren't quite verbatim but he speaks slowly, pausing as I hurriedly scribble:

> I see the vet interacting with the animals. I see him talking to the calf. His lips are pursed. I guess he is assessing its

overall behaviour, he is checking the calves over. He sees that they are fit and healthy, that they are associating with one another, and the state of the bedding, he is looking at that too. He does all this, while knowing that within a few minutes they will be shot. This brings difficult emotions. He is thinking about the loss of life. He is thinking about protecting other farms. He is thinking about doing a job to prevent disease again. This animal will not live long. But he wants to make sure that it has a peaceful life, and as peaceful as possible an end. He wants to make sure that it will be sedated, and quickly killed.

The danger, in this kind of situation, of being involved in slaughter, is you get inured to it. You get used to it. But you cannot afford to become inured to it. And then you are thinking about the pain this will cause the farmer, and the staff. He may be worrying for their sanity, wondering how they are going to go through it. And, if it were me, I would be worrying about my own sanity. Especially if I am finding it difficult to accept the policy...

And then, a sense of sadness.[12]

Objects of Care

I listen to this man, an experienced mid-career vet who has spent most of his working life in agricultural practice, and I sense his pain as he talks. Foot and mouth was not something that most farmers or vets wanted to live through, and many years on they have not forgotten it. (The small Surrey recurrence of the disease in August 2007 in the UK brought back many terrible memories). Then there's something else happening too, for like many and perhaps most field vets and farmers, Peter also thinks that the policy of contiguous slaughter was wrong. So let me tease out some of the different *aspects or objects of caring* that go into what he says, and into what Chapman tells us in words and pictures about the slaughter at Ramscliffe Farm.

Caring for the Animal

First, and most obviously, there is care for the calf itself.
Is it in distress? Is it hungry? Does it sense that something is wrong, even though the team has been careful to kill the animals at some distance removed? At any rate, it wants to suckle, and Kilby lets it do so on his finger. He talks to it too. Purses his lips, perhaps mimicking

its actions. In this set of bodily gestures, in this interaction, we might say that several of the 'five freedoms' for farm animals are being done: for instance, the freedom to express normal behaviour, and freedom from fear and distress[13]. But there's more too.

Peter also talks of the 'trained eye' of the vet. I've asked him how he knows whether an animal is in good condition when he goes to a farm. What it is that he *sees*. In response he describes how he looks for signs of ill health – the state of the feet, lameness, the condition of the animal's coat, whether it is alert or not, whether it is grazing with others. You also, he adds, need to lay hands on the animal. Then he's talked about how the stockman interacts with the animals in his care. Does he relate with them quietly and confidently? Does he or she reveal a gentle confidence? These are good signs. Or does he shout at them? This is less good. Then he's talked about the state of the bedding, about whether the animals are interacting with one another. And he likes what he can see in the photos of Ramscliffe. It looks as if the bedding is good and the animals are associating with one another.

And yet the calf will shortly be killed. This isn't cruelty, which is what a sentimental urban world might imagine. For caring for the calf is also, and crucially, a matter of a good death. Peter:

> 'It is part of the responsibility of the vet to ensure that [farm animals] lead as good a life as possible, but then to give them a good death at the end of that life... If there is slaughtering, this should be humane, done in a respectful manner. And it is important that the animal should be in a fit state for slaughter.'

Slaughter in foot and mouth was dramatic, traumatic, and unusual because it was conducted en-masse, on the farm. But stock-rearing is about slaughter anyway. So if the team at Ramscliffe is doing its job well then the animals will die a 'good death'. One that is (an interesting term) 'humane'. And we've seen how this is done. Encouraged first into the parlour with extra feed. Sedated. Coaxed or carried to the place of slaughter. Killed, and pithed. Of course this makes it all sound rather easy if a bit grisly. As we write about it we're glossing the messy materialities and embodiments, and most of the complexities and specificities. Chapman:

> As the clamp filled with sedated cows I was shocked to see one cow walk over to another lying motionless on the floor. She sniffed for recognition, staring at the body as if in disbelief.

> It was chillingly human. Another came in and did exactly the same and they both stood there rooted to the spot.[14]

Writing catches something and simultaneously loses almost everything. This is what it *does* as it moves away from the farm. But what the team is attempting, very seriously and very professionally, is to achieve a good death: humane and respectful. *Care for the animal in life, and care for the animal in the process of killing*. This is a first part of caring for the vet.

Caring for the Farmer

But then there are people who work on the farm including the farmer. Again the practical is intertwined with the emotional or the 'personal'. Peter:

> Veterinary practices have their business focus, but there is also a pastoral side. If you forget about the pastoral side then you lose the trust and loyalty of clients.

At Ramscliffe it is most unlikely that the vet has any business connection with the farmer: so far as we know they have never met. In normal times the State Veterinary Service sends a vet to each farm every so often to check the welfare of the animals and renew (or occasionally not) the licence to hold stock. This is a stressful and serious business for the farmer. First it is time-consuming and therefore costly.[15] Second, the farm may fail the inspection: *in extremis* a state vet can put a farmer out of business. In this volume Vicky Singleton details some of the increasing strains for livestock holders in the UK as stock records and tags are checked in addition to the welfare of the animals.[16] Indeed the Ramscliffe farmer, Lake, has an inspection-related panic before the slaughter team arrives and rushes off to clear the slurry tank.[17]

But if the state vet is caring for the welfare of the stock and, as a part of this, has power over the farmer, the latter is often also moderated by care and concern. First, the vets creatively adapt the rules. For instance, the state vet responsible for the pig finishing unit, Burnside Farm, where the foot and mouth epidemic started, reports that when he made his twice-yearly visit in the summer of 2000 he discovered that the welfare of the pigs was at serious risk. Barriers between the pens had been broken down by large boars, there was unregulated sexual activity, there were pregnant sows, farrowing, fighting between boars, slurry was overflowing, and two dead sows were located in pens alongside the living.

> I rang [the pig farmer] and told him I was shocked and disgusted by what I had seen ... I told him that ... I was going to pretend that morning's visit hadn't happened and that I would return to the farm early the following week, when I expected to see all problems resolved.[18]

Here he tempered justice with mercy. The people in question were not the best farmers in the world, and were bending various rules with consequences that turned out to be disastrous. But they were already in serious trouble anyway because the market was depressed, and they couldn't sell their pigs for a decent price (hence the size of the boars). So he gave them one last chance.

Returning to Ramscliffe, for Philip Lake and his parents the slaughter is dreadfully painful. I've already quoted Peter who suggests that Kilby may be '...be worrying for their sanity, wondering how they are going to go through it'. Peter goes on to describe how he himself identified foot and mouth on one farm:

> He had been called because the farmer suspected hypomagnesium, this is lack of magnesium and causes what farmers call the 'staggers'. He reported [the fact that the problem was really foot and mouth] to the farmer, who didn't believe it. 'Rubbish' [said the farmer]. 'Sorry',... said [the vet] 'but I think it's foot and mouth'. The diagnosis was confirmed by a visit from the State Veterinary Service. Then he talked about what would happen, and they made arrangements to get the children off the farm. 'It was terribly traumatic. The loss of the herd and the grief of the family had a considerable effect.'

This is a story that repeated itself hundreds of times up and down the country in 2001. And though there were complaints of incompetent and careless slaughtering teams, such stories are far outnumbered by the compliments about a horrible and difficult job sensitively undertaken. Peter reported that when he saw them at work the slaughtermen were 'efficient and caring', and the official 'Lessons to be Learned' report published after the epidemic observes that:

> in the majority of cases an unpleasant task was conducted effectively, often in very difficult conditions. Many farmers praised the manner in which the slaughtermen did their job. One submission said 'there were Government inadequacies in every area bar slaughter.[19]

CHAPTER 3

We move, then, beyond the caring by the vets as individuals to the caring practised by the team as a whole. Caring for the herd in the killing was also to do with caring for the farmers, for trying to preserve their sanity.

Caring for the Self

And then also important is the care of the self. I've already quoted Peter on this. Peter Frost-Pennington, a poet and temporary state veterinary officer in 2001, writes:

> This is not what I trained for: I hope familiarity will never make me immune from the trauma of killing
> But I do hope – for the animals' sake – to be good at it.[20]

There are two dangers: on the one hand to be caught up and immobilised by the pain; but then, on the other, there is another kind of horror. What kind of person would one become if one became used to killing? Care of the self, then is a double move. First it has to do with protecting the capacity, the propensity, to experience the possible suffering of the animals to be killed. One would not want be the kind of person who was indifferent to killing, who didn't care that this caused suffering.[21] And then, the second move, the identification with the task at hand, and especially the animal, needs to be moderated. Care, here, is about responding, but not responding too much. It is about being there, about sensitivity, and yet it is also about distance. It is precisely about self-protection.

Learning how to balance empathy and distance is part of a professional training. Caring for the animal and caring for the self go together. It is set of practices for retaining sanity. We don't know what Robert Kilby is thinking. However, the way he acts is consistent with this, because he doesn't want to talk about the contiguous cull with Chapman. Indeed, he doesn't really want to engage with him much at all. This is not a moment for talk. He is in work mode. I'm guessing that the need for concentration was partly practical, to do with doing the task well. But I'm guessing that it was also defensive: limiting his self-exposure to the loss of life and livelihood. Care for the animals, care for the farmer, and care for the self, here at least it seems that the three went together.

Caring for the Bigger Picture

But then there are larger units too. As Kilby puts it tersely in his response to Chapman, 'You have to look at the bigger picture'. Peter spells the logic out. 'He is thinking about protecting other farms. He is thinking about doing a job to prevent disease again.' But this unpacks itself in various ways because there are different versions of the bigger picture.

First, for instance, there is *the disease and the animals around the country*. Poet-vet Frost-Pennington:

> But don't get me wrong
> I have seen plenty of this plague-
> And it is no common cold.
> The animals suffer horribly,
> as the skin of their tongues peels off
> And their feet fall apart.
> We must try to kill them quick and clean,
> As soon as it appears in a herd or flock.[22]

He's talking of animal suffering. It is the vet's duty of care to minimise the individual but also the collective suffering of animals – which means eradicating the virus from the UK.

Then, second, there are *human groups* in a variety of shapes and sizes. Killing may care for the *neighbours*, for a version of locality. Chapman describes the argy-bargy between a Devon farm and the Ministry of Agriculture, Food and Fisheries, MAFF, through a series of visits and phone calls. The farm, untouched by foot and mouth despite the presence of the disease on nearby holdings, was trying to save its livestock:

> One insensitive MAFF official even had the audacity to ask the question: 'OK, so we let your animals live. How will you feel if FMD then spreads to the rest of Dartmoor.[23]

You can *see* the neighbours, or at least you can go and visit them. But there are more abstract or at least geographically-distributed versions of the bigger picture. So, for instance foot and mouth was damaging to the meat trade and to the national economy for a mix of social and biological reasons. Biologically, the disease reduces the productivity of animals as they lose weight and produce less milk. It can also be catastrophic in the South where it is often endemic. Here is an FAO animal health officer:

> Three weeks ago, I met a farmer in Bangladesh who owns eight cows. When FMD hit, their milk yield dropped by over 70 per cent in just a couple of days. Last year, when FMD struck, four out of his eight cows aborted. Of the four calves that were born, three died.[24]

Many, including Peter, argue that it should be eradicated in the South.[25] So the collective here is biological but also geographical, economic and human. It is both abstract – it isn't there at Ramscliffe to be seen or visited – and made real. It *matters*. And the argument applies to that abstraction, the UK. This is an economic actor too. With foot and mouth disease in the country the UK cannot export meat or live animals to its most profitable overseas markets. So here we have a pressing reason for eradicating it – and indeed eradicating it by slaughter rather than vaccination in combination with slaughter. Under the EU and WTO regime in 2001 export restrictions would be (and were) lifted more quickly if no recourse was made to vaccination.

So this is a fourth object of care. As Kilby works, he also cares for the 'bigger picture'. Except, here's the complication, the character of that bigger picture is on the move. Animals and their suffering? Neighbours and their life's work? The economic interests of the meat trade? The economic well-being of the country as a whole? Or, in some versions, the partisan political interests of a government keen to eradicate the disease and win a general election? It is very easy to imagine ways in which these different 'bigger pictures' don't map onto one another. And this mismatched mapping was very real in 2001. This is why there were so many arguments about the contiguous cull.

Choreography and Tinkering

I have listed four objects of care. In 2001 care for the animal, care for the farmer, care for the self, and care for various versions of the collectivity – all of these were present. All were overlapping. But this list is a convenience. In practice the multiplicity is much larger. In the work of Kilby and his team at Ramscliffe and that of the other vets up and down the country, they cared: for the animals in life, the animals at the point of death, and the animals after death; pastorally, for the farmers; for their own sensitivity to slaughter and suffering, and the necessary self-protection that goes along with this in order to retain sanity; for an abstract collectivity, the national herd; for the neighbours; perhaps for the meat trade, for the national economy, and on some versions, the political fate of the government. This, then, is care multiple. So how does it work? How is it managed? And when and how does it break down?

The contributors to this volume emphasise that care is best understood as a set of materially heterogeneous practices involving not simply particular kinds of subjectivities, but also instruments, and technologies together with other material elements, texts and inscriptions. Again, the contributions assembled in this volume imply that care may be understood as *choreography*. This term was introduced to social studies of science by Charis Cussins[26] who used it to draw attention to the intricate organisation that goes into the routines of practice:

> I use the word 'choreography'... as the dominant ontological/political metaphor throughout, to invoke materiality, structural constraint, performativity, discipline, co-dependence of setting and performers, and movement.[27]

Her particular interest was in the complexities of patient subjectivities in the context of infertility treatment. But the process of veterinary caring is choreographed in analogous ways. It too involves the intricate ordering and distribution of bodies, technologies, architectures, texts, gestures and subjectivities. And the metaphor of choreography also reminds us of the extreme degree of *effort* that goes into that organisation: what may sometimes appear simple from the outside is never that way in practice.

Crucial to the ordering of choreography, including the choreography of care, is the arrangement and distribution of events and actors in space and time. It is obvious that there are moments when good care requires that particular elements be brought together: the straw and the silage clamp; the fingers of the vet and the calf; the bodies of the cows and the pithing rod. If, as Mol has argued[28] argued, care is an unfolding embodied and material process, then the space-time choreography of these moments of juxtaposition and contact is central to its organisation. At the same time it is also important to understand that this organisation is more or less local, for the precise structure of contact cannot be predicted. Care depends not so much on a formula as a repertoire that allows situated action.

However, in the present context even more significant for my argument are the separations and distances that are also entailed in care. We have seen the importance of a number of these. There is, for instance, the isolation of the farm from the outside world: no-one is to come onto or to leave the premises while the slaughter is taking place. There is the moment when Lake, the farmer, abandons Kilby's team to return to his kitchen because he cannot bear to watch the slaughter of his animals. We have Peter's account of the arrangements to move the children off the farm before the slaughter team arrives. There is the physical organisation of the slaughter of the cows: care is taken to ensure that the calves, no doubt already disturbed, are not close by while this takes place. Then, and differently, there is Kilby's refusal to talk about the contiguous cull with Chapman. All of these are examples of the choreography of separation. And all are crucial to good care.

Why? One answer is that caring takes the form of spatially and temporally segregated events. First this has to be done, then that, and then something else. But another answer is that if it is the case, as I hope I have shown, that veterinary care is care multiple – if multiple objects are simultaneously being cared for – then the coherence, consistency, or compatibility of the practices that care for those objects is chronically uncertain. Indeed, more strongly, it is chronically problematic. Quite simply, caring for a good life and practising a good death do not necessarily go together, not, at any rate, at the same time and the same place. Care of the self and care for the calf may be, and quite likely are, in tension. Somehow or other, distance between the two needs to be practised. Care for the individual farmer and care for the national collectivity may fit together, but possibly they do not. The choreography of care multiple – and care, I'm hinting, is probably always multiple – necessarily depends on the organisation of separations. Let me insist, too that it necessarily depends on the *unfolding* of separations. And this is the final piece in the puzzle: for, as I briefly mentioned above, it also follows that such separations cannot be planned and orchestrated beforehand.

Literally read, choreography refers to the writing of dance. More usually the term is used to refer to a space-time set of rules or practices which shape but do not determine the actions of the bodies of the dancers. As we have seen, Cussins extends the term to refer to the complex subjectivities of women undergoing fertility treatment. If we apply this to veterinary care then we need to say that the latter rests upon routines for ordering complex objectivities and subjectivities. Then we need to add that since the objects of care are multiple it depends, in particular, upon routines for separating moments and objects of care and (possibly even more important) the subjectivities that go with them. And then finally we need to add that those routines are also and essentially experimental. They grow out of the routines and repertoires of past practice – but they are themselves also a form of trial and error, involving the creation of new practices for separating and handling tensions between different subjectivities and objectivities.

This, surely, is what Kilby is engaged in when he refuses to talk about the contiguous cull with Chapman. His terse comment is a self-protective improvisation that reflects the need for self care. Again, and surely, this is what he allows to happen when he lets the calf to suckle on his fingers. For this too is an improvisation: it was not built into the rules that define the proper slaughter on farm premises – or indeed the proper care of farm animals. Annemarie Mol talks of the importance of tinkering in medical care. She treats the latter as a set of constantly unfolding and only partially routinised practices for holding together that which does not necessarily hold together. And this is the nature of veterinary care too: it can be understood as an improvised and experimental choreography for holding together and holding apart different and relatively non-coherent versions of care, their objects, and their subjectivities. It is the art of holding all those versions of care in the air without letting them collapse into collision.

Acknowledgments

All work is collective, and I am grateful to Nick Bingham, Steve Hinchliffe, Annemarie Mol, Ingunn Moser, Jeannette Pols, Vicky Singleton and Helen Verran for comments, resistance, and long-term support. I am most grateful to 'Peter' for talking with me at length about veterinary practice in the context of foot and mouth disease. And I am also very grateful to Chris Chapman and James Crowden for their document, *Silence at Ramscliffe* (Oxford, the Bardwell Press, 2005). The book is extraordinary, and they have kindly let me borrow from it.

Notes

1. Chapman had been commissioned by Beaford Arts and the Devon County Council to document foot and mouth in Devon.
2. BBC Online Devon (2002).
3. Foot and Mouth Disease 2001: Lessons to be Learned Inquiry (2002).
4. Chapman (2005, 44).
5. Chapman (2005, 44).
6. Chapman (2005, 66).
7. Chapman (2005, 53).
8. Chapman (2005, 52).
9. Chapman (2005, 44-52).
10. Chapman (2005, 51).
11. Mercer (2002, 2).
12. Interview with vet, 7th March 2007. All the quotations from Peter are from this interview.
13. Farm Animal Welfare Council (2007).
14. Chapman (2005, 52).
15. The costs of monitoring and inspection are a continual concern for the farming industry, and there are continual tussles around the issue. For an example in the context of animal welfare certification see Keeling (2007, 26).
16. Singleton (2007).
17. Chapman (2005, 42).
18. Dring (2001, 7).
19. Foot and Mouth Disease 2001: Lessons to be Learned Inquiry (2002, 76).
20. Frost-Pennington (2001, 8)
21. The care of the self with respect to moral worth, goes back in the context of animals at least as far as the early modern period, and was arguably separate from any idea of moral or ethical worth of animals themselves. For this argument see Fudge (2006).
22. Frost-Pennington (2001, 7).
23. Chapman (2005, 25). The farm's attempts to save its animals failed.
24. Roeder (2001).
25. For discussion of this, see Kitching *et al.* (2007).
26. Cussins (1998).
27. Cussins (1996, footnote 14, page 604).
28. Mol (2008).

References

BBC Online Devon (2002), 'Photos tell Graphic Tale of FMD Tragedy', BBC, http://www.bbc.co.uk/devon/culture/2002/photos_fmd.shtml, (accessed 29 April 2007).

Chapman, Chris, and James Crowden (2005), *Silence at Ramscliffe: Foot and Mouth in Devon*, Oxford: The Bardwell Press.

Cussins, Charis M. (1996), 'Ontological Choreography: Agency through Objectification in Infertility Clinics', *Social Studies of Science*, 26: (3), 575-610.

Cussins, Charis M. (1998), 'Ontological Choreography: Agency for Women Patients in an Infertility Clinic', pages 166-201 in Marc Berg and Annemarie Mol (eds), *Differences in Medicine: Unravelling Practices, Techniques and Bodies*, Durham, N.Ca. and London: Duke University Press.

Dring, Jim (2001), 'My Involvement with the Waughs', London: DEFRA, http://www.defra.gov.uk/footandmouth/pdf/dringstatement.pdf, updated 16th March 2004, (accessed 9th August 2004).

Farm Animal Welfare Council (2007), 'Five Freedoms', London: Farm Animal Welfare Council, http://www.fawc.org.uk/freedoms.htm, (accessed 8 November 2007).

Foot and Mouth Disease 2001: Lessons to be Learned Inquiry (2002), 'Report', London: London, The Stationery Office, http://213.121.214.218/fmd/report/index.htm, (accessed 28th August, 2003).

Frost-Pennington, Peter (2001), 'Into the Valleys of Death', pages 7-8 in Caz Graham (ed.), Foot and Mouth: *Heart and Soul. A Collection of Personal Accounts of the Foot and Mouth Outbreak in Cumbria 2001*, Carlisle: BBC Radio Cumbria.

Fudge, Erica (2006), 'Two Ethics: Killing Animals in the Past and the Present', pages 99-119 in The Animal Studies Group (ed.), *Animal Killings*, Urbana and Chicago: University of Illinois Press.

Keeling, Linda, and Bettina Bock (2007), 'Turning Welfare Principles into Practice. approach followed in Welfare Quality®', paper delivered at the Second Welfare Quality® Stakeholder Conference, Federal Institute for Risk Assessment, Berlin, 3-4 May, 2007, 25-28.

Kitching, Paul et.al. (2007), 'Global FMD control-Is it an option?' *Vaccine*, 25, 5660-5664.

Mercer, Ian (2002), *Crisis and Opportunity: Devon Foot and Mouth Inquiry 2001*, Tiverton, Devon Books, http://www.devon.gov.uk/fminquiry/finalreport/, (accessed 28th August, 2003).

Mol, Annemarie (2008), *The Logic of Care: Health and the Problem of Patient Choice*, London: Routledge.

Roeder, Peter (2001), 'The 'hidden' Epidemic of Foot-and-Mouth Disease', Food and Agricultural Organisation, http://www.fao.org/News/2001/010508-e.htm, updated 29 May 2007, (accessed 8 November 2007).

Singleton, Vicky (2007), 'Irresponsible Accountability? Tracing Cattle, Moving Practices', in The Social and Material Practices of Agriculture, Farming and Food Production, Lancaster: Centre for Science Studies.

How to become a guardian angel
Providing safety in a home telecare service

Daniel López, Blanca Callén, Francisco Tirado and Miquel Domènech

Introduction

> Home Telecare is specially designed for those people who, for reasons of health, disability or isolation, require continuous attention. It is also for those people who want to enjoy independence without renouncing their safety (Red Cross Telecare Service pamphlet).

The Catalan Red Cross Home Telecare Service presents itself as a safety provider. That is the promise. It supplies elderly people with a technical solution to balance living independently at home with the possibility of urgently needing care. Governments are fostering technical solutions like these since they are cheaper than institutional and home care, and users and relatives like them because they do not require dramatic changes of lifestyle. Simply by fitting a few small devices to the house of the person in need – a pendant to be worn around the neck and a special telephone – they can be linked up with the Red Cross teleoperators and provided with a feeling of safety. One of our informants, an elderly lady using the Telecare Service we studied, put it succinctly when we asked her why she decided to link up:

> Because I was left on my own. And I found out about it from other friends. And I thought: 'Hey! Why should I be alone in a five-bedroom flat! As, well, it's a bit scary. Although things can happen to anybody… But when you reach a certain age, it's only natural that something could happen to you! So I thought: 'Well, yes, yes. So my family are now nice and calm in their house. And I sometimes even think: 'If anything ever happened to me, I would not call them, right? My children, you know? Me and you [the Red Cross telecare service]! You would take me to a hospital and then notify them, wouldn't you? So with you, I'm not scared and thinking: Oh no, I'm alone! No, no, no. I have the Red Cross, don't I? It's as if I had a guardian angel! (Telecare User 5:751-45:49).

Chapter 4

Providing safety is supposed to be a way to make people less dependent on their relatives. However, it is a complex thing to do. It not only depends on a telecare device and the service behind it, but also on the support this service can mobilise by calling upon relatives, neighbours and healthcare resources. The service provides safety by coordinating heterogeneous resources, from ambulances to neighbours, and by managing unforeseen situations and irreducible risks. Compared with care settings in which either formal or informal caregivers are always present, telecare entails dealing from a distance with a huge variety of users, daily routines, domestic spaces and care resources. A good telecare service, then, is far more than just a hotline. It provides people with 'whatever is required', and is able to manage any kind of situation. However, as long as it is not called upon, it remains hidden in the background and does not interfere with anyone's daily life. It is this remarkable way of being present and absent at the same time that makes the Telecare Service a 'guardian angel'.

Drawing on ethnographic research carried out in a Catalan Home Telecare Service, in this chapter we explore how safety is provided and how, in practice, the status of a 'guardian angel' is achieved. We particularly focus on the work of the telecare operator. The operator, as we will demonstrate, engages in two kinds of practices. On the one hand, there are what are known as *securing practices*. These make the system efficient and reliable while seeking to produce guarantees and to achieve a clear sense of continuity between what users need and the resources mobilised to meet these needs. However, complete 'securing' is impossible. So, rather than seeking to avoid all risks, it is better to work on the assumption that incidents and unforeseeable situations are normal. Instead of negating what does not quite fit by defining it as an exception, an accident, or an 'unsuitable demand', the service has to deal with it. This calls for another type of practice: *caring practices*. These caring practices constantly challenge the protocols and codes of the system. They attune to what lies in between the lines by 'active listening'. The securing practices and caring practices provided by the Telecare Service, vital as they are to providing safety, should not be considered the planned actions of a skilful subject. Rather, they both emerge when different demands and different events link up with different understandings of what it means to *properly* attend to a call. In this chapter, we will outline how, in practice, this takes shape through different materialities and how, at the same time, a certain kind of safety is provided.

Answering calls, managing needs

The Home Telecare Service[1] that we studied covers most of the Catalan territory. It was set up for elderly people who want to keep living alone in their homes and was designed to help their relatives balance their work, leisure and caring time. Rather than directly offering physical help, it acts as a mediator between the person in need of care (called 'the user') and the available carers (called 'the resources'), such as relatives, neighbours, ambulances, doctors, fire brigades, police forces, volunteers, social assistants, etc. The service works by means of a phone line that is connected to a domestic terminal and a slightly adapted telephone, through which the user can communicate with an alarm centre without leaving home. Instead, all that users have to do is press the red button on their telephones, or that of the pendant around their neck, to get in touch with a teleoperator. They can then ask the teleoperator for immediate help, or talk about anything, even if not particularly urgent. If help is needed, the teleoperator will call the most appropriate resource. In order to decide who this might be, teleoperators have access to a database that contains all the medical and personal details of the user. Hence, 'safety' depends on the way teleoperators in the alarm centre manage incoming calls.

At first glance, a telecare service alarm centre resembles the control cabin of a submarine. This is not only because of the profusion of screens, lights and gadgets, but also because, like submarines, the alarm centre is sealed off from what is happening in its immediate surroundings, while trying to capture and interpret only those sounds that may indicate what is happening to the users. The service's operating system is simple. The user or client's terminal is connected to the alarm centre. When a button is pressed or a routine is activated – for example because a user has not complied with the condition of pressing a green button every 12 hours – the terminal sends a seven-digit code to the centre. This causes the user's data to appear on the operator's screen. This means that when operators take a call they have all the user's personal information available on-screen, ranging from clinical diagnoses to notes left by other operators, and including treatments received, prescribed medication, the name of the healthcare professionals attending to the user, the names of the relevant relatives, or the user's call history. With this information at their disposal, in addition to what the user does or does not tell them, including the sounds that accompany the call or the occasional disconcerting silence, operators should be able to define the situation and decide how the service should respond. Therefore, the starting point for the mobilisation – or not - of other resources is the encoding of the call.

Encoding is so important that when operators take a call, even before they have spoken with the user, have already opened a menu on their computer screen and entered a preliminary code that allows them to encode the call. The most common codes for calls are: 'A33: activated by error'; 'A37: courtesy call'; 'A01: social emergency'; 'A02: health emergency' or 'B04: unannounced absence'. More experienced operators are able to correctly encode a call as soon as the user starts speaking. The exercise is surprising to an external observer. Simply upon hearing 'oops, I've made a mist…', an experienced operator encodes the call as 'A33: activated by error'. If what they hear is an apology accompanied by a long explanation, they encode the call as 'A37: courtesy call'.

Clearly, the more difficult situations are those in which the user says that something serious has happened. This is how one operator proceeded in such a case:

> Elena[2] receives an alarm call.
> -'Hello, Maria'.
> The user responds after a few seconds, but it is difficult to hear her. She is distant.
> -'Have you fallen over? Can you hear me? Have you fallen over?' repeats the operator.
> Maria seems to answer from a distance that she has,
> -'I have fallen over, I'm bleeding'.
> Elena opens the call encoding menu and under 'reason' selects 'A02 health emergency'. She turns round and tells Rubén, the coordinator:
> -'A fall in Barcelona and her head is bleeding'.
> The shift coordinator tells her to call 061. Elena shouts:
> -'Stay calm, Maria, I'm going to call your son and send an ambulance!'
> Elena clicks on the mouse and the computer dials 061.

In this case, the operator must decide whether this is an A01 or an A02. The former would mobilise social resources (family members, or other contacts) and the latter health care resources. The dilemma is resolved as soon as the user says that she is bleeding. With this statement the medical emergency protocol has to be followed, which includes the following actions: 1) ascertain the situation of the user; 2) mobilise the user's social resources – preferably those with keys to enter the home before notifying other family members; 3) mobilise health care resources; in the event that entry cannot be gained because there are no keys available, mobilise the fire brigade or police; 4) maintain constant verbal contact with the user to keep her/him informed and provide her/him with a sense of security and company; 5) do not close the call until it is certain that the user has been attended to, and continue attempts to contact family members and other contacts in the event that this has not been possible; 6) complete the alarm report with a description of actions that have been undertaken. If the user is admitted to hospital, open a diary to monitor her/his situation.

Telecare operators are faced with the task of encoding every time they receive a call. The database has 45 possible codes that refer to protocols. The chosen code should activate the protocol that best meets the needs of the user. This gives us the first answer to the question of what the telecare service is. It is, in practice, the provision of safety. It is a matter of translating what users ask for into well placed requests to the proper care resource. It is a matter of linking up specific 'types of calls' with the 'appropriate resources' to meet the users' needs.

Securing practices

The Home Telecare Service is a manager of resources and must refer users' problems as quickly and efficiently as possible to the pertinent resources, whether these are ambulances or family members. To make this possible, the tasks and processes involved have become more and more standardised. (Winthereik et al., 2007; Winthereik and Vikkelsø, 2005). Files, databases, guidelines for interaction and protocols for action have become homogenised. The safety of the users has been linked to a proliferation of more and more control mechanisms that must ensure that the information is transmitted fully and efficiently. As a part of this process, it has become possible to audit the practice of taking calls.

The security thus achieved is not a simple matter. It depends on the alignment of a wide range of elements: telephone lines connected to a hub that selects and transmits them to terminals; registry mechanisms such as databases and the reports filled in by operators; DVD recorders that register everything happening on a telephone line; protocols that outline courses of action; operator training programmes; practices for searching for information in databases; discourses about family solidarity, care of the elderly, welfare, autonomy and quality of life; and conversational skills, such as the ability to ask the right questions and know when and how to close a conversation. So, providing security depends on an extensive socio-technical arrangement (Berg, 1999). This arrangement not only needs to be in place, various elements also have to be attuned to and aligned with each other. The following example helps to illustrate this:

> On a summer Sunday at 1 p.m., a user's daughter arrived at her mother's home to take her for lunch, and find her mother lying on the living room floor. As the mother was delirious and had hypothermia, the daughter immediately called an ambulance to take her to hospital. Shortly afterwards, the telecare service received a complaint. The complaint triggered a procedure called 'Non-compliance'. This ascertains whether the care outlined in the service's protocols and quality manual has been offered or not and whether the codes, the records written by the operator, the recording of the conversation and the protocol all correspond with one another. In other words, it implies a check as to whether all of these elements were correctly aligned. The person responsible for this quality check started by retracing the call history, and looking at the codes that were registered to find out what happened on this occasion. What incoming calls were made (their codes begin with A), what outgoing calls were made (their codes begin with S) and what the operator did (the action codes, which are simply numbers). The present user had an extended service policy. This meant that she was supposed to notify the centre by pressing the green button on the terminal every 12 hours or at most every 24 hours. If the button was not pressed, an alarm was activated. When the records were checked, it turned out that a B01 call [mobility check – user at home] was made on Saturday at 9.00 a.m. According to this, the user had pressed the button to notify that she was at home and fine. However, at 9:00 p.m., when she was supposed to press her button again, no call was received and therefore at 9.00 a.m. on the following day, 24 hours after the last okay signal, the mobility check alarm was automatically activated. The operator called and coded a B01 (mobility check – user at home). This means that the operator had spoken with the user and made sure that she was all right. The codes thus indicated that the user had simply forgotten to make the call, but was found to be all right.

However, the process of 'non-compliance' did not end here. A second check was necessary, the person responsible had to listen to the recording of the call in order to be certain that it really was a B01 and not something else. And indeed, by listening to the call, it was possible to verify that the user had said she had not been able to make the second call due to a fall, but that she was all right now and had managed to reach her bed and lie down. After this, one could hear the operator asking three times whether the user wanted her to call a family member or whether she required help. Three times the user responded in the negative. Given all of the above, the person responsible concluded that the operation had been faultless: 'She asks her three times if she needs anything', we are told. The service could refute the complaint made by the user's daughter.

This process of 'non-compliance' clearly demonstrates how the security mechanisms work to guarantee that information is transmitted correctly. If all is well, the encoding of the call, the implementation of the action protocols corresponding to it and the interaction between user and operator are articulated in such a way that each one inevitably refers to the other (see Latour, 1999). Codes, protocols and interactions should be perfectly matched. The code sequence that appears in a call history must represent the actions stipulated in the action protocols while also representing the interactions the operator has actually made with users, family members or other resources.

Clearly, this perfect alignment is difficult to achieve. For this to happen, different elements must collaborate. The database encoding system is crucial, as it lays down the patterns. It is a homogenising device that obliges all operators, whatever the call, to select a call code (incoming, outgoing and action) before hanging up.[3] It also fulfils another function. Together with the system for recording calls and the protocols, the encoding system allows for a constant assessment of what operators do. It makes it possible to evaluate whether their work meets the quality standards of the service. Sometimes, if necessary, it also helps to generate new protocols or codes. However, as an interface between users and resources, protocols and coding systems are not enough. Equally crucial is a specific manner of taking calls, a style of answering the phone. The telecare service operators must gather pieces of evidence in a curious, detective-like way. As we saw in the 'non-compliance' process above, the user's statements are highly relevant pieces of evidence. Through the repetition of questions such as 'Are you alright?', 'Do you need help?', 'Do you want me to call a family member?' it is the user who is made to decide what is happening to him/her and what should be done. The operator acts as a simple intermediary.

But not only the declarations of users are taken as evidence. So, too, are assessments made by third parties, such as family members, neighbours or doctors. This introduces the idea that it is necessary to construct a socio-technical network – an *assembly of guarantees* – in which statements by users, family members or doctors are perfectly articulated with incoming, outgoing and action call codes, as well as protocols.

Nevertheless, every single call is a challenge to this assembly of guarantees. Will the teleoperator find the proper code? Will the user clearly express what he or she needs? Will the resources be available and on time? As there are many possible setbacks, good telecare depends on something more than the protocols and standards that the telecare service has put in place. As a result, one of the most valued abilities is that of improvisation. As the director of the centre puts it: 'Our ability to improvise is constantly increasing because the number of surprises we have dealt with is constantly increasing, too'. Teleoperators have to go beyond codes and protocols and always expect the unexpected. They must be aware that surprises, even if they are not foreseen, are not at all unusual. Quite the contrary, they occur all the time. Therefore, they should not be treated as exceptions but should be fluidly accommodated. In order to achieve this, codes and protocols must continually be challenged. The art is to obey them while at the same time betraying them. We shall now examine this tension, which is so characteristic of the work of teleoperators as they encode and mobilise aid resources.

Unreliable codes

When a call is made, a code is assigned to it as seems fit. But the codes that appear in the records are always treated with caution. There may be more to them than meets the eye. Take, for example, an A33, a courtesy call. According to the protocols, a call is to be encoded as 'courtesy' when all the user wants is to talk for a while. But the use of this code does not completely define a call. An operator who finds one in the records, may, by relating this code to other codes in the call history as well as to personal data and what the user, family members or doctors say, come to further specify the meaning of an A33. This specific A33 might actually mean abandonment by the family and a user who feels lonely, but another might mean that a user is feeling better, engaging in more activities and eager to tell other people about them. A third option could be that the user does not trust the telecare service and wants to check whether there really is somebody at the other end of the line should he or she need them. Therefore, although in each of these cases an A33 appears in the call history, operators must, as the director of the centre says, look beyond the code. Codes do not represent simple pieces of evidence. And while it is right to encode a call as A33 (courtesy call) when a user merely wants to talk for a while, the operator must look beyond the code to know how to react. This is achieved by linking the code to other codes in the call history, other user data and conversations with the user, their family members or professional carers. The use of such diverse data leads to a form of triangulation, and opens up new meanings.

Rebel resources

The tension between what is clear-cut and what is adaptable also emerges when (as a call comes in) a user's care resources appear on the screen. Take the user's main contacts. These resources are called upon in times of social emergencies as well in times of health emergencies, as these tend to be people (usually family members) close to the user, who care about the user, are able to mobilise themselves quickly and have access to the home. According to the protocol they serve various functions: for example, they may calm and care for the user and supply the operator with a first assessment of the situation. When required, they may provide other resources (ambulances, doctors, fire brigade...) access the user's house. In practice, however, 'main contact' is a term that can include anyone from family members who would do anything for their relatives (some even act as rivals to the service by offering greater care, for example calling several times a day and taking the user to the doctor if necessary without telling the service), to relatives who want nothing to do with them at all and who delegate any responsibility for the users to the service (even getting angry when the service notifies them that their relative is not well). And although they are far more regulated, a similar fluidity characterises such health resources as ambulances, health transportation and the fire service. For example, the ambulance service is sometimes unable to cope with the demand, whereupon operators are obliged to quickly find alternatives. Sometimes, too, there are discrepancies between the operator and a doctor about the need to send an ambulance. Although operators must activate the resources as stipulated in the protocol, they must do so assuming that these resources will not always behave as expected. Providing a user with safety, therefore, depends on the assumption that neither the situation nor the people involved are pre-defined. Instead, they define themselves, and are defined, as things develop.

Caring practices

In order to provide safety, reliability is needed as well as something else. To put this 'something else' into words: safety not only depends on securing practices, it also depends on caring practices. When we talk about caring practices we are not implying that operators must be affectionate, sympathetic or kind to users. Care is not a nice wrapping, a decoration that makes attending to users more pleasant and humane. Instead, care refers to a series of practices in which bodies, knowledge and technology are attuned to one another in a way that takes the unaccountable into account, that is attentive to the indeterminate (see also Mol, 2008). As has been highlighted by Tronto (1993), the semantics of the concept of 'care' lead us to the notion of limit. To care for something means being concerned about what threatens or might transform the limits that define it. For an operator, therefore, caring for a user means being concerned about everything that does not fit in with their routines and may change the situations they expect in everyday life. This is not fully captured by the guidelines and the information displayed onscreen and it is not part of the closed list of options the codes allow for. In contrast with securing practices, caring practices do not start with what is defined, controlled and standardised (codes, protocols, etc.), but from unforeseen events and the uncertainty that comes about when unforeseen events occur in users' everyday lives. Caring, therefore, is characterised by practices that strive to attend to what should not have been possible.

The management of care consists of allowing the indeterminacy of events to affect the service in a productive way. This implies being receptive to events before trying to fit them into a closed pattern, such as a protocol. So, while security is a practice of protection, care is a practice of risk. The openness required to care well depends on a teleoperator's willingness to ignore all rules and regulations. After all, this is how it is possible to go beyond the normalisation and closure implied by securing practices. So, providing safety requires a fine balance between collective experience as encrypted in rules, and a constant openness to the unpredictable or unlikely. This reminds us of the concept of 'belief' proposed by Despret (2004) in her analysis of Rosenthal's classic experiments on 'the effect of the experimenter'. Despret proposes that belief is 'what makes entities available to events' and experimenters open to the 'becoming' of 'the other'. This 'becoming' includes resistance, upsets and unexpected singularities. In her words, 'someone who cares' is 'someone who trusts, moreover, someone who was interested, someone it interests (*inter-esse*, to make a link)'. Similarly to the experimenters, teleoperators, too, must be open in such a way, not to their experimental subjects, but to the call and the user's specific situation. In their case, then, caring is mediating, i.e. constructing a singular link between the user's call and the resources.

However, telecare work is not only about care. Rather, it is located in the tension between security and care, constantly evaluated according to whether rules are followed and protocols adhered to, while also constantly being challenged by singularities and unforeseen events. There is, again in Despret's words, a persistent tension that emerges from 'the contrast between the manner of addressing oneself to the system, on the one hand as a care-taker, as somebody interested in its possible becoming, and on the other hand, as a judge or a master' (Despret, 2004: 124). When operators explain how they handle this, how they take charge of what should not have been possible, how they incorporate the indeterminate in their assessment of the situation and the way in which they mobilise resources, they refer to experience and intuition.

> Also sometimes, for example, you can find a case where, for example, there are old people who call you but don't ask for anything because they don't want to bother you, right? So, if you're getting to know them, well maybe because of their tone of voice you say, I have a feeling something is not right with them, but they don't want to say anything (Teleoperator 7:17-85:105).

> You also sense a lot of things. Because I remember in the beginning, last year when I was just starting out, I had no idea, I was always handing over the headphones because I didn't ... and the others, who had been doing it longer, they knew what they wanted ... it's experience... (Teleoperator 7:4-37:49).

So experience and intuition are important. But it must be cautioned that experience and intuition are not acquired individually, eventually becoming internal capabilities. Instead, they are practices developed in operators' everyday work.[4] So when we talk about the experiences of teleoperators, we are not referring to the knowledge each of them accumulates, as if it is their personal property. Rather, we are referring to a shared practice, one which consists of going beyond apparent logic and common sense and which depends on an attitude of unfamiliarity with the familiar.[5] It all has to do with questioning assumptions and challenging the call history, the user's data, and what the users themselves, their family members and other professionals say. This practice just might help one to produce a new and short-lived 'singular' meaning, one that is just enough to provide an appropriate reply. It takes a lot of time to become acquainted with this practice of caring.

The teleoperators at the Catalan Red Cross centre are deliberately given job stability. This not only allows them to learn how to use different registry systems and protocols, but also to let go of them and never discount a possibility as being 'impossible' because it does not fit. All user information always has to be 'handled with care'. This implies that it is good to know the habits of a user who calls every day to chat for a while, while, at the same time, it is important to treat each call as if it was the first of its kind. As the operators say, 'It's like actors in a play and each time, every day, the text changes a little. Well this is the same. You have to change.' (7:7-629:641) Having experience means being able to use the codes and the protocols in an individualised way to offer specific care to each user, in each case. That is why rules are not conceived as exterior and fixed working patterns to be applied automatically to a call. On the contrary, codes and protocols are to be used in a flexible, modular way and small 'tools of knowledge' should be suitably combined. This exercise of particularisation depends on being able to not take anything that happens for granted. But it also depends on other operators, the supervisor and specific objects. Like securing practices, caring practices involve a wide range of heterogeneous elements:

> Juanito is talking to the daughter of a user who has fallen and is being attended to by Juanito's colleague Miquel. While Miquel is talking to the 061 doctor for an assessment and requesting an ambulance, Juanito informs the daughter of what has happened. He explains that an ambulance is going to come and pick up her mother and asks her to go to her mother's house. As the daughter sets off, Miquel takes full responsibility for the call again and Juanito takes another one that his colleague Sol (sitting behind the next computer screen) has left on hold. Before putting on the headphones, however, he turns to Sol and complains jokingly that he doesn't understand the note she has attached

to the code. Sol explains that the call concerns a user who
goes for dialysis everyday but has not done so today and
wants to go, which means she needs an ambulance.

This is a common enough occurrence: operators take calls collectively, in coordination with each other. They make notes in the computer files that they attach not only to the call codes, but also to all types of information recorded in the database: main resources, user, etc. The technician in charge of the maintenance of the database is proud of its adaptability: 'There are many open fields that you can fill in as you like. I mean, it's not a completely closed program, but rather one that can be adapted to every need'. (3:41-133:133) Although the open fields allow for the addition of further verbal information and cannot be used to enter, for example, statistics or photographs, their relative openness is still essential because, as one operator puts it: 'It allows others to do their work without going crazy'. (3:42-133:133) The open fields in the database therefore act as sites to which teleoperators can turn in order to find out anything that cannot be recorded in the closed fields of the database. They are essential for individualising codes and sharing the specific nature of each situation. For instance, a B04 code [not notified absence] changes meaning when a note is attached that says *Hairdresser's*. The operator understands that it is highly unlikely that there is a problem. Instead, the user has not pressed the green button because she has gone to the hairdresser's and forgotten to do it.

As we can see, the operators' work is not only co-ordinated through a system of encoding, forms and standardised protocols. In addition, there are flexible technologies – open fields, notes, scratch papers – which help to coordinate care and make it specific and individual.[6] They make it possible to share aspects that do not fit in forms, and that, in a totally secured world, would remain invisible. This fluid data, imperceptible in the 'closed response' fields, interferes with the tight referential relations among codes, protocols and actions taken. However, they allow telecare operators to specify any arising situation in such a way that it may be dealt with down to the last detail.[7] This means that when one follows the work of a telecare operator, one observes a wide range of practices that always involve third parties, people as well as technologies. These include talking with a user whose data appears onscreen; listening to what is happening on the other end of the line; attending to what the other operators are doing; or keeping an eye on the 'on hold' tray in order to know which calls are being attended to. All the while, the teleoperator must also code and attach notes about everything relevant to the case. If done well, taken in unison, all of these practices are what they need to be doing: caring.

Entangling security and care to provide safety

Providing telecare users with safety is a complex matter. It involves reliability and efficiency, as well as the capacity to manage all manner of imponderables. It requires a complex system of highly protocolised and audited work in which every action is sequenced and planned according to standards, whilst at the same time depending on improvisation and the capacity to attend to the specific elements of each case. This is nothing new. It again underlines something that has also been demonstrated in earlier studies on protocols and care practices (Winthereik *et al.*, 2007). The implementation of protocols and accountability systems in health care settings requires, either explicitly and planned or implicitly and improvised, a whole series of adaptable practices that are difficult to audit because they are heterogeneous, contingent and local (Singleton, 1998).

One of the most interesting aspects of the telecare service is that taking calls involves playing the security game and the care game while respecting the rules of each, despite the fact that they are very different. In the service, this dual game, so crucial to the work carried out at the alarm centre, is known as 'active listening'. In explaining the 'activated by error' code, the director of the service puts it like this:

> Well, what is fundamental for us is active listening, right? That is, you understand what the user is telling you, they are telling you they have made a mistake, right? But they carry on and on, etc, etc. What is required then is not an 'activated by error' code, what is needed is something that you are not giving them. They want conversation, to feel safe, they want something more intangible, to put it that way, and that is not found in a protocol, right? (Director of the Call Centre 2:27-75:95).

The director insists that it is essential to correctly identify the call code, but that something else is needed as well. Something more, something that goes beyond according with the accountability system. A good telecare operator is sensitive to nuances and to the hidden needs behind the words. A good telecare operator engages in security practices but also adds caring practices. The ideal of 'active listening' is only achieved when codes and protocols align perfectly and are individualised so as to specifically attune to the case at hand. Active listening is therefore not just a matter of merely transmitting information so as to put users in contact with the necessary resources. However, the teleoperator is also not a strong agent who must assess and decide what the user needs. Instead, active listening is a matter of being two different things simultaneously: an intermediary and a mediator (Latour, 1996).

The safety provided to users does not therefore stem solely from the reliability, efficiency and speed with which the service encodes the call and mobilises the relevant resources. It also comes from the attentiveness of the operators, the ability to perceive the nuances of each call and their flexibility in responding to them. The telecare service can make people feel safe thanks to an active listening process by which security practices and care practices become entangled.[8]

The etymology of the word 'security' could have taught us so much. Security comes from the Latin securitas, which means *sine cura*, careless. Therefore, security refers to a state in which one is freed from all concerns that might hold one's attention. Security implies disregarding, reducing one's attention for 'what should not be possible'. Providing security implies aligning codes and protocols in such a way that each one refers to the next and the space for what should not be possible is reduced to the minimum. However, providing security is only a partial way of relating to the insecurity of existence (Dillon, 1996). It is not enough to simply combat insecurity and reduce it to a minimum. As operators know all too well, there are always unexpected events. In order to deal with these it is necessary to improvise and challenge the standards and procedures of the service. That is why operators must both comply with the rules and at the same time never be completely certain about a situation. They need to be unconcerned but not negligent.[9] It is crucial to stay alert. For this reason, regulations do not annul the operators' concern, but rather construct a care threshold that focuses them. Thus there is not necessarily any opposition between security and care, between protocolised and non-protocolised practices or between an abstract reason and a practical reason (Berg, 1997). Instead, 'active listening' draws them together, rather than opposing them. The space in which the meaning of codes is cast in doubt, the precepts of protocols are betrayed, and the different aid resources are articulated individually, at the same time still depends on them. It would be as negligent to never make a rule or a standard or never guarantee anything as it would be to try to eliminate any type of insecurity. Caring depends on some form of security.

This, then, is how one can become a guardian angel. It is a process of becoming, but one never quite gets there, as the safety provided by the home telecare service is always emerging, but never reached. It depends on an entanglement between providing security and giving care. That is to say, it depends on practices, technologies and bodies that follow different logics – security and care – at the same time, in a delicate balance. Or, put in yet another way, user safety emerges from the productive combination of practices that seek to close the space of what should not be possible and practices that attempt to incorporate the unlikely and deal with it in an attentive way.

Acknowledgments

This paper was written as part of the PhD Social Psychology Program at the Autonomous University of Barcelona (UAB) in the context of a project on the 'Psychosocial Impact of Technoscientific Innovations', funded by the Ministerio de Ciencia y Tecnologia.

Notes

1 The average user of this Home Telecare Service is a woman of eighty-two who lives alone in the city and hires a basic telealarm device that only works when the alarm is pressed voluntarily.

2 All names are fictitious in order to preserve the anonymity of those involved.

3 The system used is very similar to the NHS Clinical Assessment System (CAS), as it shares the same logic. Users feel secure if responses are consistent, quick and based on the statistically most significant and problematic cases (Hanlon et al., 2005).

4 Elsewhere, we have called these practices ex-inscriptions (López and Domènech, 2008) in talking about the deliverance of immediate attention in a home telecare service.

5 This attitude emerges when intimate knowledge is achieved (Mackenzie, 2001) and defines a kind of taste, a way of being sensitive to something. 'It is an active way of putting oneself in such a state that something may happen to oneself' (Hennion, 2007:109).

6 Besides face-to-face communication (Schubert, 2003), such soft technologies are essential in these work spaces, where it is essential to organise improvisation (Whalen et.al., 2002).

7 The use of these flexible technologies is essential in promoting greater intimacy. As Bowker and Leigh-Star (1999) explain, 'A manageable classification system (for whomever) does not only require the system to classify the same things across sites and times but also to uncover invisible work; this affects the data recordings. The combination of these two thus requires compromise. Finally, to keep a level of intimacy in the classification system, control is a trade-off against the requirement to make everything visible. These trade-offs become areas of negotiation and sometimes of conflict' (Bowker and Star, 1999: 232-233).

8 In a similar way, in a case study focused on anaesthesia practices, Maggie Mort et al. (2005) have shown how safety also necessarily entails dealing with changing boundaries between consciousness/unconsciousness, human/machine frontiers and expert/lay knowledge.

9 As Dillon (1996) explains, securitas for the classic world was both a valued asset and an evil which made man negligent.

References

Berg, Marc. (1999). Patient care information systems and health care work: a sociotechnical approach. *International Journal of Medical Informatics*, 55(2), 87-101.

Berg, Marc. (1997). *Rationalizing medical work: decision-support techniques and medical practices*. Cambridge, Mass.: MIT Press.

Bowker, Geoffrey C. and Star, Susan Leigh. (1999). *Sorting things out: classification and its consequences*. Cambridge, Mass.: MIT Press.

Despret, Vinciane. (2004). The Body We Care For: Figures of Anthropo-Zoo-Genesis. *Body and Society*, 10(2-3), 111-134.

Dillon, Michael. (1996). *Politics of security: towards a political philosophy of continental thought*. London; New York: Routledge.

Hanlon, Gerard, Strangleman, Tim, Goode, Jackie, Luff, Donna, O'Cathain, Alicia, and Greatbatch, David. (2005). Knowledge, technology and nursing: The case of NHS direct. *Human Relations*, 58(2), 147-171.

Hennion, Antoine. (2007). Those Things That Hold Us Together: Taste and Sociology. Cultural Sociology, 1, 97.

Latour, Bruno. (1996). Trains of thought – Piaget, formalism and the fifth dimension. *Common Knowledge(3)*, 170-191.

Latour, Bruno. (1999). *Pandora's Hope: Essays on the Reality of Science Studies*. London: Harvard University Press.

López, Daniel and Domènech, Miquel (2008). On inscriptions and ex-inscriptions: the production of immediacy in a home telecare service. Environment and Planning D: Society and Space, 26:663-675.

MacKenzie, Donald A. (2001). *Mechanizing proof: computing, risk, and trust*. Cambridge, Mass.: MIT Press.

Mol, Annemarie. (2008). *The logic of care. Active patients and the limits of choice*. New York: Routledge.

Mort, Maggie, Goodwin, Dawn, Smith, Andrew F., and Pope, Catherine. (2005). Safe asleep? Human-machine relations in medical practice. *Social Science & Medicine*, 61(9), 2027-2037.

Shubert, Cornelius. (2003). *Patient safety and the practice of anaesthesia: how hybrid networks of cooperation live and breathe*. Berlin: Technische Universität (Institut für Soziologie).

Singleton, Vicky. (1998). Stabilizing Instabilities: The Role of the Laboratory in the United Kingdom Cervical Screening Programme. A M. Berg and A. Mol (Eds.), *Differences in Medicine: unraveling practices, techniques, and bodies* (pp. 86-105). Durham N. C.: Duke University Press.

Tronto, Joan C. (1993). *Moral boundaries: a political argument for an ethic of care*. New York: Routledge.

Whalen, Jack, Whalen, Marilyn, and Henderson, Kathryn. (2002). Improvisational choreography in teleservice work. *The British Journal of Sociology*, 53(2), 239-258.

Winthereik, Brit Ross, van der Ploeg, Irma, and Berg, Marc. (2007). The electronic patient record as a meaningful audit tool – Accountability and autonomy in general practitioner work. *Science Technology & Human Values*, 32(1), 6-25.

Winthereik, Brit Ross and Vikkelsø, Signe. (2005). ICT and Integrated Care: Some Dilemmas of Standardising Inter-Organisational Communication. *Computer Supported Cooperative Work (CSCW)*, 14(1), 43.

Care and disability
Practices of experimenting, tinkering with, and arranging people and technical aids

Myriam Winance

In order to examine the question of care practices in the field of disability, I will start with the contradiction that emerges when one compares two approaches: the *Disability Studies approach*, developed by some disabled researchers and activists, and the 'ethics of care' approach developed by certain feminists in the early 1980s in Anglo-Saxon countries. *Disability Studies* is linked to the *Disability Movement* created by disabled persons in the United States and Great Britain in the 1970s (Barton & Oliver, 1997; Oliver & Barnes, 1998; Scotch, 1988). Although it takes different forms in the two countries, the starting point is the same: criticising existing practices such as re-education and rehabilitation, which are interpreted as implementations of a medical model. This medical model defines disability as something that results from an individual, pathological or functional causality and focuses the action on the individual to be 'rehabilitated'; this model is also linked to practices of institutionalisation. In the 1970s, disabled people reformulated their experience not as being an experience of being 'maladjusted to society', but as an experience of being 'excluded from society'. They became aware that their disability is the result of architectural, social and cultural barriers that society imposes upon people with impairments. This awareness is the basis for what we now call the 'social model' of disability, which defines disability as being the result of a social causality. From this, Disability Studies went on to develop the demand that practices and society be changed in order to make it possible for disabled people to participate. The people committed to this movement fight for the ability to control their lives and to decide for themselves what they need. They oppose existing practices that are seen as oppressive and infantilising. From this standpoint they criticise the notion of care (2001; Keith, 1992), inasmuch as relationships of care place those who receive it in a position of dependence and passivity. They defend the implementation of a formalised and functional relationship of help to the exclusion of any emotional dimension. To designate this relationship, researchers use terms such as 'help', 'support' or 'personal assistance', rejecting that of 'care' in order to stress the desire for control and autonomy that disabled people are looking for in their everyday lives.

The beginning of the 1980s in the United States saw the emergence of another movement now identified by the term 'ethics of care', which includes different works (Brugère, 2006; Feder Kittay & Feder, 2003; Paperman, 2004, 2005; Tronto, 1993, 2005). What these works have in common is that they look to revise the practices and values relating to care, in order to build an ethic of care as opposed to an ethic of justice. These works begin with a criticism of the autonomous rational subject (the modern Cartesian subject) and demonstrate a relational, affective, emotional me who is built and supported by relationships of care. They thus place the accent on vulnerability and dependence[1] (constitutive for everybody, whoever he/she may be), on the ensuing need for care relationships and on the asymmetry and affective dimension of these relationships. In their opinion, everyone is, at a given moment in his/her life, involved in relationships of care, either as the one who is caring or as the one who is being cared for. The aim of these works is then as follows: to consider the moral norms that allow the development of relationships of care (conceived as relationships of dependency), which although asymmetrical are not relationships of domination. 'An ethics of care may be one way to understand the moral commitments and relations that arise among the persons unequally positioned in relations of dependency.' p. 3 (Feder Kittay & Feder, 2003).

I am not going to discuss these works any further, but only wish to stress the opposition between the two approaches.[2] On the one hand, Disability Studies researchers demonstrate that a disabled person is not a person who is 'constitutively or essentially dependent', but that his/her dependence results from social organisation. They therefore demand the ability to choose and control their own lives, including the possibility to develop a relationship not of care, but of assistance or support, a symmetrical relationship. On the other hand, the theorists of care believe that we are all dependent upon one another, and that we are all involved in affective and asymmetrical relationships of care; independence is a fiction, an illusion.

The aim of this article is to escape from this opposition by making a methodological shift, towards the examination of particular situations of care, that is, the practices and techniques for compensating for inabilities. These techniques encompass recourse to technical aids as well as rehabilitation and re-education practices. In this paper, I will analyse such techniques through four cases taken from two ethnographical studies. The first study involved observing wheelchair tests that took place at a test centre located inside a major hospital. Approximately 120 models of manual and electric wheelchairs, on loan from the manufacturers, were exhibited in a room measuring 350m². Benoît, a physiotherapist, received patients (from the hospital or from the outside) who had made appointments and who needed a wheelchair. He showed the patients one or more wheelchairs and allowed them to try them out.[3] I was able to observe 34 tests, including those made by Mrs. Sabin, Serge and André that I will discuss in this paper. The other, final example that I use, that of Martine, is taken from an ethnographical study carried out at a day hospital in a re-education and functional rehabilitation centre. My examination of these practical care situations will lead me to make a theoretical shift with regard to the notion of care. Whilst Disability Studies and ethics of care researchers have different conceptions of the person (either as dependent or independent), they both base themselves on the same conception of care in terms of a relationship of aid going from one person, a carer, to another, the cared for; the former – active – helps and supports the latter – passive. The description of the wheelchair tests and the rehabilitation practices will lead me to offer a conception of care in terms of shared work, dispersed in a collective of humans and non-humans (Callon & Law, 1995), each person in the collective being simultaneously an object and a subject of care. I will describe this work as empirical tinkering (Mol, 2006; Pols, 2004), the purpose of which, for the people involved, is to empirically shape an arrangement between the persons and the chair that suits them and that causes the emergence of movement sensations, possibilities and abilities for everyone.

Spotting what works and what does not

Mrs. Sabin, aged 60, has a cerebral motor deficiency. Two or three years ago, she lost the ability to walk. At first she rented a manual wheelchair. When the rental continued, French social security forced her to buy her own wheelchair, without giving her any warning. She therefore had to buy a wheelchair very quickly from a catalogue, without being able to test it, and this is the wheelchair she currently uses. It is a basic wheelchair, with a metal chassis covered with a blue waxed material, high square armrests, and two detachable footrests. It is heavy and not very manoeuvrable. Mrs. Sabin is small and her wheelchair is far too big for her. It is very uncomfortable and she quickly gets back pain when sitting in it. It is also difficult for her to move it on her own. She has decided to buy a new wheelchair, and accompanied by her husband she has come to the test centre to try out a new chair, the SP, which one of her friends uses. During the tests she tries three light top-of-the-range chairs, and finally chooses the SP.

> *Benoît*: You saw Mrs. X with her SP, and you want to try the same model?
> *Mrs. Sabin*: Yes, hers seems more comfortable, you get better back support. In this one my back and my feet hurt, and the two footrests are no good, my feet get stuck between them and it hurts. I want a wheelchair with a single footrest. With two, I get stuck.
> *Benoît*: Are you always in your chair? Have you walked before?
> *Mrs. S*: Yes, I'm going to walk. They are going to operate on me and I hope I'll be able to walk again.
> *Benoît* [repeating and insisting]: Have you walked before?
> *Mrs. S*: Yes, until two or three years ago.
> *Benoît*: And are you in your chair all day long?
> *Mrs. S*: Yes.
> *Mr. S*: Yes, or on the sofa, because she can't cope with being in this all the time.
> *Mrs. S*: This one is uncomfortable and when I have spasticity attacks,… it's impossible, I end up spending all day lying down, it's impossible to do anything else.
> *Benoît*: And can you move on your own, or does your husband always push you?
> *Mr. S*: Inside, she moves around on her own, but when we go out I push her. Because, well, she has trouble moving on her own. Inside she manages, more or less.
> *Benoît*: Yes.
> *Mrs. S*: For me it's hard to push myself because it's too wide and too big.
> *Benoît*: The main problem is the back, it's too high.
> *Mrs. S*: I'd be better off with a junior model, because I'm really not very big!
> *Benoît*: We no longer work in terms of adult/child. Because at the end of the day it's a question of size […]. You need a small size. So I see you put your bag next to you… that's important for you… you want to always be able to do that?
> *Mrs. S*: Yes, I want to be able to put it next to me.
> *Benoît*: Do you sometimes stand up?
> *Mrs. S*: No.

> *Benoît*: How do you go about getting onto the sofa?
> *Mrs. S*: I remain seated. I stay seated and I move from one to the other.
> *Mr. S*: Yes, but you put your weight on one foot.
> *Benoît*: Do you lift up the footrest?
> *Mrs. S*: Yes, often. I often lift them up.
> (Test Centre, June 1999)

At the start of the test, the centre manager and Mr. Sabin are next to Mrs. Sabin in her wheelchair, and look at her. Benoît asks Mrs. Sabin questions about what she does or does not do, how she feels in her wheelchair and how she uses it. Mrs. Sabin and her husband both reply to his questions. The research is done in a joint manner. Mrs. Sabin explains what *she does not like*: she gets back pain and her feet slip between the two footrests. She cannot move the wheelchair on her own. Mr. Sabin speaks up to give further details about how she uses or does not use the chair, and how she feels when sitting in it. He points out that she is unable to spend all day in the wheelchair and that when moving to the sofa she puts her weight on one foot. The actors also look at what *she likes*; for example, being able to have her bag next to her. Furthermore, in their analysis they always relate what Mrs. Sabin can or cannot do to the characteristics of the wheelchair. They link actions to wheelchair characteristics; for example, Mrs. Sabin relates her difficulty in using the wheelchair on her own to the size of the chair, whilst Benoît relates it to the height of the back. In this way, through their conversation and by watching how Mrs. Sabin is seated in her chair, they gradually see what is right or wrong with the current chair, and furthermore they do this in terms of the characteristics needed for the new wheelchair: it must be light, small, have a single footrest and a low back, be easy to manoeuvre and comfortable. As the test continues, so does this analysis, taking the form of a physical confrontation between the person and the various different wheelchairs, and of a tinkering with the ways in which they suit one another.

Trying a chair, experimenting, groping, handling

After exploring what a new chair will need, the second stage is to fit the person and the wheelchair together. For one, two or even three hours, the actors experiment, test and successively touch the person, the chair and the 'person-in-his/her-chair'; they look, they examine each and every characteristic of the chair and the way in which the person is seated. They explore the position of each limb and/or whether a given action will be possible. Here the research into what works and what does not takes the form of an exchange of perceptions. The test is long and slow; patience is needed. To care is to take one's time, to 'quibble' over details, to examine together, to test, explore and feel in order to make the right adjustments.

> *Serge, aged 41, has a cerebral motor deficiency and uses a manual wheelchair with a customised seat, but he would like an electric wheelchair because his girlfriend cannot push him anymore. At first the idea is that she should be the one to drive it. He is unable to drive an electric wheelchair because he cannot control his hands and arms, which tend to make uncoordinated movements. But at the same time, they have already owned one electric wheelchair that Serge's girlfriend drove, but they had problems getting past certain obstacles and climbing slopes. Benoît therefore suggests trying to let Serge drive with a chin control. Serge, with his customised seat, is transferred onto a small electric wheelchair with a chin control.*
>
> *Benoît*: Even for someone who is used to it, this is not easy, so you mustn't be impatient; even for an accident victim who does not have these movement problems [*that is: sudden uncontrollable movements*] it is hard, the installation takes a very long time... Afterwards you know a bit more, you have a better idea of the position, but at the beginning it takes time, it's a nightmare... so you mustn't get cross if we have to experiment and if we don't get it right straight away. [...] *Benoît tries to position the control in front of Serge's chin, the difficulty being that it must not be too far, so that Serge can reach it and use it without too much effort, nor too close, so that Serge doesn't move it by mistake. He finds a position.* Can we try it like that? *Serge tries to reach the control with his chin, but does not succeed. He concentrates and tries again, but can't do it.*
>
> *Benoît*: I suggest we give ourselves fifteen minutes to experiment and to try to find the right position, and then we'll see. *He changes the position of the control, he tries to lift it higher and turn it. The control is not very flexible, which makes it hard to position it; he ends up finding another position that seems better. He then explains to Serge how it works.* When you pull down, the chair moves forward, and when you push, the chair reverses; to turn you have to push on the side.
>
> *He turns the chair on, and Serge starts to control the chair. We can see that he is concentrating to control the movements of his head and to watch where he is going. He manages to move around,*

to move forward and turn; he sometimes finds it hard to stay in the same direction, but overall he manages to use the control.
(Test Centre, June 1999)

By experimenting and tinkering in this way, the actors try to answer the question of how the person feels in this chair and what can he/she do in this chair. They explore how the person feels in his/her wheelchair, the way in which the chair makes it possible or impossible to do certain things. They 'de-scribe'[4] and deploy the characteristics of the person and those of the wheelchair. They swap perceptions and compare them, in order to try to define which body, with what sensations and what (in)abilities, is shaped by this wheelchair.

> *Mrs. Sabin is sitting in the SP*
> Benoît: Right, okay, this is a top-of-the-range chair, it's different from the one you have, which is a basic chair. The problem is finding the right size. I think this one is too big. I usually advise that one should be able to get a hand between the armrest and the buttock, but no more than that. Now, if you'd like to be able to sit next to the bag... It's important that the back of the chair properly supports your back, and if your husband pushes a lot, he has to be able to push without too much problem.
> Mrs. S: *She has already tried to move a bit and she is immediately enthusiastic* Ah yes, this is completely different, so much better, it rolls well. *She tries the chair, makes it move.*
> [...]
> Mrs. S: The canvas back is much nicer than the other.
> Benoît: It's mainly because it goes round the tubes instead of just over them. So what don't you like about this chair? What would you like to change? For me, it's the width... it's too wide, but for you it's alright?
> Mrs. S: Yes.
> Benoît: Don't you need a strap in front of your ankles to keep your feet in place?
> Mrs. S: No, my feet stay in position on their own, it's just when I flex my legs, they need a few seconds to bend, but apart from that... it's fine... they stay in place on the other chair, they are always like that. [...]
> Benoît: [...] But there are other questions... there you've got your knees bent, does that bother you?
> Mrs. S: No, no problem.
> Benoît: Because there's the same model but with a longer-

> frame, so you could have your feet further out. Your legs will be less bent.
> *Mrs. S:* No, this one's fine.
> (Test Centre, June 1999)

These extracts demonstrate the meticulous joint exploration that is done during the test; this exploration relates to the sensations that Mrs. S feels in each part of her body. Does this chair and its characteristics (wide, footrest somewhat backward, small front wheels, canvas back) suit Mrs. S who is small, who has spasticity attacks (such people usually do not like to have their legs bent backwards for too long) and severe scoliosis? In the two extracts above, from the tests carried out by Serge and Mrs. Sabin, we see a 'disassembly' of the body and of the wheelchair. The person's body and the wheelchair are not considered as wholes, but in terms of their parts, with each part being capable of its own particular action. There is thus the issue of whether Mrs. Sabin's feet will stay on the footrest or whether they will suddenly lift up. In Serge's case, there is the question of the sudden uncoordinated movements of his limbs and head. Here, the body is an overflowing body. It has resistance, tested by the actors. The purpose of the joint work done throughout the test is to bring out a 'body-in-a-wheelchair'. The actors tinker together to come up with an arrangement between the person and the chair that suits them.

Shaping what works: defining an arrangement between person and chair

The exploration and exchange of perceptions transform the person and the chair. The search for a suitable position, which the person finds comfortable and which allows him/her to act, involves a gradual shaping of person and chair: one moves an arm or a leg, and then one changes the width of the chair, one adjusts a cushion, a headrest, etc. From the very outset, the manufacturer sees the wheelchair as an object that can be customised, changed and tinkered with to suit the person who will be using it and to suit his/her sensations and (in)abilities.[5] During the tests, the actors constantly change and adjust the settings of the chair and the position of the person.

> *André, who has Duchenne myopathy, has just been transferred into the TWS, an electric wheelchair, and is telling his mother and the test centre manager how he is feeling, what is okay and what is not, and how he needs to be positioned in order to feel more comfortable.*
> *André:* inaudible:... my right-hand side...

Benoît: Who has understood that André needs to be recentred in the chair because he has the impression he is going to fall. It's the armrests? You want me to bring them closer [to the seat]?
André: No, it's fine. Mummy! I'm going to fall!
Mother: No, we are holding you... when he doesn't have the table he panics. It's because he has nothing to hold on to.
Father: Yes.
Benoît: But... it's a bit too wide at the sides. Maybe it will be better if I pull the whole thing closer together. I'm going to pull the whole thing closer to the seat *Benoît brings the armrests closer to the seat.*
André: You need to push me further back. *His mother then pulls him from behind.*
Mother: Shall I pull your leg?
André: Yes? *Very gently, his mother pulls his leg forward, following André's instructions, until he says stop.*
Benoît: Does the back need to be more upright?
André: I need a headrest. *Benoît goes to get one and positions it.*
Mother: I'll do something so that it pulls less on your legs. *She moves his legs.*
André: Unintelligible
Mother: *She has understood and she repeats.* 'I can't do my movements and swing to get back into position...' No, I can see that.
[...]
André: I'm too far back. [...] At home we've added some foam padding.
Mother: Yes... at home we have made our own cushion, and so it is just the right shape and doesn't push on your legs: it's round. The one from the distributor is straighter. I buy foam, cut it and cover it. On your chair there are two cushions, and we've added a bit at the front so that it doesn't pull on your legs... But the cushion doesn't matter, we can make another one.
(Test Centre, June 1999)

The actors gradually shape a person-in-a-wheelchair; they tinker around to make an arrangement. To achieve this, they experiment, they test, they pay attention to details and they try to adapt. The back is 'a tad too upright', the hand is placed 'a millimetre' too far from the wheelchair control. The actors act on the materiality of the person and the chair in an attempt to make them suit one another. They adapt, they make adjustments to person and chair to try to find how they can 'fit one another', how they can 'come to an arrangement'. And every time they find an arrangement, they assess it by once again exploring the sensations of the 'person-in-a-wheelchair', looking to see to what extent 'it works'. This process is what I have called the process of adjustment (Winance, 2006b, 2006a, 2007b). Through this exploration and shaping, through this process of adjustment, a position emerges that suits the person, a position in which he/she feels comfortable, in which there is less pain and in which new actions are possible.[6]

To care is to tinker and to doctor. To care is to 'quibble', to handle, to adjust, to experiment, to change tiny details in order to see if it works, to see if the person and the wheelchair can come to an arrangement and if they might get along with one another. Wheelchair tests bring to bare that care implies work on the body as well as on what is felt and may be felt by the various members of the collective involved in it. Here, care bespeaks a sensitivity shared and distributed among the actors. The object of care is not one single person but a collective. The work of caring involves attention that is built by the collective and directed towards the sensations and possibilities of action that emerge for the person concerned. This attention is 'material'; it includes the object, the wheelchair. The actors touch and watch in order to shape a 'person-in-a-wheelchair' capable of certain actions, in order to enable him/her and to give him/her more (or new) mobility (Winance, 2003). Mobility here refers to the ability to make links: to move in the world *and* be moved by it or by the others.

To enable the person: making him/her move and be moved

Pain prevents action; it immobilises people by focusing their attention on what is hurting. A dual breakdown takes place. On the one hand between the person and this body that hurts, on the other hand between the person and his/her environment. Someone who is in pain withdraws; he/she is unable to act (Leder, 1990; Scarry, 1985). If a person is not sitting properly and is in pain in his/her chair, he/she cannot do anything; he/she is paralysed. To move becomes difficult for him/her; to be moved also. By adjusting and adapting the 'person-in-a-wheelchair', the actors are acting on this dual breakdown (Winance, 2006b, 2007b). Working on a person's sensations changes both these sensations and the person's (in)abilities; it opens possibilities for the person by transforming the relations that shape him/her; it once again gives him/her the possibility to get to the world; it allows him/her to move and be moved, to create different relations with his/her environment. This is the final goal not just of wheelchair tests, but also of re-education practices, of which I would like to give the following example:

> On the first day of my stay at the re-education centre, I attended Dr. Ramon's consultations [Dr. Ramon works in re-education and rehabilitation]. It is the turn of a young woman, Martine, who has been a paraplegic since her road accident. She comes with her husband and children. She now lives at home, but continues to have her consultations at the re-education centre. Her physiotherapist also attends the consultation. For some time now, they have been working on learning to walk again. In order to be able to walk, Martine has to wear articulated splints on her knees and ankles, to give her support up to her pelvis. She then stands between parallel bars on which she leans for support. The doctor asks her to show him how she walks, so that he can assess her progress. Martine stands up between the bars, concentrating in order to remain upright. She takes her weight with her arms and takes a first 'step'; she slowly moves her two legs forwards, placing them in front of her, then moves her hands on the bars. Martine has lost the use of her legs, it is impossible for her to put one leg in front of the other. 'Walking' involves taking her weight with her arms, and swinging the body forwards. Before each movement she thinks carefully and concentrates on what she must do. The physiotherapist explains to me that the problem is that she has no feeling below the pelvis; she can no longer feel her legs, they are a dead weight. She must replace feeling with thinking in order to keep her balance and make a movement. Walking is a movement in four stages that uses the entire body; when we walk, we move a leg forward, then an arm, then the other leg and finally the other arm. The purpose of the exercise is not really to learn to walk again, as it is very unlikely that Martine will ever use this method to get around; it will always be far more laborious than using a wheelchair, and will only be useful for certain transfers or short distances. Yet this exercise allows Martine to use all her body, to be aware of her entire body in movement, even if she has to think about it to regain confidence and realise that certain things remain possible. At the end of the consultation, Martine tells me: 'I know I will never walk again, and that the wheelchair is more practical, but

with these exercises I can have new sensations' (Re-education centre, consultation, 23/06/99).

This consultation instantly spoke to me. Some authors (Barnes, Mercer, & al., 1999; Oliver, 1990) (Ebersold, 1997; Stiker, 1999) have criticised re-education practices and the ideal of normalisation that they implement.[7] Here, normalisation means alignment with the social and functional norm of being able-bodied. Yet this consultation seemed to fit this criticism. Martine will never walk again, the lesion of the spinal column is definitive. Yet she is working with her physiotherapist to learn to walk again. Re-reading my notes, I underlined the physiotherapist's and Martine's comments at the end of the consultation. They know that Martine will never walk again. And they anticipate the criticism of normalisation.

The aim of learning to walk again is not to re-establish a functionality that has been lost or that is considered to be normal; it is to teach Martine to feel her body and her legs in a different way. Martine 'lost *her* legs' in the accident, they became a dead weight, they have become *legs*. During the exercise, she is relearning to feel *her* legs, she is learning that they can once again be *her* body, but in a different way. In other words, through this exercise she is doing and performing her body (Mol & Law, 2004), her body that has legs, *her* legs. But because Martine can no longer directly feel her legs (as the able-bodied can), she is learning to feel them through the intermediary of reflection, of her other senses (sight), and, above all, through the intermediary of a technique (splints and parallel bars). This technique is part of her body. It plays the role of mediator (Latour, 2004) by defining Martine's experience of her body. Yet in fact, the splints remain separate from Martine.

In the case of a wheelchair, a common materiality and common sensations emerge from the work done.[8] Not only is the person's perception of his/her body transformed by the chair, but he/she gradually learns to 'feel' the wheelchair, which becomes 'his/hers', which constitutes 'his/her body' and which enables him/her to act.[9] In this way Serge, who has never driven an electric wheelchair, gradually learns to feel the chair's movements and to feel these movements as movements of his chin and of his entire body. His girlfriend points out that, 'It's good for him to control with his chin, it makes him use all his muscles', while pointing to his abdominals. She adds, 'When he is driving, I can see he uses them all, it's great'. And a little later: 'It gives him more freedom, it won't always be like that and in any case not outside, but if he wants to move around he'll be able to do it, it's good. [...] Because he really wants that; inside he'll be able to move around on his own, he just needs to ask, we'll position it and he can move... but of course, outside, he never goes out alone, he'll always have someone with him'. The wheelchair is not just a means of getting around, compensating for a loss of mobility, a means to an end. Thanks to this technique (chair and chin control), Serge will be able to 'move by himself'. In his case, 'moving by himself' means being able to move from room to room when he is bored, when someone is annoying him or when he wants to change activities. With his chair, Serge will also be able to move around outside, without someone having to push him, but instead driving the wheelchair using a second control; this will make it possible to go for longer walks. This means more freedom for Serge, greater freedom of movement. It is also the sensation of a different body, a body that can move around, a body that can build up muscle, a body that can work. The technical object, the wheelchair, is a source of pleasure (or/and displeasure), of possibilities (or/and impossibilities). For Mrs. Sabin, her new wheelchair will mean more mobility because she will be able to move it herself, greater comfort and well-being, and a lower number of transfers because she will be able to remain in her chair all day long. To care is to enable, to open up new possibilities of action for the person. Throughout the wheelchair test, the issue of the possibilities of action[10] available to the person is explored by the actors from empirical, material and emotional points of view, i.e. by working on the relations that link the person to his/her chair and by making the person into a 'person-in-his/her-chair'. More broadly speaking, new sensations and new actions are made possible by the collective of which the person is a part. So the object of care is not directly the person, but his/her sensations and abilities for action that appear through the relationship – the attachment – between the person and his/her wheelchair. In this case, care is not a relationship of assistance between an active carer and a passive care receiver, but a collective attention to the sensations and actions that emerge for the person in question; it is an attention to the nature of the relationship that develops between the person and the chair, and, more broadly, to the nature of the relationships that exist within the collective. To care is to organise and to tinker with the different entities of a collective so that they adapt to one another, so that they might live together, so that each might get something out of it, might start to move and be moved by the others.

From collective care to care for the collective

I have shown above that care is given to the person's sensations and possibilities of action. But what person are we talking about? Are we only talking about the disabled person, the person who we intuitively consider to be the receiver of care? Let us return to the case of Mrs. Sabin.

> *Benoît*: okay ... so what about the height of the back?
> *Mr. S*: *who has tried pushing Mrs. S in her chair.* Can't we lift the handles up higher?
> *Benoît*: Yes, we can, this is a 35cm back, so we can go up to 37cm, or else we can take the 40cm back which can go up to 43cm.
> *Mr. S*: Yes, I have to bend over a bit with this one, it would be better if it were a bit higher...
> *Benoît*: Okay, the monoblock footrest is good; the back is a bit low, it's easy to get a 40cm back. But Mrs. Sabin, won't that be uncomfortable for you when you move? *He puts his fingers higher up against Mrs. Sabin's back.* There, move, I'll be the higher back... how's that?
> *Mrs. S*: It's okay...
> *Benoît*: It's not uncomfortable? Move without my hand and then with it... *He places his hand then removes it, repeating the process several times.*
> *Mrs. S*: Ah, that's better.
> *Benoît*: Without?
> *Mrs. S*: Yes, it's better without.
> *Benoît*: Yes... so a higher back will be a problem for her.
> *Mrs. S*: Yes, it's better without your hand.
> *Mr. S*: Why?
> *Mrs. S*: You see, with his hand it's uncomfortable.
> *Benoît*: The solution is to pull the handles up, like this one *He shows a chair with higher handles.* You pull the handle out. from the back. But it's a lot of money to achieve very little.
> *Mr. S*: I'll make do with these. I'm a little bent forward, but well... [...] As I do a lot of pushing, I'd like bigger front wheels, it's easier.
> *Benoît*: A good compromise would be these wheels here. They are a bit bigger than your wheels and the ones on the chair at the moment, and as they are hard they roll better.

Attention is not directed solely to Mrs. Sabin and how she feels in the chair, but also to Mr. Sabin and how he feels when he pushes the chair. In other words, the object of care is not 'Mrs. Sabin-in-her-chair' but 'Mr. Sabin-who-pushes-Mrs. Sabin-in-her-chair'. The actors' attention is focused on the sensations and possibilities of action for each person. Hence the search for an arrangement which suits everyone. In Mrs. Sabin's test there is a dilemma. Easier handling for Mrs. Sabin means discomfort for Mr. Sabin, who often has to push. It seems to be difficult to reconcile handling that will be comfortable for both of them, especially as the two handling situations relate to opposing qualities of the wheelchair (a low back for Mrs. Sabin, but high handles for her husband). A compromise is needed between the possibilities of action for Mr. Sabin and the possibilities of action for his wife. Such a compromise means adapting the chair: they keep the low back and low handles and replace the front wheels with slightly bigger ones.[11] Attention is thus shared because it is focused on the collective, on all of the individuals comprising it, on the sensations, on the possibilities of action for each separate individual and for everyone together and finally on the nature of the relationships that unite them.

André, his wheelchair and his mother are then linked by relationships of strong dependency resulting from a temporal evolution: the illness getting worse, the wheelchair becoming old and worn, etc. At the moment, André cannot do anything without his mother; she has to be with him constantly, whether it is to move him or to drive the wheelchair for him, both inside and outside. The decision to change the chair comes just as much (if not more) from the mother as from André himself. To give André the chance to drive his chair, even if only to a limited extent, is to change their relationship, to reduce their *feeling* of dependency, to make it possible for both him and his mother to regain some freedom of movement.

In my fieldwork I have noticed that the request for technical aid (wheelchair, bath seat, adapted shower, etc.) comes just as often from the carer (whether a member of the family, a friend or a professional) as from the person requiring care. For the carer, technical aid means the chance to change his/her relationship of care with the disabled person, to 'reverse the direction of care', and to make it understood that he/she also needs care and is not just a carer, but must also be helped, particularly in the provision of care. He/she must be helped to help. When one includes the mediation of a technical aid in the relationship of care, one is caring both for the carer and for the disabled person. The technical object makes it possible to share the care among the members of the collective, be they the disabled person, family or professionals. It changes their sensations and their (in)abilities. It modifies the relationships of dependency between them; it adds distance or proximity, and may be the source of freedom of movement for them. People in the collective are thus at the same time objects and subjects of care. Furthermore, they are also all responsible for the quality of care given in the collective, even if they hold different positions and have different abilities. People may find themselves in asymmetrical positions because they do not have the same abilities. Nevertheless, in this case of the wheelchair, the care appears to be symmetrical and shared. Symmetrical means that each person gives care to the other. Shared means that everyone in the collective is giving and receiving care. With this issue in mind, I am now going to examine the question of *good care*.

Care as a search for compromise 'Le mieux est l'ennemi du bien'[12]

> *Benoît, manager of the test centre, tells me about his job. After talking to the person and those with him/her (family, friends, professionals), he shows them one, two or three wheelchairs and lets the person try them out.* [...] The problem is that when they arrive to see me, they don't really have any criteria for making their choice, except maybe 'inexpensive' and 'the lightest'. So I try to develop criteria, to see what they want. The aim of the tests, which last between one and three hours, is to let people choose the wheelchair 'that suits them best'. While he explains his work, he tells me about what he calls his 'philosophy of things', which he sums up as being 'le mieux est l'ennemi du bien' [the perfect is the enemy of the good]. Over time, he has learned that it is sometimes necessary 'to avoid giving too much advice; giving too much advice is not a good idea [...] people have a wheelchair, the one that suits them best, but they don't know why they have that one. You need to keep things simple'.
> Wheelchair Test Centre. May 99.

In this extract, Benoît gives us the keys to understanding what 'good care' means in his practice. First of all, *good* is defined in comparison to *the perfect* (or *the better*). But what is this *good*, what is this *perfect*? To answer this, let us return to the examples. In the example of Mrs. Sabin, Benoît repeats several times that he feels the wheelchair she has chosen is too wide for her, with Mrs. Sabin replying that it is the right width because she wants to be able to have her bag next to her. In this example, the *perfect* would be a narrower chair, with the *good* being a wider chair with room for the bag. We can take the example further. Regarding the issue of double manoeuvrability, for both Mr. and Mrs. Sabin the *perfect* would be a lower back and higher handles, with the good being a low back, low handles and medium-size front wheels. The *perfect* is thus what, *'in absolute terms'*, suits the person concerned. By 'in absolute terms', we mean without taking into account all of the relationships surrounding the person which link that person to other entities, which *attach* him/her to them (Gomart & Hennion, 1999; Latour, 1999), without considering the world in which the person lives, without taking into account to what the person is attached and what attachs the person. The *good* is an arrangement of people and things that is a compromise, allowing a life together and allowing motion and emotion for all those involved in the collective. The example of André throws light on this point.

André has two problems. First, his wheelchair is old and is about to fall apart. Second, he can no longer drive it, his mother has to drive it for him and has to accompany him wherever he wants to go. This is why the family wants to buy a new wheelchair. But André's chair is a PP, which was withdrawn from the French market after a series of accidents. So André cannot buy the same model and has to change brand. The test is long and very difficult. Benoît ends up advising the family to try one final repair and adaptation of the old wheelchair. Someone good at D.I.Y. can change the control, which would avoid the need to change the wheelchair. Then, during an ethnographical course with a distributor, I learn that the PP has been modified and it is now possible to buy one. When I return to the centre I pass this information on to Benoît, who has a think, hesitates, and finally says that it is preferable to leave things as they were decided at the end of the wheelchair test, repeating that 'the perfect is the enemy of the good'. For André the *perfect* would have been to change chairs. A new wheelchair would be more reliable and safer than his old one, with recent electronics that are compatible with a wider range of controls. But this solution is the *perfect*. It does not take into account André's history with *his* chair, nor that of the collective of which he is a part. The process of adjustment continues throughout the use of the chair. A rest is added, or a strap to hold the feet, and slowly the person and the chair get used to one another. The person is taking the shape of the wheelchair, adopting a given position because the chair holds him there, while the chair is taking the shape of the person (for example, the cushion keeps the shape of the sitting position). A new wheelchair of the same brand is anything but the same as the old one. Furthermore, there are complex relationships of dependency, interdependency and *attachment* between André, *his* chair and his mother. The *attachment* is physical and affective. It is impossible to change the chair as this could destroy the collective that is holding and shaping André. For André, it would mean risking losing everything, losing comfort and the (few) activities that are made possible by this collective. This *perfect* (a new chair) might prove to be a *worse*. However, for his mother, the current arrangement has become unbearable, she feels trapped. In this case, the *good* means only changing the control of the old chair, modifying one single link in order to try to extend possibilities for everyone, to alter their relationships in a tiny way by once again giving a possibility of movement to both André, and his mother who cannot stand it any longer. The *good* is not intended to 'change the (i.e. their) world'.

To care is to be sensitive to the attachments that support people, attachments which are sources of both constraints and opportunities, which are openings and closures. The *good* is always a relative good. It relates to a given situation. What suits people is negotiated within that situation (Pattaroni, 2005; Pols, 2004); the *good* is a compromise that combines comfort and discomfort, abilities and inabilities for each person in the collective. In Serge's case, the *good* means alternating moments when he drives with moments when his girlfriend drives. The *good* reconciles his desire to drive with the recalcitrance (Latour, 2004) of his body, as demonstrated in the following quote:

> Serge's girlfriend: The problem, as I well know, is that he wants it so much that he makes a huge effort. He wants it so much... and I'm worried that afterwards things will go wrong because the effort required is too much. With the head wand (*a curved stick fixed to the forehead to allow the person to drive the wheelchair*) it was the same thing, he managed to do it, but it required such an effort that he was exhausted, he couldn't do anything afterwards. [...]
> *She then talks to Serge, who is trying to drive the chair*: Don't worry, stop trying, you're getting tired and **it's all your body that is annoying you and getting in the way**, we've seen that you've understood and that you can do it, don't tire yourself out. [...] He's tired now... Stop contracting, stop trying, **your whole body has had enough,** your whole body is tired and has given up [*She presses against his stomach and tries to unbend his arms*].

The *good* is finding the arrangement that works; the *perfect* is an arrangement that is likely to break down, with the different components falling apart, because the perfect is what suits the individual alone and apart from the others -humans or non-humans. At the end of the day, the objective of good care, through gradual shaping, is to define the way in which humans and non-humans can work together, organise themselves and *live together*. The most suitable arrangement is always a compromise, source of abilities and disabilities, source of movement for all concerned.

This arrangement, with differing degrees of duration and stability, is the permanent object of the collective's work of care. Care requires patience and time.[13] It has a fastidious and routine aspect. When André sits in the new chair, he immediately calls his mother because he is scared of falling, and she asks him how she should position him. The father interjects: 'Here we go again... it's always the same, move this, move that... it's always the same', and the mother, talking to us, says: 'Every morning it's the same nightmare, it takes over half an hour'. Then she turns to André, speaks to him, moves around him changing the position of each limb in turn. A person has to be installed in his/her chair every morning and all the adjustments have to be made, even though with the repetition of care a mutual understanding and complicity can develop. As Benoît says, the installation is always difficult, 'it's a nightmare'. After a while, 'it's a bit easier, you know the position better'.

Conclusion

The starting point of this article was the debate between Disability Studies researchers and the theorists of the ethics of care about the notion of *care*, with the former rejecting it and the latter defending it in order to construct an ethic. Whilst at first sight these two movements are in opposition to each other, they are based on an identical conception of care as a relationship of dependency between an active carer and a passive receiver of care. Analysis of the wheelchair tests opens up a different conception of care. In this case, care is a shared work, carried out jointly by the collective. It revolves around assembling and arranging the entities of a collective so that they fit together. To care is to tinker, i.e. to meticulously explore, 'quibble', test, touch, adapt, adjust, pay attention to details and change them, until a suitable arrangement (material, emotional, relational) has been reached. The work of care involves a transformation of what these entities are, of their materiality and their sensations, of what they do and, above all, of the way in which they are linked to one another.

When looking at care practices, the theorists of the ethics of care demonstrate that people are defined through their relationships with others. They reveal not an autonomous individual, but a relational me, involved in relationships of dependency. We are all undoubtedly at the centre of a network of care relationships that supports us and makes us who we are. The analysis of the wheelchair tests demonstrates the same thing. People are held and supported by their relationships with humans and non-humans. However, we hear Disability Studies researchers defending the notion of an autonomous subject. Indeed, whilst we are all part of networks of relationships, it is undeniable that some of these relationships are felt as relationships of dependency, whilst others are not. This difference must be taken into consideration and explained (Winance, 2007c). Analysis of the wheelchair tests offers certain elements of response, shifting the questions of in/dependence towards those of arrangement and movement. It suggests that through tinkering and adjustment, *care* involves *modulating* the relationship and balancing the positions of each member of the collective (simultaneously the subject and object of care). Modulating the relationship means determining the proximity or distance that separates or unites two people, distinguishing between the attachments, transforming dependencies, etc., so that people construct themselves in their relationships with other entities as people with given qualities, (in)abilities, dispositions, and, in one way or another, as people who are *independent*, who might move by themselves. In all four cases it can be seen that the purpose of the wheelchair tests and re-education practices is to define the way in which a person, by attaching him/herself to different devices, can separate him/herself from others. At the end of the day, the aim of care as shared work is to construct a person who is both *attached and detached, 'dependent' and 'independent', moving on his/her own and being moved by others*. This question about the perceived nature of the attachment outlined in this paper will need more analysis.

Acknowledgments

I would like to thank J. Barbot, E. Fillion and A. Mol for their careful reading of this article and for their suggestions for improvements. I also thank Christopher Hinton for his help in translation.

Notes

1 These works distinguish between different types of dependency: inevitable dependencies caused by disability, growing old or childhood, and avoidable dependencies resulting from social arrangements. (Feder Kittay & Feder, 2003).

2 Certain authors combine the two approaches, in particular Hughes, Mckie, Hopkins, & Watson, 2005; Watson, Mckie, Hughes, Hopkins, & Gregory, 2004.

3 This test centre is one of just two that exist in France. Elsewhere wheelchair tests are done either in a re-education centre or at home – either by home help services who ask distributors to bring some chairs to test, or by the distributors themselves. Test practices are thus relatively unequal, depending on who is doing them and under what conditions. A test centre is an ideal place for observation, because the manager has acquired skills specific to the matter in hand. I nevertheless observed that other professionals possess the same skills. For example, I was able to observe one distributor and a regional department for aid and information – part of the French myopathy association – whose practices and skills proved to be similar to those of the test centre manager.

4 Here their descriptive work is very similar to a sociologist's work of description, as defined by the sociology of sciences and techniques (Akrich, 1992), with the difference that it is material.

5 The extent to which a wheelchair can be customised depends on the model and the price.

6 On the question of (in)abilities as performances emerging through a heterogeneous network, see also Moser, 1999; Moser & Law, 1998.

7 For an analysis of the performativity of approaches and their normalising effects, see Moser, 2000. On its historical and political aspect, see Winance, 2007a.

8 S. Kurzman (Kurzman, 2002) analyses the process through which an orthesis becomes something that makes one's body. More precisely, he focuses on the way in which patients and orthoprothesists develop a common language that allows them to understand how to align and adjust the orthesis to the body. He does a detailed analysis of the constant process of translating the sensations felt by the actors and the mobilisation of different norms of reference (subjective experience, 'normal walking', biomechanics, etc.).

9 In other words, the process of adjustment shifts the separation between what is one's body and what is one's environment. It is a process of constitution, of personalisation (inasmuch as the wheelchair shapes the person, his/her qualities and (in)abilities), and not a process of familiarity (Thévenot, 1994) that leaves unchanged the distinction between what is/makes one's body and what is the world.

10 New possibilities of action go with new impossibilities. The wheelchair testing is a trial that forces people to make concessions, to evaluate what constraints they accept for regaining some freedom. About this process of concessions in the case of people with muscular dystrophy, see Callon and Rabeharisoa, 1998.

11 Wheels with a small diameter make it easier for the person in the wheelchair to manoeuvre the chair, especially when turning around.

12 Literally, this expression might be translated: 'the perfect is the enemy of the good'. The dictionary's translation will be 'it's better to let well alone'. This last translation does not exactly correspond to the French expression. It is why I keep the literal translation.
13 Care has different temporalities. Care is generally associated with the notion of a duration, but analysis of the wheelchair tests shows a more one-off aspect of care in the case of Benoît. I would like to thank Janine Barbot for drawing my attention to this point.

References

(2001). 'Rethinking Care' from different perspectives., *Global Conference on Rethinking Care*. Oslo.

Akrich, M. (1992). The De-scription of technical objects. In W. Bijker, & J. Law (Eds.), *Shaping technology, building society: studies in sociotechnical changes* (pp. 105-224). Cambridge: MIT Press.

Barnes, C., Mercer, G., & al. (1999). *Exploring Disability. A Sociological Introduction*. Cambridge: Polity Press.

Barton, L., & Oliver, M. (1997). Disability Studies: Past, Present and Future (p. 294). Leeds: The Disability Press.

Brugère, F. (2006). La sollicitude. La nouvelle donne affective des perspectives féministes. *Esprit*, 123-140.

Callon, M., & Law, J. (1995). Agency and the hybrid collectif. *South Atlantic Quaterly*, 94, 481-507.

Callon, M. and V. Rabeharisoa. (1998). Reconfiguring Trajectories: Collective Bodies and Chronic Illnesses. Paper presented at the workshop Theorizing Bodies in Medical Practices, The Paris Centre de Sociologie de l'Innovation and The Netherlands Graduate School of Science, Technology and Modern Culture, Paris, September.

Ebersold, S. (1997). *L'invention du handicap. La normalisation de l'infirme* Paris: CTNERHI.

Feder Kittay, E., & Feder, E.K. (2003). The subject of care. Feminist perspectives on dependency (p. 382). Lanham-Boulder-New-York- Oxford: Powman & littlefield publishers.

Gomart, E., & Hennion, A. (1999). A sociology of attachment: music amateurs, drug users. In J. Law, & J. Hassard (Eds.), *Actor network theory and after* (pp. 220-247). Oxford: Blackwell and the Sociological Review.

Hughes, B., Mckie, L., Hopkins, D., & Watson, N. (2005). Love's labours Lost? Feminism, the disabled people's movement and an ethic of care. *Sociology*, 39(2), 259-275.

Keith, L. (1992). Who Cares Wins? Women, caring and disability. *Disability & Society*, 7(2), 167-175.

Kurzman, S. (2002). 'There's No Language for This.' Communication and alignment in contemporary prosthetics. In K. Ott, D. Serlin, & S. Mihm (Eds.), *Artificials Parts*, Practical Lives (pp. 227-246). New York: New York university Press.

Latour, B. (1999). Factures/Fractures: from the concept of Network to the concept of Attachment. *Res*, 36, 20-31.

Latour, B. (2004). How to talk about the body? The normative dimension of science studies. *Body and Society*, 10(2-3), 205-229.

Leder, D. (1990). *The Absent Body* Chicago: University of Chicago Press.

Mol, A., & Law, J. (2004). Embodied action, enacted bodies. The example of hypoglycaemia. *Body and Society*, 10(6), 43-62.

Mol, A. (2006). Proving or Improving: On health care research as a form of self-reflection. *Qualitative Health Research*, 16(3), 405-414.

Moser, I., & Law, J. (1998). "Making voices": Disability, technology and articulation. Maastricht, The Netherlands: paper presented at Politics of Technology Conference.

Moser, I. (1999). Good passages, bad passages. In J. Law, & J. Hassard (Eds.), *Actor network theory and after* (pp. 196-219). Oxford: Blackwell.

Moser, I. (2000). Against normalisation: subverting norms of ability and disability. *Science as Culture*, 9(2), 201-240.

Oliver, M. (1990). *The Politics of Disablement* Basingstoke: Macmillan and St Martins Press.

Oliver, M., & Barnes, C. (1998). *Disabled People and Social Policy: From Exclusion to Inclusion* London and New York: Longman

Paperman, P. (2004). Perspectives féministes sur la justice. *L'Année Sociologique*, 54(2), 413-433.

Paperman, P. (2005). Les gens vulnérables n'ont rien d'exceptionnel. In P. Paperman, & S. Laugier (Eds.), *Le souci des autres. Ethique et politique du care. Raisons Pratiques* (16) (pp. 281-297). Paris: Editions de l'Ecole des Hautes Etudes en Sciences Sociales.

Pattaroni, L. (2005). Le care est-il institutionnalisable? Quand la 'politique du care' émousse son éthique. In P. Paperman, & S. Laugier (Eds.), *Le souci des autres. Ethique et politique du care. Raisons Pratiques* (16) (pp. 177-200). Paris: Editions de l'Ecole des Hautes Etudes en Sciences Sociales.

Pols, J. (2004). *Good care. Enacting a complex ideal in long-term psychiatry* Utrecht: Trimbos-instituut.

Scarry, E. (1985). *The Body in Pain. The Making and Unmaking of the World* New York and Oxford: Oxford University Press.

Scotch, R.K. (1988). Disability as the Basis for a Social Movement: Advocacy and the Politics of Definition. *Journal of Social Issues*, 44(1), 159-172.

Stiker, H.J. (1999). *A History of Disability* Ann Arbor: University of Michigan Press.

Thévenot, L. (1994). Le régime de la familiarité. Les choses en personne. *Genèse*, 17, 72-101.

Tronto, J. (1993). *Moral boundaries: A political argument for an ethic of care* New Yord: Routledge.

Tronto, J. (2005). Au-delà d'une différence de genre. Vers une théorie du care. In P. Paperman, & S. Laugier (Eds.), *Le souci des autres. Ethique et politique du care. Raisons Pratiques* (16) (pp. 25-49). Paris: Editions de l'Ecole des Hautes Etudes en Sciences Sociales.

Watson, N., Mckie, L., Hughes, B., Hopkins, D., & Gregory, S. (2004). (Inter)Dependence, Needs and Care: the potential for disability and feminist theorists to develop an Emancipatory model. *Sociology*, 38(2), 331-350.

Winance, M. (2003). La double expérience des personnes atteintes d'une maladie neuromusculaire: rétraction et extension. *Sciences Sociales et Santé*, 21(2), 5-31.

Winance, M. (2006a). Trying out wheelchair. The mutual shaping of people and devices through adjustment. *Science, Technology and Human Values*, 31(1), 52-72.

Winance, M. (2006b). Pain, Disability and Rehabilitation practices – A phenomenological perspective. *Disability and rehabilitation*, 28(18), 1109-1118.

Winance, M. (2007a). Being normally different? Changes to normalisation processes: from alignment to work on the norm. *Disability and Society*, 22(6), 625-638.

Winance, M. (2007b). Du malaise au « faire corps »: le processus d'ajustement. *Communications* (Corps et techniques, 81, dossier coordonné par T. Pillon et G. Vigarello), 31-45.

Winance, M. (2007c). Dépendance versus autonomie. De la signification et de l'imprégnation de ces notions dans les pratiques médicosociales. *Sciences Sociales et Santé*, 25(4), 83-91.

Now or later?
Individual disease and care collectives in the memory clinic

Tiago Moreira

Dementia is widely associated with irreversible loss: loss of memory, loss of independence, loss of selfhood. The image that emerges from many expert, lay and first-hand accounts of the disease is a daunting one. Adjectives used include 'insidious', 'dreadful' and 'inhuman'. In this context, dementia is predominantly framed as a disease characterised by cognitive decline. To make things worse, for quite a while the decline is not straightforward. Instead, the loss of an ordering grasp on the world tends to be intermeshed with moments of lucid, insightful perception of the disease process. Iris Murdoch exemplified this when she described her condition as one of 'sailing towards darkness'.[1] The tension is acute: only insofar as Murdoch has experienced darkness can she describe where she is going. But her ability to describe depends on the fact that she is not enclosed by darkness, but persists in her former lucidity.

A similar tension between dark and light is present in the context of scientific research and technological development. Here, the disease is pictured as dark, even sinister, and our lack of knowledge about it contributes to this. Research is supposed to illuminate our understanding of the disease and its causes and lead to the development of treatments. Because the disease is portrayed as so dreadful, it seems that scientific knowledge and technological solutions are urgently needed. However, what this hides is that depicting of dementia as a dreadful disease linked with age-associated cognitive decline is not a self evident reflection of reality. It is linked to a particular, historically contingent way of framing human aging. When senility was made into a research object in the 1970s and turned into 'Alzheimer's disease', a progressive neurological disorder, specific modes of clinical reasoning were linked up with the use of newly available visualisation instruments (notably electron microscopy). These were politically aligned, particularly in the United States, around a clear distinction between 'normal' and 'pathological ageing' (Fox 1989; Holstein 2000; Ballenger 2006). From the outset, however, Alzheimer's disease has been a contested disease category and over the years there has been a sustained debate about whether Alzheimer's is a qualitatively different disease state or an extreme within a cognitive continuum (Brody 1982; Brayne and Calloway 1988; Whitehouse and Brodaty 2006) – alongside outright challenges to the very definition of Alzheimer's disease (Kitwood 1997). In this paper, I take these divergences and differences as a point of departure to investigate how dementia and cognitive decline can be understood, managed and experienced in different ways within the same health care setting – in this case memory clinics.

Drawing on ethnographic material gathered in a memory clinic, the paper suggests that there is a complex tension between forms of practice that individualise and those that collectivise 'early memory loss'. There are two, interrelated dimensions to this complexity. First, inspired by the work of Callon and Rabeharisoa on the relationship between knowledge, forms of embodiment and political articulation (Callon and Rabeharisoa 1998), I conceptualise *individualisation practices* as condensing 'memory loss', through a variety of representations, diagnostic classifications and techniques, into the individual's own body and thoughts and, in turn, making the individual's self correspond to the operations s/he can perform on her/his memory. By contrast, *collectivisation practices* locate memory loss within the shared context of family, home, friends, work, etc. They distribute what it is to have and to handle memory to various actors surrounding a particular person. This person may still be the one who is seen to have dementia, but this is not confined to a brain, it is distributed and managed by family, community, the clinic, drug regimes, memory groups and so forth.

If only because memory clinics were set up to do research on Alzheimer's disease and to test drugs against it, individualisation practices are particularly strongly embedded there. In order to under- stand why this is the case, it is necessary to move to a second analytical platform and draw on the concept of 'regime' – generalised modes of linking knowledge, action, objects and subjectivities through forms of justification in which people publicly legitimise their actions (Boltanski and Thevenot 1991). This is not only to avoid the scale assumptions that come attached to explaining practices in localised settings through patterns in less localised processes (biomedicine, the biomedical model, etc.) but also, and more importantly, to capture the complexity that is inherent to understanding how a plurality of regimes deploy different practices of understanding, managing and experiencing 'memory loss' in a memory clinic. The paper argues that as a drug testing site, the clinic holds together a *regime of truth* that is oriented towards the production of robust knowledge, with a *regime of hope* that fosters and flares positive expectations (Moreira and Palladino 2005). Jointly, and in tension, these regimes enrol patients into an individualising version of health care, and enrol them with a disease that they have to individually bear, face and deal with, demanding patients to effectively engage in the production of their own illness (Callon and Rabeharisoa 2004).

However, despite their research origins, memory clinics also contain practices of collectivisation that are in close relationship to another regime, the *regime of care*. The version of dementia articulated in this regime is neither underpinned by inevitable cognitive decline nor relieved by promises of an imminent therapeutic solution. Instead it is a matter of handling daily life, of making things work from one day to the next, of tinkering. Collectivisation and care are more difficult to do and to sustain in and around the memory clinic than diagnosing and treating disease in an individualising mode. This is not only due to the history of these clinics, but also the fact that 'care collectives' can only be formed by abstaining from the dark facts and positive dreams that come with the regimes of truth and hope. Thus they depend on a fragile and never quite complete process of displacement that Nietzsche called 'active forgetting' (Nietzsche 1989). This paper is ultimately an attempt to provide clues on how to prolong these moments.

Making memory loss at Greene Memory Clinic

Greene Memory Clinic, located in a (not-to-be-specified) place in Northern England, is attached to a university research centre where dementias of various types are investigated. First developed in the United States in the 1970s, memory clinics were introduced in the UK in the 1980s. They were meant to facilitate research by recruiting patients for clinical trials, clinical studies of dementia progression and other, similar projects. Recently, most have managed to establish themselves as independent specialist out-patient services for patients with early dementia and/or Mild Cognitive Impairment. However, some, like Greene, remain attached to the research institution they used to serve. This implies that patients in Greene are still enrolled in in-house research projects as well as in larger studies involving other centres in the UK, Europe and the US. The increase in the number of memory clinics has been associated with the licensing of cholinesterase inhibitors for Alzheimer's from 1997 onwards, and thus one the main functions of memory clinics such as Greene's is the formulation of pharmacological treatment plans for patients.

Typically, patients are referred to a memory clinic by a GP or a secondary care practitioner because of memory problems experienced by the patient or detected by relatives and friends. In the clinic, patients are assessed by an interview, physical examination and psychiatric evaluation, ideally complemented an interview with an 'informant' (relative, friend, etc), which is also meant to assess the burden of the main carer(s). Then there is a standardised assessment of cognitive function such as Mini Mental State Examination, and (less frequently) an assessment of non-cognitive domains, such as depression. Also important are laboratory evaluations of thyroid, renal and liver functions as well as a blood and blood glucose tests. At Greene's, patients also have a CAT scan or MRI as part of their clinical assessment, but not all clinics have swift access to such tools. As a result of all of this work, patients can be diagnosed with dementia, early dementia or Mild Cognitive Impairment and managed within the clinic. They may also be diagnosed with psychiatric conditions such as depression or anxiety, in which case they are referred to a psychiatric service or primary care. It may even happen that they are discharged with no diagnosis at all. An example[2]:

> We (consultant, nurse, psychologist and observer) are in the consulting room. There is no patient yet. The consultant opens the record of one of the 'new patients' and reads out her name: Mrs. Brennand. He also gives her address and then summarises the patient's referral letter. We learn that Mrs. Brennand's husband worries about her decreasing ability to manage both the house and a new part-time job that she took up after his retirement. Someone suggests that Mr. Brennand may be having a problem of his own: his wife's career may well be at odds with his expectations of retired life. General nodding, except for the nurse, who does not join in. There is something above and beyond this, she says. There have been incidents during the last weeks: the stove gas left on for an entire morning; bills left unpaid; a medical appointment forgotten. Mrs. Brennand blames these incidents on herself. She is also unhappy about her performance at work. All of this suggests that there is more going on than just Mr. Brennand complaining about his wife. And why would she come along if this was just his idea? The consultant guides us through his interpretation of Mrs. Brennand's MRI scans: he points to

small structural changes in the medial temporal lobe, which one would not expect to see in a woman of her age. However, the change is not impressive enough to allow him to make firm conclusions. The nurse and the psychologist leave and the consultant calls Mr. Brennand into the room.

Mr. Brennand is an articulate man, dressed in a grey suit and tie. He was a high-ranking civil servant until his retirement six years ago. When asked why he and his wife are seeking help, he concisely describes how his wife used to be focused, organised and pragmatic and how she recently became more anxious and disinterested. Has this happened since she took a job? No, she has been working for four years and has only started to change in the last year. Mr. Brennand and the consultant then explore some of the history of their married life. They met at university, she gave up work to stay at home with the children and had always wanted to return to work one day. They also touch on Mrs. Brennand's difficult relationship with her parents, which has been a burden for her whole life. A more structured assessment of Mrs. Brennand's situation – her depressive moods, her recent memory problems – follows.

At the same time, Mrs. Brennand is in another room with the psychologist. Their interaction is very regimented. The psychologist briefly explains the sort of tests that will follow. Then she asks a variety of questions about real places, events and people and about pictures she puts on display. She asks for words, numbers, and names of places, then she wants to know about the use of objects and the order of things such as animals or numbers. She also presents Mrs. Brennand with math tasks: counting and then adding and subtracting numbers. Then Mrs. Brennand is requested to draw a clock and its arms and to copy a few figures. During this time, the psychologist tries to avoid responding to all comments and requests for assistance. Instead, she repeats the question or silently waits for an answer. When Mrs. Brennand is finished and comes out of the psychologist's room, Mr. Brennand has just left the consultant. As they meet, she tells him, frustrated, that the tests made her feel stupid. The nurse tries to calm her. Meanwhile, the psychologist takes a few minutes to calculate the results. Back with the consultant, she reports that Mrs. Brennand's overall scores are slightly below the average scores for her age group and that she does least well in tests with time limits.

Invited back into the consultant's room, Mrs. Brennand immediately asks about her scores. Rather than answering that question, the consultant re-opens the conversation by asking her how she is doing. Mrs. Brennand tells about the recent domestic incidents and how upset they make her. The consultant tries to move away from what makes her anxious, but fails: Mrs. Brennand asks about her scores again. The consultant counters by asking if she is perhaps expecting too much on herself. He also tries to present the consultation as being about helping her, not making her life more difficult. She is only half convinced, but says that she feels things are not like they were. From there, the consultant explores her life history with her. It does not differ much from the version presented by her husband. However, there are a few differences, the most important one being that Mrs. Brennand says that she needs her job for herself; for her own wellbeing. Only then does the consultant tell her about her scores and MRI results. He suggests that if she wants to achieve her goals, she might need help. She seems to accept that. He then presents her with three possibilities: one, that she enrols in one of the 'memory groups' (self help groups organised by the clinic's nurse where small groups of patients talk about daily life and how to practically handle it, as well as about the emotional consequences of memory loss); two, that she tries cholinesterase inhibitors, drugs that ameliorate symptoms of cognitive decline; or three, that she gets a more thorough assessment of her depressive symptoms.

Mrs. Brennand doesn't ask further questions but immediately picks up on the second possibility: she has heard about these drugs from a friend whose husband is taking them. The report was positive. She had also read about them in the papers and hoped that they might be a solution for her. The consultant is not so enthusiastic. He sees cholinesterase inhibitors as part of a package. On their own they are likely to be of limited value. Nonetheless Mrs. Brennand wants to try them. She says she will think about the other suggestions. The consultant seems to conclude that on this occasion he can't reach a further compromise, and asks Mrs. Brennand to make an appointment with the nurse for a follow up visit two to three weeks after she has started taking the drugs. At this point Mr. Brennand is called in and informed of the plan. He looks pleased with the result, and says that he, too, has heard good things about these drugs and was hoping that they would be prescribed to his wife. The couple leaves re-assured and smiling.

This story exemplifies the typical process of assessment I observed at Greene's clinic. As the meeting starts, only the nurse has met the patient before. The clinical staff's discussion is oriented towards documents – the GP's letter, patient records, lab tests, MRIs, a report from the neuroradiologist. The aim of this is to frame the various interactions with the patient and carer/informant that will follow. The GP letter/referral letter is pivotal to this, because it supplies the narrative structure of the request for help. Typically, however, this narrative structure is deconstructed in an atmosphere of measured scepticism and an alternative narrative is put forward. In our case, the possibility of Mrs. Brennand really having memory problems is put into doubt by the suggestion that Mr. Brennand's expectations of retirement are not being met. The two contrasting narratives are then both confronted with interpretations of various brain images and, sometimes, with information collected by the nurse. This comparison enables the staff to test the strength of the request for help and to organise their diagnostic work. In Mrs. Brennand's case, we see this when, once they meet, the consultant tries to differentiate between the husband's possible desire to have his wife at home and her 'actual' clinical need.

When people first visit a memory clinic, 'memory problems', whether experienced by the patient or detected by relatives, are unclearly defined and fuzzy. In addition to this, they are entangled with a variety of emotional and practical issues and embedded in mundane activities of everyday life. The work of memory clinic staff consists of defining the 'memory problems' by disentangling them from a complex array of episodes, stories, worries and expectations. The clinical interview with the patient and the carer/informant are crucial to this. In this interview, the clinician, usually an old age psychiatrist, asks questions in such a way that the patient and the carer/informant come to tell stories of recognisable patterns of memory loss: tasks, names, words and appointments forgotten. The clinician then seeks to evaluate how these losses interfere with the patient and carer's daily lives. Corroboration of the patient's account by the carer/informant is an important element of moving from a 'subjective complaint' to an 'objective symptom'.

This process continues with the gathering and standardised calculation of the results of neuropsychological tests. Here the patient's performance is evaluated in relation to the performance of individuals of the same age and education. The standardised assessment of cognitive function adds to the picture and may confirm or contradict the psychiatrist's clinical impression. The composition of 'objective memory loss' is sharpened with the visual inspection of the brain scans, during which the psychiatrist look for sign of lesions or atrophy in regions associated with 'memory loss'.[3] If the blood investigations cannot detect any other 'organic cause' for cognitive malfunction and thus decline is confirmed at every level of the assessment, the patient is diagnosed with a 'memory impairment'.

The diagnostic practices deployed in the memory clinic can be seen as attempts to disentangle or purify 'memory': they detach, for *good clinical reasons*, the mundane forgetfulness from the contexts where it was originally experienced. Through successive procedures of inscription, what was fuzzy, ill-defined and ungraspable at first is gradually mapped onto the patient's brain. This, then, is what we may call a trajectory of individualisation. In Mrs. Brennand's case such individualisation is clearly taking place: falling short of the statistically informed expectations, memory comes to be located in her organic flesh. Not only the diagnosis is individualising: this individualisation is reinforced by the exploration of possible solutions. As a strategy, this correspond with a reinforcement of her need for control; analytically, it amounts to a concentration of agency on a small list of actors: Mrs. Brennand, the drugs and, intermittently, the staff at the memory clinic. In Callon and Rabeharisoa's (1998) terms, this corresponds to an emphasis on the somatisation of embodiment, where knowledge and action enact the body as an 'object' to be handled and managed by an autonomous and accountable subject. It is up to Mrs. Brennand as an individual to manage medication schedules, take the drugs and monitor both their intended and 'side' effects. She must remember to take the drugs. It is her who must remember the details about the onset of the drugs' effects, their progression and development. She must report them skilfully to visiting nurses or consultants in clinic. Her life will be absorbed by the work of managing the myriad of components that come attached to drugs.[4]

Early Dementia: Truth and Hope

Why would someone like Mrs. Brennand be willing to do all this work and assume the responsibilities that come with taking drugs such as cholinesterase inhibitors? One answer is that she hopes that this will allow her to regain control over her life. However, the very idea that 'taking control of her life' is what she needs to do only arises because so many things around her (both inside and outside the clinic) already point in this direction. It is as if her trajectory was framed by an 'architecture of individualism' from the very beginning. The knowledge, technologies and expectations that are involved all work together to enact Mrs. Brennand as a separate being, who, at least as long as she is capable, is able, autonomous and accountable. How is this enactment supported, how is it 'equipped?' In thinking about this, it may help to mobilise the concept of 'regime' such as it was coined by Boltanski and Thévenot (1991). Their 'regimes' are modes of linking knowledge, action, objects and subjectivities. They are neither small nor large, but infuse practices regardless of their scale. And they do not necessarily appear in pure form, but, in actual practices, may come together, co-exist, and interfere (Law and Mol 2002).

One way of viewing Mrs. Brennand's story is through the interaction between what she and her husband desire and how clinical staff at the Greene clinic manage expectations by working through the uncertainties that are inherent to the diagnosis of early dementia. In the memory clinic, two regimes jointly and in tension, sustain the individualising process described above: the *regime of truth* and the *regime of hope*. The latter, the regime of hope, we may recognise as being at work in the expectations with which the Brennands come to the clinic. These expectations only emerge towards the end of the story, but they were there all along. Like many other people, the Brennands heard about dementia drugs long before they came to the clinic and they were optimistic about them. The existence of these drugs fed into their reasons to seek medical care to begin with. This is not all that surprising as since the 1980s (at least in a countries like Britain or the United States), public health campaigns about dementia (whether in the form of Alzheimer's disease or of related disorders) have generated and fuelled positive expectations of therapeutic solutions that may soon be 'rationally derived' from scientific knowledge about the basic disease mechanisms.[5] When cholinesterase inhibitors became available at the end of the 1990s, this appeared to be part of the hoped for breakthrough. The expectations then took the form of a demand for diagnosis and treatment of early dementia.

Memory clinics came to be seen as privileged institutions for mediating – or rationing – access to these drugs.

But how to go about such rationing? It is here that a regime of truth comes into play. As there are no tests or other instruments that can help to clearly differentiate between the 'worried well' and those who might benefit from further diagnosis and perhaps pharmaceutical therapy, standardised assessments can only be used in conjunction with clinical judgement. Take the case of cognitive tests. Cognitive tests depend on comparison with the performances, on the same test, of people of a similar age and educational background. Or, as professionals would say, diagnosing someone as suffering from Mild Cognitive Impairment requires that an 'objective memory impairment for age and education' be identified (Petersen, Stevens et al. 2001).[6] Thus the practice of testing depends on 'normative data' against which an evaluation of any new individual can be made. These normative data did not exist from the start: they had to be crafted. The need to craft them was made explicit in 1984, when a consensus conference organised by the US National Institute of Neurological and Communicative Diseases and Stroke and the Alzheimer's Disease and Related Disorders Association published clinical criteria for the diagnosis of Alzheimer's. They could not do so quite as accurately as they wanted. Although neuropsychological tests were available at that time, 'there [were] no normative population standards for many of these tests' (McKhann, Drachman et al. 1984). The consensus group made an appeal to the National Institute of Aging (NIA) to fund studies that would help craft population standards. The NIA was itself invested in promoting an optimist view of ageing, not only through a differentiation between 'normal' and 'abnormal' ageing (Holstein 2000), but also by championing basic research on the biochemical or neuropsychological mechanism of age-related diseases (Ballenger 2006). The establishment of 'normative data' on cognitive function would at the same time materialise the ideal of 'normal ageing' as well as enable the identification of abnormal cognitive function in the elderly.

The particular regime of truth that got thus established is infused with a 'will to know' about a person's cognitive ability that has been actively disentangled from its daily life situation at home and even from the comparatively more 'natural' situation of the clinical interview. The artificiality of this test's set-up is intentional and it involves a lot of effort. The psychologist in the clinic often commented on the importance of 'not giving clues' about the answers of the test through non-verbal behaviour. At one point in my field work, an outgoing elderly man managed to consistently resist the interaction rules of the tests. His test results were immediately seen as useless by the clinical staff because his interactions with the psychologist undermined comparison with the other test subjects, who had accepted the interaction rules of the cognitive test. And however much distress the test itself and the neutral, non-responsive attitude of the psychologist may cause (as Mrs. Brennand's story, like many others, underlines) they are crucial to its function.[7]

The regime of truth not only surfaces in the tests and in the setting of normative data, in which the memory clinics have played a large role. It is also apparent in the other main research line of these clinics: testing the effectiveness of cholinesterase inhibitors. The clinics do this jointly with hospitals and universities and in collaboration with the pharmaceutical industry, which means that the drugs are actually at the centre of research focused on Alzheimer's disease. And in evaluating the effects of these drugs on people's performances in cognitive tests, a particular 'will to know' is linked up with a particular set of therapeutic expectations. A regime of truth and a regime of hope come together. One could say that together these two allow for the very existence of these clinics. Both of them help to shape the practices of individualisation that one encounters there. They put someone like Mrs. Brennand in the position of an isolated individual who may have an impaired brain and now hopes for 'the best'. It is this hope that makes her willing to submit herself to tests, however exerting, and that to a certain extent keep her motivated in her work of being a patient (Strauss, Fagerhaugh *et al.* 1982). And if the 'result' of the tests are below the standards set, Mrs. Brennand might even decide to take it upon herself to meticulously engage in her own treatment, by swallowing the drugs and monitoring their effects.

Unmaking memory loss at Greene's Memory Clinic

Is this all? Does the memory clinic only allow one to personally embody and take responsibility over one's illness? My fieldwork suggests that there might be a different way of managing and living with early memory loss. Again, the best way to start making sense of this alternative is through a case story:

> The nurse, the consultant and I are in the main room of the clinic. The nurse tells about a home visit she did the day before. She went to see Mr. and Mrs. Fenwick.
> Mr. Fenwick had first come to the clinic a few years ago because he and his wife noticed that he was becoming more

'absent-minded'. He had always been an introspective person, but in the months before the first appointment he had found himself 'switching off' during social occasions such as family reunions or Sunday dinners. At that point, the clinic's assessment concluded that he was suffering from Mild Cognitive Impairment, but the decision was made that he would return for another assessment six months later. And so he did. Mr. Fenwick's second assessment revealed a deterioration in his ability to remember information that he had been supplied with during the cognitive test. He also complained that sometimes he would forget small bits of messages given to him by his wife, or directions given to him on the street. That there were bits missing was all the more upsetting as they were missing from a wider picture that he could recall. The decision was made for Mr. Fenwick to start taking drugs and going to a memory group. Unfortunately, he did not respond very well to cholinesterase inhibitors and he suffered from stomach problems, one of their common side effects. However, he found the memory group activities very helpful. He and his wife developed a complex system of prompts and reminders that would help him not to forget, for example, to take the rubbish bin in on Monday morning after she had gone shopping. His wife had convinced members of the wider family to also use some of these techniques, so that there was a 'system' in place that did not need to be adapted when Mr. Fenwick came along. As the nurse tells the story, I can see that she admires the way the couple have dealt with the situation.

Three years later, both Mr. Fenwick's memory and his mood had gotten worse. The consultant suggested that he might try taking the drugs again. He did so and kept taking them even though he once again suffered from their side effects, because both he and his wife thought that the drugs were slowing down his deterioration. The consultant and the nurse thought so, too. In the mean time, the Fen-wicks had also bought a new house, and moved from the city suburbs to the village where Mrs. Fenwick's sister lived. The new house had a smaller garden, but more trees, which Mr. Fenwick particularly enjoyed. Recently, almost two years since he started on the drugs and moved house, another assessment led to the conclusion that Mr. Fenwick was again declining. Various solutions were explored, from trying a higher dose of drugs to getting a more intensive type of home support. No decision was taken in the consulting room, because the Fenwicks wanted to think about the various possibilities. The nurse went to visit them to check on their decision. They had decided to only increase the amount of house cleaning help. The consultant asks if they are not the least bit daunted by the new situation. 'No', the nurse replies, 'they're just getting on with it'.

The nurse's remark beautifully encapsulates the way in which the Fenwicks, their family, the clinical staff, the diagnostic tools, drugs and less high-tech aides had been moving along together in the past 6 years. 'To get on with it' is an English expression that means to pursue one's course, to move forward. It usually means that things are being done without too much reflection or determination. One *just* continues to do what needs to be done. Of course, this *just* is a gesture towards our shared understanding of the complexity of doing exactly this. It also signals that there is no attempt to capture or control this complexity. No fuss, no big claims, no overarching plans or hopes.

The Fenwicks and those around them had come to take each new situation as a small shift, to be handled by making a few small adjustments. They were able to do this by concentrating on the specific situation at hand, without worrying too much about what might happen in the future. As they did not focus on a probable trajectory of cognitive decline, they were not daunted by it either, and did not look for definitive solutions. Thus the story of the Fenwicks is about practices of collectivisation of early memory loss. Here, memory loss is not so much located within a single brain, but in shared contexts (of family, home, friends, work, etc.). Dealing with it, too, is spread out over various actors around the designated patient (family, community, the clinic, drug regimes, memory groups and so forth). Practices of collectivisation tend to have an open dynamic: there is a continuous mutual tuning between members of the collective and if frictions occur or new situations arise, new members may be sought. Importantly, the Fenwicks and their collective are able to organise life in a way that enables their enjoyment of gardening and other outside activities. Yes, Mr. Fenwick's body and brain are, at times, framed, discussed and managed as flesh, but only to enable him to do things with his body (and brain), even if it is just sitting in the garden looking at wind-brushed trees. In Callon and Rabeharisoa's (1998) terms, this means that they have been able to organise a continuous alternation between 'having' and 'being' a body, open to a variety possible worlds where Mr. Fenwick can participate (rubbish collection, family life, gardening, etc.).[8]

It thus seems we have left the order of the clinic where a regime of truth and a regime of hope jointly and in tension structure what is going on. The Fenwicks, instead, much to the liking of the nurse who went to visit them, live along the lines of a regime of care.

Early dementia: Care and its difficult enactment

In the memory clinic people like the Fenwicks are an exception. Most patients and carers oscillate between engaging in care and wanting to find definitive solutions. The nurse, however, admires them, not because they do anything heroic or out of the ordinary, but because by 'just getting on' they exemplify how it is possible, even in a clinical world dominated by the truth of cognitive decline and the hope of a cure against it, to build a world of care. But *how* is this possible? What does it take to build an ever-provisional care world beyond, but also along with, this other world, present not just in the clinic but in the press, in talk with one's friends? How can we deal with an ongoing emphasis on individuals, their brains and their memories?

In order to answer this, it helps to look into the *regime of care*. Pivotal is that this regime reconfigures the most dire consequence of the joined regimes of hope and truth in dementia research and clinical work: the fear of losing one's memory, independence and selfhood. This fear is particularly significant in Mild Cognitive Impairment (or so-called pre-clinical dementia), where the real impact of memory loss on everyday activities, social roles and identity is limited but the anxiety created by a horizon of further cognitive decline can be large and impairing (Corner and Bond 2006). The *regime of care* formulates a version of the self that is collectively arranged and always evolving. It does not insist on identifying the origin of the change experienced by the collective, and does not fuel the hope that a 'causal intervention' might prevent further change. Crucially, it focuses on the specific situation in which people find themselves, and trusts that small re-arrangements will produce a new and workable ways of doing things. It brackets off the horizon of cognitive decline as something that simply does not *belong* to any specific situation. It is no part of the actual (or, for that matter, any future actual) 'here and now'.
In the clinic itself, the regime of care is most notably visible in the work of memory groups. These are fora where patients meet to discuss their cognitive difficulties, to provide mutual support, and to

gain an understanding of their illness and strategies that help them cope (Zarit, Femia *et al.* 2004). Memory groups clearly work along the collectivisation pole of the memory clinic. This is obvious in the way experiences are shared among the group. In fact, because only rarely is one member's experience of early dementia unique, accounts of these experiences are assembled together in group sessions by various group members. In this way, memory groups promote a 'community of experience' that members come to belong to. They are also important instruments of discursive elaboration of experience for persons who might be experiencing 'difficulties with words'. From this point of view, they help to make sense of the illness through storytelling, which provides a provisional sense of collective order to selves that have been significantly altered.

Secondly, memory groups are also a platform where memory management techniques are exchanged and discussed. One particularly successful technique is 'putting it in writing', a technique that tries to replace reliance on short term memory with written notes and letters. There is, however, quite a lot of ambiguity about what kinds of information should be put in writing and, furthermore, this is likely to be different for different persons. Are we talking about routine everyday tasks, such as checking that the heating is working, or should one also write down the reasons why moving house was a good idea? What is put in writing also changes with time. Groups thus frequently discuss how best to adjust this technique to the circumstances of the person at that moment. In this, the group becomes a medium through which patients construct an evolving form of 'collective expertise' that is recursively used and changed as new experiences are shared in the group.

This 'collective expertise' also concerns strategies of coping with the illness. One important aspect of these discussions is how to relate to others. Memory group members are encouraged to maintain occupational roles and leisure activities. In these contexts, disclosure of a diagnosis of memory loss is likely to provoke discomfort or stigma. However, giving access to this information to key persons involved in these activities might be beneficial, because it might enhance the chances of continuing to take part in those contexts. In discussions about who should be involved and how best to engage them with the best interests of the patient, the group also draws on and re-articulates the moral and political boundaries of the patient collective (Callon and Rabeharisoa, 1998). Decisions on whether or not a person should be 'in the know' entail redrawing distinctions between types of persons, e.g., those previously categorised as 'friends' will sometimes have to be subdivided according to the kind of support they might be able to give in an activity, regardless of the strength of emotional ties forged in the past. Such discussions are political, not only because participation and access to spheres of social life comes to be seen as dependent on mundane alliances with others (Bartlett and O'Connor 2007), but also because each new alliance will constrains the amount of control the person has over the whole collective. For this reason, only a few people are typically brought in.

The work of memory groups is strikingly pragmatic. Stories about one's experiences, techniques for dealing with memorising and the drawing of boundaries around one's care collective are all valued according to the effects they produce. All changes in the collective management of daily life are evaluated by attending to whether or not they produce a fit between patient, carer(s) and the social and material environments he or she lives in. As memory loss comes with change, achieving this fit is a complex issue. To address this complexity, the staff present in memory groups tries to control the number of issues that are discussed in support sessions. This is in stark contrast with what goes on in individual assessment sessions. There, as many issues as possible are teased out and all kinds of uncertainties are explored. But in support sessions (with their productive time constraints), patients and carers are always asked to focus on one or two prominent issues at a time, just those that happen to be causing the most anxiety or that bring along acute frustration.

The specific regulation of uncertainty present in the advice to 'deal with one problem at a time', sometimes extends to the patient's home. It is here that care's organisation of collectives is put to the test. Patients and carers see themselves faced with the task of translating what they learned in the memory group to their everyday routines. To support this translation work, nurses or social workers may make home visits. However the patient and the carer still have to do most of the work. This may include moving house, calling in help, or making agreements within the family (as we saw above in the case of the Fenwicks). Most of the time, however, translation work is not so much about setting up entirely new arrangements as about shifting elements or relations within existing arrangements. It is about continuous adjustment, about 'tinkering'.[9]

Tinkering as a concept helps think about the collective arrangements set up in dealing with dementia, because it encapsulates both how arrangements are repaired and how these repairs are provisional. The story of the Fenwicks gives a good example of this in their decision to raise the amount of house cleaning help. This small shift allows Mrs. Fenwick to support her husband in the activities he values most, in particular gardening. There is an impressive creativity involved in tinkering. Having been offered a variety of ways to handle Mr. Fenwick's decreasing cognitive status, he and his wife come up with a modest alternative that surprises the consultant. This alternative is not intended as a durable solution, but increasing the dose of the drug would not have been a durable solution either. What it does do is shift the attention away from the patient, while further extending the collectivisation of the care. The creativity at work here is not that of the genius-type, individual kind, evoked by the late 'ribbon paintings' that the painter Willem De Kooning produced when he was suffering from early-to-mild dementia (Espinel 1996). By contrast, the creativity that belongs to the regime of care, the creativity of tinkering, involves the collective. It shifts and fosters the distributed links that make it possible to 'get on with it'. It allows the patient collective to, once again but in a slightly different way, be collectively capable of action because it renders the patient collective as a 'dispositif' for action (Jullien 1992; Gomart and Hennion 1999). Here perception as well as action are directed towards the mundane. This is crucial in order to keep the horizon of cognitive decline at bay that, elsewhere in the clinic, is persistently evoked through the interaction between 'truth' and 'hope'.

Care's orientation towards the mundane, towards 'just this, now', underpins the disentanglement from the horizon of cognitive decline because it enables a collective's 'active forgetting' about individual memory loss. Nietzsche proposed the concept of active forgetting in contrast to the dominant view of forgetting that had (and has) dominated philosophy since Plato.[10] Instead of an inevitable, time-driven erasure of the traces left by events that remembering attempts to oppose, Nietzsche considers how the act of forgetting might be fundamental to the continuous unfolding of difference in the world (Ricoeur 2004). Forgetting is essential 'to make place for the new' (Nietzsche 1989). This generative aspect of forgetting is intimately linked with how it *detaches* the present event from its history, how it *dismembers as it assembles* in specific, tinkering ways.[11] In this, active forgetting is not so much about erasure but mostly about a displacement, a re-direction of the focus of perception and action. We know, however, that this is difficult to achieve.

One of the main reasons for this is that memory clinics rely heavily on the flow of resources generated by the interaction between truth and hope. Thus, when in March 2005 the UK's National Institute for Health and Clinical Excellence recommended that anti-dementia drugs should not longer be available on the National Health Service (NHS), one of the main concerns for clinicians was that such restrictions would undermine the provision of other, care-oriented services that had grown out of the availability of cholinesterase inhibitors – such as memory groups. In the memory clinic, this link between the hope-truth body and its care limb, so to speak, is institutionalised in the standardised requirement to produce regular assessments of patients' progression/deterioration. Such assessments reinforce the subjective demands for accountability, requiring the patient and carer to join in the enterprise of reproducing Alzheimer's disease. Returning to the regime of care entails actively forgetting this link, without totally severing or erasing it. And to achieve such balance, one *just* has to 'get on with it'.

Forgetting

In this chapter, I have used two case stories to exemplify two sets of practices that organise 'early memory loss' in memory clinics. I have suggested that the tension between individualising and collectivising practices is mapped onto a space in which the mutually reinforcing opposition between the regimes of truth and hope is orthogonally crossed by the regime of care. The paper traces the reasons why the regimes of hope and truth are so entrenched within memory clinics and provides clues into the fragile processes that sustain enactments of care collectives in this context.

From this, the chapter also suggests that the regime of care and its collective handling of memory loss provide us with an alternative to the portrayal of cognitive decline offered by Iris Murdoch, quoted at the beginning of the paper. In this alternative care world, memory loss does not loom above the horizon, as one does not live with one's eyes focussed on something so far away. Instead, care is a matter of tinkering, here and now. Stronger still, forgetting itself may not necessarily always be a bad thing. Remembering everything can be horrendous, too. As Nietzsche put it:

> There could be no happiness, cheerfulness, hope, pride, no present, without forgetfulness. The [person] in whom this apparatus of suppression is damaged so that it stops working, can be compared [...] to a dyspeptic; he cannot 'have done' with anything. (Nietzsche, 1989: 58).

Nietzsche's digestive analogy, if perhaps impolite, underlines that shedding is integral to living. Thus Nietzsche presents us with a view of forgetting that is the opposite of Murdoch's. Where Murdoch gestures towards a downwards dynamic between clarity and darkness, Nietzsche's evokes the tension between enabling fruitful presents and the forgetting that underpins them. This firm entrenchment in the present makes space – or makes a space/time – for pragmatism and creative tinkering. Such tension is also significant in understanding how care can survive next to the individualising practices within hope and truth. It does not promise to produce anything at all through the disposal of memory, nor does it ask for this shedding to be taken into account: 'just get on with it'.

But is this a recipe for the co-existence of care, truth and hope within dementia clinics? The answer to this question depends on the extent to which my analysis is valid and applicable to other institutions. Memory clinics are specifically designed to address and manage 'early memory problems' (see above). In many respects, one of their aims is the elaboration of scenarios of cognitive decline and the facilitation of strategies that help patients regain control over their lives. This is underpinned by an understanding of dementia as a progressive, staged condition (Blennow, de Leon *et al.* 2006), where early dementia is conceived of as a period where individuals can still manage their condition. As the condition progresses, and without therapeutic strategies to halt this progression, individuals are seen to be less capable of 'being in control' and a variety of caring, collectivising strategies are put in place.

What appears to be happening is that as the patient moves along such 'natural stages' of the disease, care gains more centrality and recognition. We do not understand, however, what effects the recognition of care has on the interaction between truth and hope. If in the memory clinic the maintenance of care collectives depends on their active disentanglement from individualising practices, what is the role of care collectives in the management of moderate or severe dementia patients? Is care an alternative to or a reinforcement of the individualising forces later on in the dementing process? Such questions require research that takes into consideration the relationship between the configuration of standardised stages of cognitive decline, the institutions that are designed to manage patients at different stages and the diversity of strategies that together enact such management at different times in the trajectories of patients.

Notes

1 See Bayley, J. (1999). *Elegy for Iris*. London, St Martin's Press.

2 The ethnographic stories in this paper are intended as 'plausible fictions', also known as ethnographic fiction, due to the ethical framework in which the research was developed For a useful use of this 'device', see Latour, B. (2002). *La Fabrique du Droit: Une ethnographie du Conseil d'Etat*. Paris, La Decouverte. and also Rinehart, R. (1998). "Fictional Methods in Ethnography: Believability, Specks of Glass, and Chekhov " *Qualitative Inquiry* 4(2): 200-224.

3 In early dementia, these are the transentorhinal area, hippocampus and medial temporal lobes. See, for example, Nestor, P. J., P. Scheltens, *et al.* (2004). 'Advances in the early detection of Alzheimer's disease.' *Nature Medicine* 10 Suppl: S34-41.

4 See also the analysis in Akrich, M.(1996). 'Le medicament comme object technique'. *Revue Internationale dePsychopathologie* 21: 135-58.

5 See for this history Moreira, T. (2009). Testing Promises: Truth and Hope in Drug Development and Evaluation in Alzheimer's Disease. *Do We Have a Pill for That: Interdisciplinary Perspectives on the Development, Use and Evaluation of Drugs in the Treatment of Dementia*. J. Ballenger, P. Whitehouse, C. Lyketsos, P. Rabins and J. Karlawish. Baltimore, Johns Hopkins University Press: 210-230.

6 In the delayed recall test, for example, performances below 1.5 standard deviations are considered worthy of further attention. They do not immediately and directly give reason to diagnose someone, or, as the researchers involved put it, 'this level of performance is not used as a cutoff score' (Petersen, R. C., Ed. (2003). *Mild Cognitve Impairment: Aging to Alzheimer's Disease*. New York, Oxford University Press: 20). Rather than isolated scores, profiles of memory impairment have become the diagnostic standard.

7 This is not to say that these tests are beyond criticism. Not just Mrs. Brennand, but quite a few research commentators are critical about the whole procedure, all the more where the accuracy of the test outcome is not deemed to be good enough. See Corner, L. and J. Bond (2004). 'Being at risk of dementia: fears and anxieties of older adults.' *Journal of Aging Studies* 18: 143-155.

8 See also Mol, A. and J. Law (2004). 'Embodied Action, Enacted Bodies: the Example of Hypoglycaemia.' *Body and Society* 10(2-3): 43-62.

9 Tinkering, according to Mol, characterises practice in the logic of care Mol. Mol, A. (2008). The Logic of Care, London, Routledge.

10 For a different use of Nietzsche's concept, see Shenk, D. (2001) The Forgetting, London, Flamingo.

11 For an exposition of this dynamic see Callon, M. (1999). 'Ni Intellectuel Engag', Ni Intellectuel D'gag': La Double Strat'gie de L'Attachement et du D'tachement.' *Sociologie du Travail* 41(1): 65-78.

References

Akrich, M. (1996). 'Le medicament comme object technique.' *Revue Internationale de Psychopathologie* 21: 135-58.

Ballenger, J. F. (2006). *Self, Senility, and Alzheimer's Disease in Modern America: A History*. Baltimore, Johns Hopkins University Press.

Bartlett, R. and D. O'Connor (2007). 'From personhood to citizenship: Broadening the lens for dementia practice and research.' *Journal of Aging Studies* 21(2): 107-118.

Bayley, J. (1999). *Elegy for Iris*. London, St Martin's Press.

Blennow, K., M. J. de Leon, *et al*. (2006). 'Alzheimer's disease.' *The Lancet* 368(9533): 387-403.

Boltanski, L. and L. Thevenot (1991). *De La Justification. Les Economies de La Grandeur*. Paris, Gallimard.

Brayne, C. and P. Calloway (1988). 'Normal Aging, Impaired Cognitive Function, and Senile Dementia of the Alzheimers Type – a Continuum.' *Lancet* 1(8597): 1265-1267.

Brody, J. A. (1982). 'An epidemiologist views senile dementia: facts and fragments' *American Journal of Epidemiology* 115(2): 155-162.

Callon, M. (1999). 'Ni Intellectuel Engagé, Ni Intellectuel Dégagé: La Double Stratégie de L'Attachement et du Détachement.' *Sociologie du Travail* 41(1): 65-78.

Callon, M. and V. Rabeharisoa (1998). *Reconfiguring Trajectories: Agencies, Bodies and Political Articulations: The Case of Muscular Distrophies*, Centre de Sociologie de L'Innovation, -cole des Mines de Paris.

Callon, M. and V. Rabeharisoa (2004). 'Gino's lesson on humanity: genetics, mutual entanglements and the sociologist's role.' *Economy and Society* 33(1): 1-27.

Corner, L. and J. Bond (2004). 'Being at risk of dementia: fears and anxieties of older adults.' *Journal of Aging Studies* 18: 143-155.

Corner, L. and J. Bond (2006). 'The Impact of the Label of Mild Cognitive Impairment on the Individual's Sense of Self' *Philosophy, Psychiatry, & Psychology* 13(1): 3-12.

Espinel, C. H. (1996). 'de Kooning's late colours and forms: dementia, creativity, and the healing power of art.' *Lancet* 347(9008): 1096-8.

Fox, P. (1989). 'From Senility to Alzheimer's Disease: The Rise of the Alzheimer's Disease Movement.' *The Milbank Quarterly* 67(1): 58-102.

Gomart, E. and A. Hennion (1999). A Sociology of Attachment: Music Amateurs, Drug Addicts. *Actor-Network Theory and After*. J. Law and J. Hassard. Oxford, Blackwell: 220-247.

Holstein, M. (2000). Aging, Culture and the Framing of Alzheimer's Disease. *Concepts of Alzheimer's Disease*. P. Whitehouse, K. Maurer and J. Ballenger. Baltimore, Johns Hopkins University Press.

Jullien, F. (1992). *La Propension des choses*. Paris, Seuil.

Latour, B. (2002). *La Fabrique du Droit: Une ethnographie du Conseil d'Etat*. Paris, La Decouverte.

Law, J. and A. Mol, Eds. (2002). *Complexities: Social Studies of Knowledge Practices*. Durham NC, Duke University Press.

Kitwood, T. (1997). *Dementia reconsidered*. Philadelphia, Open University Press.

McKhann, G., D. Drachman, *et al.* (1984). 'Clinical-Diagnosis of Alzheimers-Disease – Report of the NINCDS-ADRDA Work Group under the Auspices of Department-of-Health-and-Human-Services Task-Force on Alzheimers-Disease.' *Neurology* 34(7): 939-944.

Mol, A. (2008). *The Logic of Care* London, Routledge.

Mol, A. and J. Law (2004). 'Embodied Action, Enacted Bodies: the Example of Hypoglycaemia.' *Body and Society* 10(2-3): 43-62.

Moreira, T. (2009). Testing Promises: Truth and Hope in Drug Development and Evaluation in Alzheimer's Disease. Do *We Have a Pill for That: Interdisciplinary Perspectives on the Development, Use and Evaluation of Drugs in the Treatment of Dementia*. J. Ballenger, P. Whitehouse, C. Lyketsos, P. Rabins and J. Karlawish. Baltimore, Johns Hopkins University Press: 210-230.

Moreira, T. and P. Palladino (2005). 'Between truth and hope: on Parkinson's disease, neurotransplantation and the production of the 'self'.' *History of the Human Sciences* 18(3): 55-82.

Nestor, P. J., P. Scheltens, *et al.* (2004). 'Advances in the early detection of Alzheimer's disease.' *Nature Medicine* 10 Suppl: S34-41.

Nietzsche, F. (1989). *On the Genealogy of Morals and Ecce Homo*. New York, Vintage.

Petersen, R. C., Ed. (2003). *Mild Cognitve Impairment: Aging to Alzheimer's Disease*. New York, Oxford University Press.

Petersen, R. C., J. C. Stevens, *et al.* (2001). 'Practice parameter: early detection of dementia: mild cognitive impairment (an evidence-based review). Report of the Quality Standards Subcommittee of the American Academy of *Neurology*. [see comment].' Neurology. 56(9): 1133.

Ricoeur, P. (2004). *Memory, History, Forgetting*. Chicago, University of Chicago Press.

Rinehart, R. (1998). 'Fictional Methods in Ethnography: Believability, Specks of Glass, and Chekhov'" *Qualitative Inquiry* 4(2): 200-224.

Shenk, D. (2001) The Forgetting, London, Flamingo.

Strauss, A., S. Fagerhaugh, *et al.* (1982). 'The work of hospitalised patients.' *Social Science & Medicine* 16(9): 977-86.

Whitehouse, P. and H. Brodaty (2006). 'Mild cognitive impairment. [see comment] [comment].' *Lancet* 367(9527): 1979.

Zarit, S. H., E. E. Femia, *et al.* (2004). Memory Club: A Group Intervention for People With Early-Stage Dementia and Their Care Partners. 44: 262-269.

Animal farm love stories
About care and economy

Hans Harbers

Summer 2000

It is half-past one in the morning. I have just finished Jan Siebelink's *Mijn Leven met Tikker* (*My Life with Tikker*), about fourteen years of intense companionship between the author and his chum Tikker. In the last chapter, Tikker, the dog, dies. The story is over. Sleep won't come. Feeling a bit sad. Have to think about Romke, my own dog, who is asleep downstairs. At least, I hope so. Sooner or later, he will die too. But surely not yet? I get up, go downstairs, and nestle beside him on the sofa. He rolls onto his back, stretches his four legs into the air and sighs deeply. What an intense mutual pleasure.

April 2004

The time has come: Romke has died from a heart complaint. He breathed his last in the garden, with his head on my son's legs, just two hours before that last merciful injection, which had already been scheduled. I arrived home ten minutes too late to see him go. I still regret it — all the more because my wife had the firm impression that he was looking for me, waiting for me.

December 2004

Bought a new dog. What a word! You don't simply 'buy' a dog, as if it's a new bike! We were dogless for about six months. Didn't want a new one right away, not only so we could experience life without a dog, but also because it would have felt like a betrayal of Romke. It turned out that we couldn't live without one. So now we have Joppe — another Frisian pointer.

April 2006

The puppy courses have all been completed successfully. But Joppe still remains a bit anxious, a little nervous. So we sign up for an extra course: an agility course in which he learns to perform all kinds of exercises and tricks. This seems to be good for his self-confidence. An alternative therapy, we are told, would be to have him castrated. I can't find the heart for it — well... heart? The hurt is somewhere deeper. During the first lesson, when I intervene in a conflict with another dog — how stupid can I be? — he bites off the top of my finger. Friends are shocked. 'Your dog is still alive — didn't you have him put down?' they ask. Pure ignorance! Joppe couldn't help it. It was my fault, and his fight. What was I doing there, getting involved? Our relationship doesn't suffer. On the contrary, in fact. Sometimes I surrender to him completely. On Sundays, for example, when he carefully licks off my sweat after a game of football. Or after an exhausting day when he massages my toes with his tongue.

Introduction

There is no shortage of care for animals – at least, for domestic pets in middle-class families living in the centre of town like mine. When we consider the billions spent in the domestic pet industry, this care starts looking excessive – my own dogs not excluded. There is the food branch for cats and dogs, with its increasingly advanced feeding programmes, and the medical sector in which the facilities for pets in the West are better than those for people in Third World countries. We even take part-time jobs to pay for the expensive operations of our household favourites[1], not to mention the world of burial ceremonies for our beloved quadrupeds, or the baby-sit centres, walkies services, dress shops, and even dog-washing machines.

This exorbitant level of care for domestic pets is echoed in public reactions to crises in the bio-industry such as 'mad cow disease' (BSE), outbreaks of swine flu, salmonella in chickens, and the regular recurrence of foot-and-mouth disease. Such crises are accompanied by the mass slaughter of animals, cranes that heave dead animals into lorries, carcass disposal plants that work overtime or, in an emergency, gigantic funeral pyres of livestock in the open air. And all of it is presented in vivid pictures in the media. The reaction of the citizen at home with a cat on his/her lap is, 'What a shame! How can we treat animals this way?'[2] Accordingly, standards for the treatment of animals are transferred form one context to another: from pets to livestock, i.e. from the city to the countryside, from citizens to farmers, from leisure time to means of existence. In general, there is nothing wrong with that. On the contrary, such a transfer of standards can have a critical, signalling function – in this case with regard to animal degradation in the bio-industry. Divergent contexts of interaction between humans and animals can inform and enrich one another.[3] However, in the light of a domestic pet industry that is getting out of hand, an all-too-sentimental reaction to bio-industrial practices begs the question as to whether this type of switch between practices, this categorical swap between domestic pet and production animal, is at all realistic – in both factual and normative respects. Can and should we treat the pig in its sty in the same way as the cat on our laps? 'Yes!' is the response of analytical animal ethicists interested in universal principles. 'No!' say historians, phenomenologists and ethnographers of human-animal relationships, interested as they are in contextual differences.

The standard animal-ethical argument in terms of animal welfare, animal rights and the intrinsic value of animals attempts to formulate universal principles for the way we treat animals – regardless of species and the historically and culturally different practices of human-animal relationships.[4] Consequently, this discourse is characterised by a high degree of abstraction and universality and, paradoxically, by a specific form of objectification. The sympathetic aim of these ethicists is to overcome Immanuel Kant's exclusively human-oriented philosophy by allowing animals into the circle of morally relevant actors. Animals are assigned the status of moral subject instead of instrumental object – of persons instead of property.[5] In their ethical-philosophical writings, however, one does not recognise all that much of this 'subjectification' of animals. On the contrary, animals are actually objectified here in two ways. First, each animal species becomes the object of scientific research in order to establish whether or not it fulfils criteria that allow it to be admitted to the circle of morally relevant actors – such as experiencing pleasure and pain, or exhibiting consciousness. Second, those animals of which it has been proven that they possess the quality in question are elevated to an object of moral regulation, in which case they are attributed certain rights. Thus, animal ethicists are much more Kantian than their condemnation of Kantianism might suggest. Despite their objections to Kant's anthropocentric dichotomy between humans and animals (called *speciesism*), and their consistency of speaking of 'human animals' when referring to human beings, their arguments remain pre-eminently humanistic, *human-centred*. In these ethical theories, animals play no part other than that of the passive entity waiting to be sheltered under the wings of human clemency and loving kindness.[6] In other words, we are faced here with a downright rationalistic and scientistic discourse. By formulating a universally valid system of values for dealing with animals, by performing scientific research on the topic, i.e. the animal in question, then logically compelling conclusions on how to act can be drawn from this input. The sum of universal values (moral truth) and objective facts (cognitive truth) automatically leads to a judgement, a directive for human action. It's as simple as ABC.

Of course, it isn't really, as is shown by the internal controversies within this discourse – controversies about the relationship between animal welfare and animal rights, about the issue of which criteria for moral relevance should be applied, or about the scientific operationalisation of such criteria. In addition, there often turns out to be a considerable gap between a conclusive philosophical argument and its practical application. On the basis of similar reasoning, various authors within this animal-ethics discourse present rather different, occasionally contrasting answers to concrete questions – for example, such as whether or not we ought to be vegetarians.[7] The customary call for more refined moral theories and even more scientific research will not be much use here, I'm afraid. This would add only fuel to the flame. A different style of moral research is necessary – a style in which the gap between unambiguous theory and ambiguous practice is not ingrained right from the outset; a style, moreover, in which animals play an active role instead of passively waiting for their rights.

The above-mentioned historians, phenomenologists and ethnographers exhibit this type of different style. Their cultural-historical and geographic studies of the changing relationships between humans and animals, or their more hermeneutically-oriented narratives on these relationships, are much less abstract, less universalist and pay more attention to differences, whether historical, cultural or biological.[8] Crucially, these studies treat the animal as a subject, as a relational being. They examine precisely this relational nature of the liaison between humans and animals: the human and the animal establish one another in this liaison, in their interaction. What humans are, and what animals are (person, property, machine, creature with consciousness or feeling – whatever) is not predefined but is given shape in this interaction. The animal is not an inactive object of scientific research and of a subsequent attribution of rights, but is an active subject, a partner in the dance of joint existence.[9] Morality, i.e., animal ethics, is not something imposed from above, a framework for evaluating actions, but is something that emanates from within – a product of interaction, something that arises from concrete action. Animal ethics is thus not a logical algorithm, cognitively and morally compelling, but rather an ongoing search for mutual respect, perhaps even love. *Morality-in-action* instead *of morality-about-actions*. The rationalistic approach of animal ethicists does well in the context of policy and legal rules – at the point where clear boundaries must be drawn between what animals can be subjected to, about what is permissible and what is punishable. In contrast, the more relational approach is of decisive importance in understanding (moral) human-animal relationships.

Nevertheless, regardless of how pleasant and cultivated the cultural-historical and phenomenological narratives may be, I observe one particular and notable absentee: the production animal. The examples given almost always refer to pets (dogs, cats, hamsters, rabbits), sporting animals (horses, racing dogs) or wild animals (apes, wolves). They seldom include production animals, in other words, animals with a primarily economic function to their keeper: cows, pigs, chickens, sheep, workhorses, etc.[10] Why is this narrative style of moral research not applied to situations in which humans and animals are inextricably linked in an economic respect – on the farm for instance? Is it inconceivable that a respectful, loving relationship can exist between humans and animals in such a setting? This appears to me to be a rather simplified judgement, an all-too-rapid compliance with the sentimental lament expressed by Joe Public. It presupposes that the relationship between humans and animals in the livestock industry should be regarded as purely instrumental, and thus morally empty or even perverse. As if economy and morality are mutually exclusive categories. To illustrate that the situation is not quite as uncomplicated as it may appear, I shall take myself back to the farm where I grew up.

Our farm

The farm on which I was raised by my parents in the 1950s and 60s, along with my two brothers and my sister, was a small, so-called 'mixed farm' with both crops and livestock in the north-east of the Netherlands. It remained mixed until the farm was shut down after the death of my father in 1971, although the accent gradually shifted from crops to livestock breeding in the intervening period. The disposal of land was economically compensated by the construction of pigpens – see the sheds behind the farmhouse in the picture below.

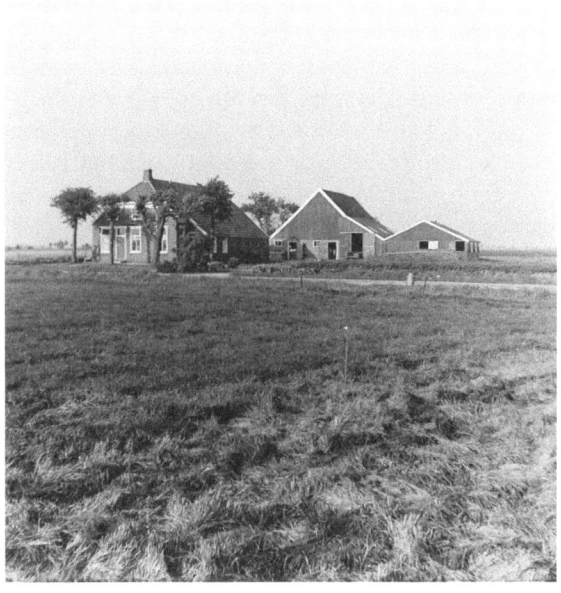

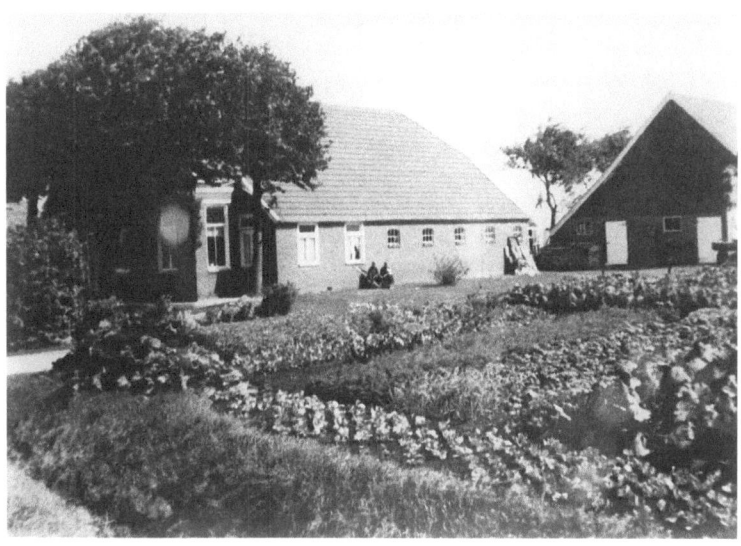

So, we kept more animals on less land. And more different kinds of animals: besides cows and chickens, there were now pigs in various sorts and sizes. The right-hand shed accommodated the breeding pigs: one boar and a range of sows who ensured a steady stream of piglets as porkers into the shed on the left-hand side.

What constitutes an adequate description of life on our farm? A warm and close family life, perhaps? A continuous struggle to survive, balancing on the edge of a minimum existence – and occasionally stumbling? Something from bygone days for which one can only cherish nostalgic yearning? Or maybe it was a precursor of the bio-industry – regardless of how small-scale, unproductive and inefficient, certainly by present-day standards, it may have been. Each of these descriptions would be adequate, and many stories could be told in each of these contexts. Nevertheless, I remember the farm primarily as an economic system; as a source of income in an indirect sense, and of our own food supply in a direct sense – beef and pork from our own animals, eggs from the chickens, fresh milk from the cows, and vegetables from our own garden.

But what does it mean, the farm as an economic system? It doesn't mean that it was a closed entity. On the contrary, it was subjected to all kinds of influences: rural culture, the authority of the church, the government, European regulations. And the economic character of the activities should not be limited to the strict sense of the market,

Chapter 7

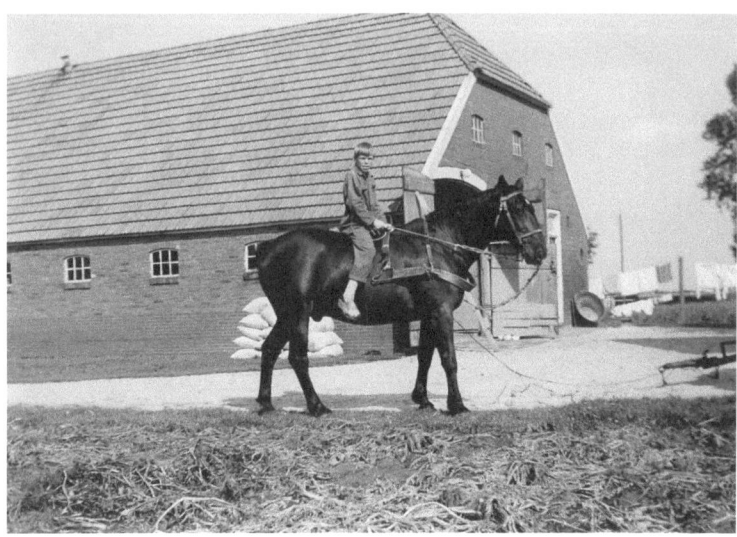

only competition and profit making – although these did play a role, of course. Above all, it was a style of life – of survival.

Farm life formed a miniature society – a network in which people, animals, plants and things co-existed, a hybrid collective in which the diverse constituent elements relationally defined and determined one another.[11] This network required permanent attention and maintenance in order to ensure continuation – unremitting *care* in the dual sense of the word: protection and concern. Being a good farmer was a question of endless care, in various modes and degrees – care relating to the animals, the plants, the crops, the buildings, the tools, the drainage, etc. Taking *care of* was always coupled with having to *care about* diverse factors – the health of a particular cow, the next day's weather if the harvest was going to be brought in, the price of pigfeed, the risks involved in that essential new investment. And there was always concern about our school results, with an eye to a future without the farm. Caring for and caring about always materialised in the context of self-preservation, the preservation of that network, that way of life.

Caring for the farm network as a whole implied care for the life and welfare of its various constituent elements. Whereas at a macro-level that care can simply be interpreted in terms of economic necessity, care at a micro-level cannot. Here, care comes in diverse forms and formats. Take, for example, the great variety of human-animal relationships on our farm – the domain to which I limit myself in this article. This variety required a kaleidoscope of different care relations – however much each individual care relationship was framed again by care for the whole, by that drive for economic survival.

Animals as partners

Let me start with Max, our horse. It is no coincidence that I mention his name – a personal name. The chickens and pigs had no names. Max did. He was the hub of the wheel. Max was literally the driving force, the farm's tractive power – we did not have a tractor at that time. We catered to his every need. We brushed him, we stroked, caressed and hugged him. Sometimes we even gave him sugar cubes – when he had hauled the annual crop of hay and straw on large wagons into the barn, for example. These wagons were so broadly stacked that he couldn't get past them to get out of the barn. He had to go through our living area, right through our kitchen and out the front door – an immense, solid horse. Well done, Max! Good boy! He deserved his reward. Yes, we loved our horse. Emma, Max's female predecessor, once bit my brother quite severely. But he never held it against her. She had a foal at that time and was protecting her offspring. Who wouldn't? Nevertheless, that love and understanding was not endless: we sold Max to a horse trader when we bought a tractor. He had become economically superfluous and Max was downsized under the butcher's knife. That's the way things go...

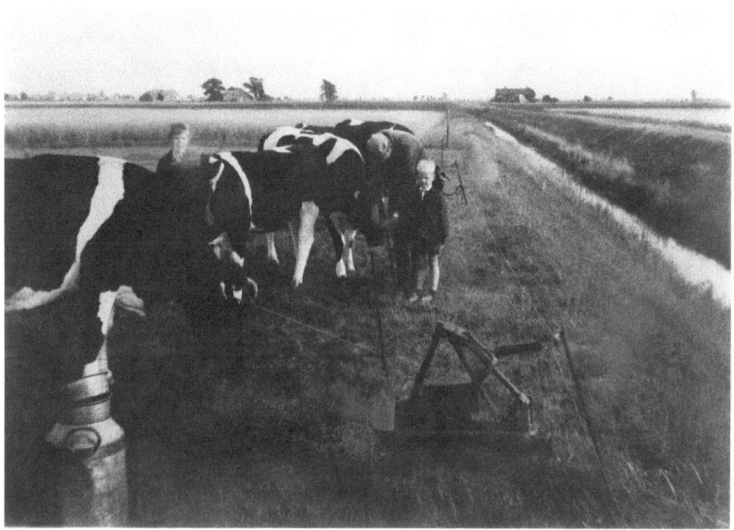

We also had a similar almost-personal relationship with the cows. They, too, had their own names – although these were perhaps less unique and individual: the daughter of Jacoba 3 was simply called Jacoba 4. But we did know every individual cow, and we knew that each cow had a different character and consequently had to be approached differently. We also knew their mutual hierarchy, which was (re)established every year in springtime when they were first released into the meadow after a winter in the cowshed. They determined through their own power struggle who was the boss, and we acknowledged the result – by recognising it and adjusting our actions accordingly. Sometimes we deliberately breached the hierarchy: by keeping the leader away from the water pump, for example, so that those further down the ranks also had the opportunity to quench their thirst. Caring well for the animals was not determined exclusively by us humans on the basis of elevated moral principles taken from animal ethics – such as welfare or fundamental rights. On the contrary, good care arose in everyday practice, in interaction with the behaviour of the animals themselves. This behaviour also contained an element of care- mutual care, which did not involve us humans. If a cow had to calve in the shed (it was always a highlight, the advent of new life), the other cows made space, and visibly showed empathy with their colleague in labour. Our care would not have been good care if it had not been attuned to this mutual care.

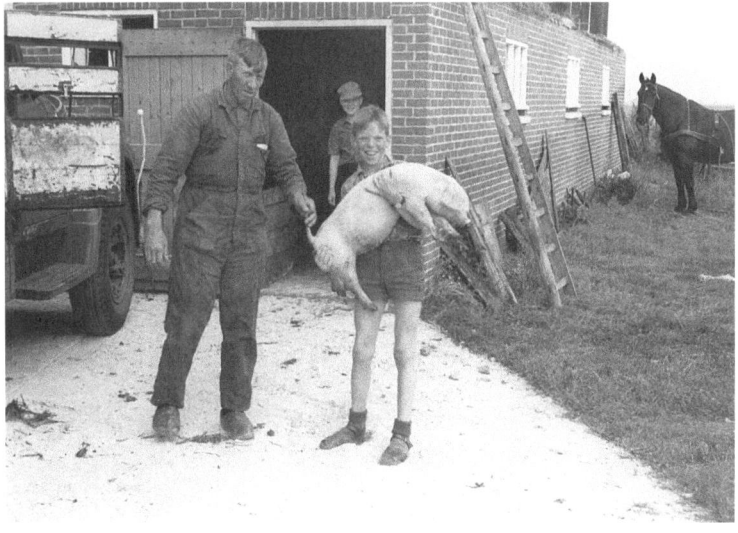

Of course, our care was ultimately devoted to the greatest possible milk production. The care with which we treated teat complaints, which mostly originated from the cows lying on their own udders on the hard concrete floor, was not only in the interest of their health and welfare, but also in the interest of our income. It could be said, somewhat ironically, that the cows worked willingly towards the increased milk flow. After all, formed and fashioned as they were by means of breeding and feeding programmes to boost the milk production, they were all the more pleased to be milked as the tension on their udders grew.

Then there were the pigs. As I mentioned, they did not have their own personal names. This does not mean that they were treated uniformly as a group, as a single category. On the contrary, we had various kinds of relationships with the different kinds of pigs. The level of attention paid to the breeding pigs – the sows, the boar and the piglets – was much higher than that given to the pork pigs. Apart from at feeding times, we were not allowed to visit them, the porkers, in the pens. They were supposed to rest, so that they could reach the right weight for the slaughter as soon as possible. No entrance, do not disturb!

The pigpen for the breeding pigs was a completely different story. It was always fun there. I played with the boar, sometimes riding on his back. His enormous testicles always impressed me. My father helped him service the sows by guiding, with bare hands, his spiral-shaped penis to the right place. There was nothing better – although my elder brother, who had less affinity with the farm, held a different opinion – than 'being on duty' when a sow gave birth to piglets. One of us stayed there to help bring as many living pigs into the world as possible. We removed the membrane that wrapped every individual piglet (if it had not ruptured of its own accord), and laid them down in the straw under the warm lamp. We also trimmed their razor-sharp teeth immediately after birth, so that they would not damage the teats of the sow. We helped them with their first attempts to drink from their mother – something for which, when they were a little older, they always thanked her by purring in her ear afterwards. The sow steadfastly responded with a contented grunt.

The more pigs, the more pleasure. Of course, this had an economic basis, but at that very moment there was also a great deal of pleasure in the abundance of life in itself. Just as we always had a competition to try and dig up the most potatoes from a single plant during the potato harvest – a rather boring job in itself, done manually at that time – we also had a competition about who 'delivered' the

Chapter 7

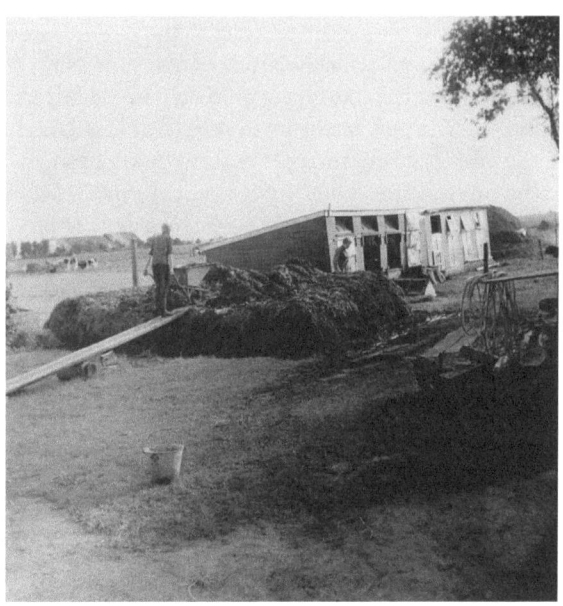

most piglets in one litter. When I was a little older, I also allowed myself a glass of beer for every piglet more than 12. When the 18th arrived, I was assured of an outstanding evening.

Chickens were also a line of business – although we only had a few hundred, in a couple of rickety wooden sheds behind the dung heap shown on the photo. Our relationship with them was much more anonymous. A chicken is only a chicken – good for producing eggs. To stimulate this production, we burned off a piece of their beaks, or they received metal blinkers, a kind of spectacles, with a wire through their beak. Then they could no longer peck one another's feathers or bodies until they bled or even died. This too was a form of care – regardless of how cruel it may sound nowadays, and how much it was framed within a certain economic context. As soon as they stopped laying, even this limited care came to an abrupt end. They were slaughtered and we would enjoy a weekend of chicken soup and drumsticks, fighting about who would get the heart – a delicacy.

Cows, pigs, chickens – those were our production animals, our partners in the system. Max, although he was not a direct supplier of a product, formed an indispensable link to all these production processes. You could summarise the logic of our farm as follows: the more they, the animals, cared for us, the better we, the humans, cared for them –

the more individually as well. In a banal version, this 'caring for us' could be read as caring for our wallet. However, this would be a little too banal. It was more a matter of dealing with their contribution to the economic system in the sense I mentioned above: the maintenance of that network of people, animals, plants and objects, the farm as a miniature society. It was not only our wallet that was at stake, but farming life itself – the freedom it brought, living and working with nature, the pleasure of dealing with livestock; in short, the whole way of life. I say this without irony, knowing all the possible objections. What can I mean by 'freedom', when we were tied up economically? What can I mean by 'nature', when we used fertilizer and pesticides? What can I mean by 'dealing with livestock', when we exploited and killed them? These objections may have a grain of truth, but if it had only been a matter of economy, my father would have done better by relinquishing the farm and getting a job as a postman. And he deliberately chose not to do so. He loved his occupation too much, loved the farm, the animals. Animals gave him much more than post packages. There was nothing more beautiful than the contentment of pigs when they had received clean straw in their pen, or of cows when we gave them fresh hay. The pleasure of the animal, the contentment and gratitude that radiated from them at such moments, was a significant component of the pleasure of the farmer – and of his children, like me. *Animal farm love*.

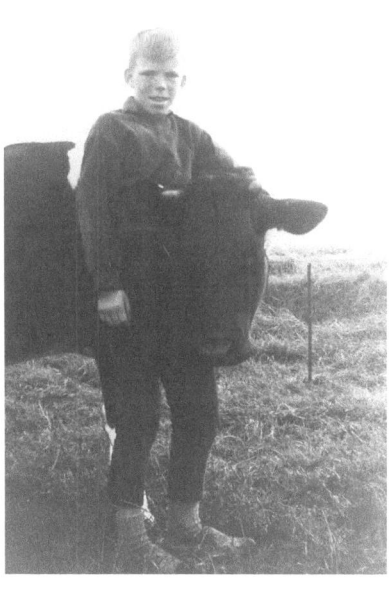

Chapter 7

Animals as enemies

The more they cared for us, the more we cared for them. But the reverse was also true. The more threatening they – other kinds of animals and species – were to us, meaning us people and the animals on the farm, the more effort we made to keep them out of our system. We tried to avoid them, keep them at bay or kill them. Rats and mice, for example. We caught, poisoned and killed as many as we could. They spread disease and gnawed on everything, from the cheese in the food cupboard and the clothes in the wardrobe to the grain in the barn and the feed for the production animals. They were enemies of the system. A great deal of care was spent on ensuring their extermination.

Or take the stoat. At first sight it is a beautiful creature, with a high 'caressability' one might say. Look at the pictures on Google. But still, it is a predator and, to us, a true enemy. On hot summer days, we removed a couple of planks at the back of the chicken sheds to give the chickens a little more fresh air. That's how the stoat could get in. She attacked the chickens like a pedigreed vampire, biting their throats and drinking their blood. We couldn't catch, kill or poison her. It was impossible among all those chickens. The only solution was to put the planks back, to keep her literally outside the system – even if the heat stunned the chickens. That was at least better (i.e. less bad) than being savaged by the stoat. Caring was also a matter of permanent consideration of the pros and cons of a certain situation.

That consideration was occasionally a very complicated issue. When do you help an animal out of its misery? Euthanasia on animals, a reasonably regular phenomenon on the farm, is also a form of good care – but when, where and how? It was easier to wring a sick chicken's neck than to kill a cow. But it remained a painful matter. At least, inasmuch as it concerned animals as partners.

When dealing with enemies, the choice between life and death was made more easily. In fact, there was no choice at all; extermination was a bitter necessity. To resist the enemy, we applied our weapons ruthlessly – pesticides for example. Every summer, we called in a small plane to fly over our potato fields. It sprayed the plants with a poisonous fluid to protect them against phytophthora – an extremely destructive potato disease. OK, you might say, this is all about potatoes and fungi: these are 'only' plants, we were discussing animals. But we also used pesticides against animals. For example, we coated the walls of the cowshed and pigpens with a blue liquid, the name of

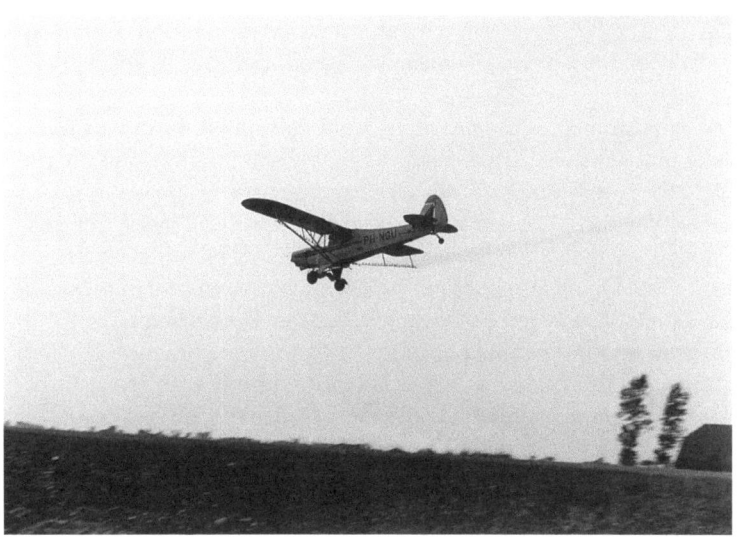

which I cannot remember, to combat flies and other insects. And in the dining room, we suspended a rollout sticky tape on the ceiling, near the lamp. Flies and mosquitoes were attracted to this, got stuck, and died a slow agonizing death. Or we would close all the windows, spray the room with the 'flash spray' (a hand spray containing poisonous liquid, long since forbidden not for animal-ethical reasons but for human health reasons), quickly leave the room, and return half an hour later to sweep up all the dead insects. We never experienced a single moral qualm. On the contrary, every dead fly was a triumph! The fly swat was always within arm's reach and was applied with concentrated enthusiasm.

Economy of care

Animals as partners and animals as enemies. Care was devoted to both, although the care was of a completely different nature – both between categories (positive and negative care) and within categories (the intensity and individuality of the care taken). But in both cases it was a matter of system-related care – care for the maintenance and optimisation of the farm as an economic system. Formulated in this way, the primacy lies with the economy, care being subordinate. That sounds familiar: *Erst kommt das Fressen, dann die Moral*. Was Marx right after all – and with him countless present-day radical animal protectionists, who find that the rules for the welfare of production animals are only scribblings in the margin? Can you genuinely speak of care in such a context – let alone sincere care? Or is it a mere palliative – a moral veil over the economic instrumentalisation of animals? It all depends on what you mean by '(good) care'.

The care we paid to the production animals on our farm was something quite different from the care I now devote to my domestic pets. Every form of sentimentalism was foreign to us.[12] Care was not something 'soft', but firmly anchored in economic activity. But this is not to say that economy was the determining factor 'in the last instance'. As I mentioned before, good farming is a matter of good caring. Economy does not precede care, but care is a substantial component of the farming economy. Economy implies care. Or, even stronger: in this case, economy is care; our farm was an economy of care. For example, annual prizes were awarded for the best cow. This was, of course, the cow that produced the most milk, preferably also with the highest fat content. But the prize was also for the healthiest, strongest, best looking, most beautiful cow – in short, the best-cared-for cow. And the farmer who won that prize was not only happy with the economic profit that he gained with his cow, but also with the cow itself, just as a dog breeder is proud of a champion dog. The cow was not only an instrument, a means, but also a goal in itself. In this sense we were more Kantian than Kant. More than that, we went far beyond Kant: the man and animal, farmer and cow, took their value from their mutual relationship – not from each one's autonomous, intrinsic worth.

Thus, care and economy were not opposing entities but rather two sides of the same coin. This means, in this particular case, that economy was coupled to care, it required care. But did it also mean that care was necessarily connected to economy? That, in the absence of any economic role (either as partner or as enemy) care became an empty category, and we thus had a licence to do what we liked with the animal in question?

It occasionally seemed that way. On Sunday afternoons we grabbed our air rifles and shot the birds from the roof – just for fun and without any (moral) scruples. Who cared? I did so due out of pure boredom, to pass the time. One of my brothers believes he may have done it on the basis of a kind of hunting instinct – just like fishing for example, something I remember as the absolute quintessence of boredom. Whatever the case, though we fished for everything that swam, we did not shoot at everything that flew. At sparrows and starlings, yes, but not at blackbirds and swallows – you left them alone. Apparently, the economy of care (implicitly) played some kind of role here. Sparrows and starlings ate the fruit on the trees and the animal feed. Blackbirds, on the contrary, could sing beautifully and swallows ate mosquitoes. So there was again a kind of economically functional differentiation between enemies and partners – even if we did not explicitly realise this. At least I can say with hindsight that I didn't. In retrospect it was also perhaps not economically necessary to pay so much attention to resisting certain enemies – the above-mentioned flies for example, or spiders and woodlice. It was my mother in particular, keen as she was on cleanliness (her responsibility and pride), who declared all these creatures to be vermin. I remember that various aunts and uncles – also farming people – had many more flies than we had in their stables, kitchens and the dining rooms. But they didn't worry about it. They must have had a higher tolerance to flies. Who your enemies were and how much you had to care was partly a matter of perception. Consequently, the economy of care was sometimes highly performative: how to act depended on one's definition of the situation. And those definitions varied considerably, resulting in different economies of care – different in time, different according to local culture, and different even per family.

The necessity of the link between care and economy can also be examined from the reverse angle. Instead of examining the decline of care when the economic role was absent, we could look at care-giving even when there was no economic reason for it. Did we have any form of care for animals on our farm that was not economically related? Or to put it even more rigorously: was there care/love for animals that could overrule the logic of economy? Yes, I believe there was – although it was extremely rare. In the 'recollection interviews' I held with my bothers in the preparation of this article, it turned out that we had difficulty in finding an example. There was the rooster that was supplied with every new delivery of chickens, just for the splendour and without any economic function. Other examples, besides being scarce, were also ambivalent and open to multiple interpretations. Take our dog, for instance.

We lived without a dog for a long time. There was no need for one. Still, after many years he arrived, our Teddy – for the children, and because my father liked the idea too. My mother wasn't so enthusiastic. At first she didn't allow Teddy into the living area at the front of the farmhouse. The idea was unacceptable, he was too dirty. He had to remain in the rear part, with the other animals. In the winter, he slept in the shed with the cows, where it didn't freeze. It was only later, when a city boy with leukaemia stayed with us for a time, that he was toler-

Chapter 7

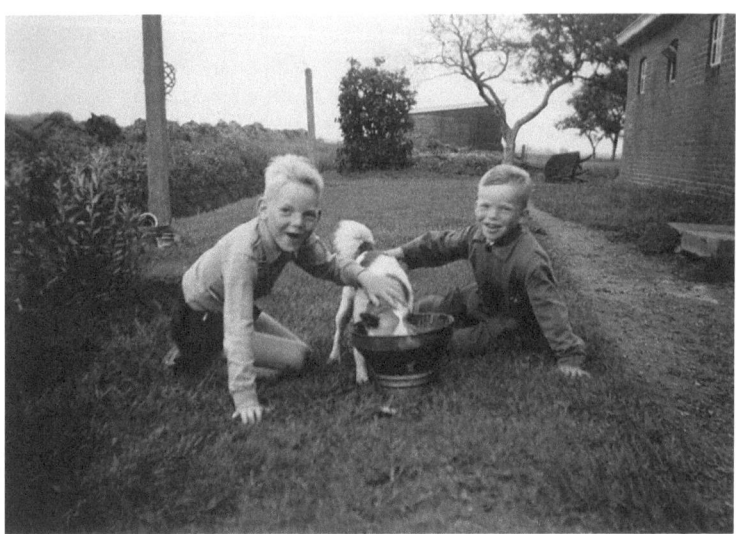

ated in the living room. And it remained that way. Teddy was the only animal to have licked his way into the exclusively human domain. Even literally: in those days too, he licked me unashamedly. He was my best friend, and my father's trusty companion. He always accompanied him to the fields and meadows, where he could care for himself very well. He wandered around for hours, seeking out rabbits and hares, without us knowing where he was. Occasionally he disappeared for several days and nights, but he always returned – to our great relief.

This wasn't the case with our third dog, Lexie, who went a-roving one day and did not return. We never saw him again. A painful experience. Likewise, I remember Teddy's death vividly. He had the habit of running after cars. Barking his head off, he would try to bite their wheels. That was his downfall one Sunday evening. He was run over and died instantly. We buried him that same evening. And it was quiet on the farm for a while.

Nevertheless, we treated our dogs differently from the way I do now, with my own dog. Traditionally, a dog on the farm had an economic function, even if it was only as a watchdog – guarding against strange people and, more importantly, against strange animals. With their barking, dogs repelled the enemies of the system I mentioned earlier. Our own dogs were not particularly watchful, but the neighbour's German shepherd really was. He ensured safety and security on that much larger farm.

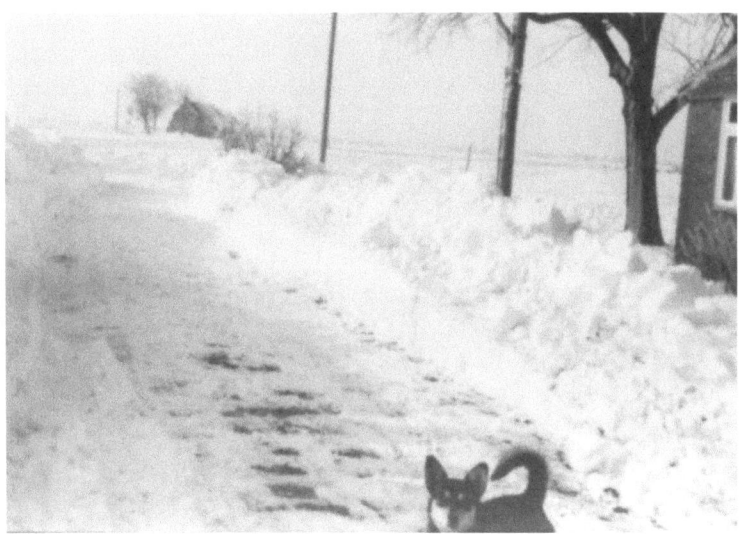

In a way, economic considerations did make their mark, even in our everyday interaction with the dogs. Teddy and Lexie did not receive special and therefore relatively expensive dog food like Romke or Joppe. They just ate what we had. And if they had fleas, they did not get a flea collar or other expensive remedies. Instead, they were drenched in petrol and ran around like mad due to the itching, after which all the fleas were dead. Money for the vet was more preferred to be spent on the cows and pigs than on the dog. Take our second dog. He was an outright failure, antisocial, ineducable, a chunk of misery. He even attacked and killed the neighbour's sheep. It was the limit. Early one morning, my father killed him by breaking his neck with one blow of a heavy stick. He had him buried before we even woke up. At the breakfast table, he announced that the dog was no longer with us. That was a shock, at least to me; especially due to the way it had occurred. I felt the stick coming down. I think my father was also uncomfortable with the situation, in view of the timing of the event and the absence of any burial ceremony as had been the case with Teddy. But those were the straightforward priorities. The animal had to go, and any other way would have meant too much of a financial drain.

Thus, although the dog had no real economic function, we took good care of him. Nevertheless, even then economic elements did somehow creep in. How complicated can the relationship between economy and care be? Care unavoidably seems to accompany economic considerations. Thus, no care without economy? That conclusion would be too quickly drawn. The margins were not great, but they did exist.

Chapter 7

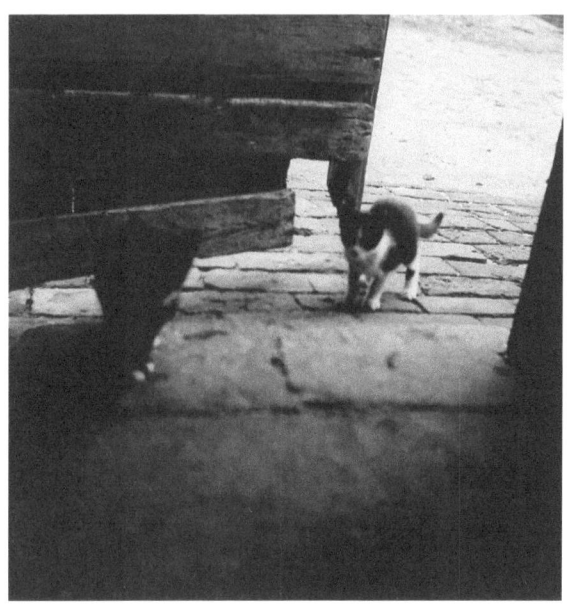

For instance, once Max had become superfluous to our needs, it still took a year before he was transported off. In strictly economic terms, this was a useless year, but not in relational terms. We procrastinated about his departure. A year of unemployment for our former hero helped considerably. It increased the distance. In the same way, Jetje, a cow with only three teats, was kept on longer than was economically responsible, just as there were more cats around than necessary to catch the mice. I cannot remember us ever doing it, but it was not unusual for people in our farming environment to drown a whole nest of kittens in cases of overpopulation. They were simply put into a bag with a heavy stone and thrown into the canal. However, if at all possible you tried to get rid of the superfluous kittens in another way, preferably by giving them away. Or by helping out natural selection: no money was spent on sick cats.

Though not in the cats' case, disease and death in general were one of those grey areas where different considerations than the strictly economical played a role. Animal suffering was not simply something that you could ignore. The question of how to react – I already mentioned the issue of euthanasia – was not decided on economic grounds alone. You received more pleasure from the birth of twelve healthy piglets than the birth of thirteen healthy piglets and a dead or sick one. A calf's broken leg was fixed, even if economic risk analysis showed it to be not particularly advisable. Once, a young calf became tangled up in the rope that bound it to a pole in the meadow, and threatened to choke. My brother hesitated when ordered by my mother to run and fetch the bread knife. Should he be loyal to her or to the calf? It was only when he realised that she did not intend to cut the calf's throat but cut the rope that he did what she had ordered.

The relational character between humans and animals manifests itself in such delicate situations between life and death, disease and suffering. An animal's suffering caused you to suffer too: you could physically feel it. Such forms of emotional involvement created boundaries and responsibilities for dealing with animals. Once, when a cow refused for the umpteenth time to stand still during milking and almost spilled a full bucket of milk, my father kicked the cow as hard as he could with his clogs – not once but many times. Although this was emotionally very understandable from his point of view (he had been grouchy the whole day), and regardless of how unfortunate it would have been economically to lose a bucketful of milk, we felt deeply ashamed – as did my father, in retrospect. One didn't do such things to cows.

But why, then, were we not ashamed to castrate our male pigs without anaesthetic, using an old-fashioned straightedge razor like the ones barbers still have? In the circles of present-day animal protectionists, this still-existent practice has become an icon of callous ani-

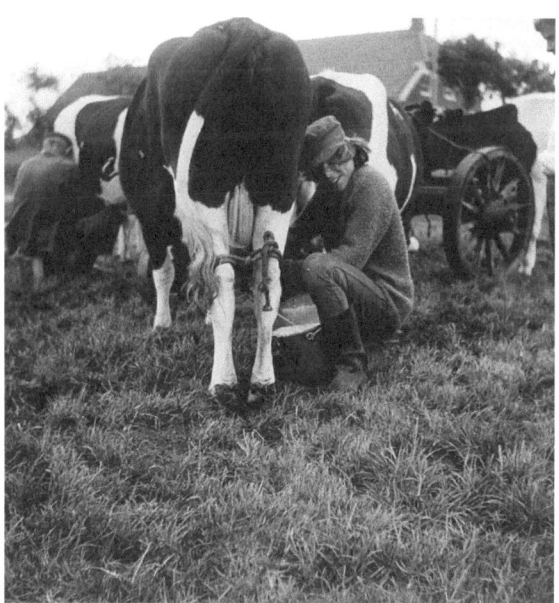

mal abuse. Particularly in urban environments, documentaries on this topic go down like hot cakes. So much cruelty evokes a passionate indignation. We didn't give it much thought at the time. It simply had to happen – to increase the tranquillity and thus the growth of the animal, to prevent sexual maturity before the pigs were ready for slaughter, and because the meat from a non-castrated pig was less popular with the consumer and therefore yielded less income. The piglets squealed like crazy, but this was mainly because their four legs were tied together and they were forced to lie on their backs so that they wouldn't move during the 'treatment'. The operation itself was no big deal: two minimal incisions, a couple of drops of vegetable oil on the wound to prevent infection, and less than a minute later the piglet was playing curly-tailed and happy in the straw with its friends. Nothing remarkable about that, was there?

And in much the same way, we had no difficulty whatsoever in slaughtering for our own consumption a self-reared pig or a cow that had something wrong with it. On the contrary, I remember this as a festive occasion. The entire farm was in a state of commotion. We slaughtered our animals on the farm – this had not yet been forbidden by law. The butcher shot the animal with a captive bolt gun, cut its throat and caught the blood that was later used to make black pudding. The animal was depilated with hot water or a burner, suspended upside down on a stepladder, cut down the middle and then its intestines were removed. The next day, the animal was processed section by section into chops, steaks, mince, soup bones and sausage – lots of sausages, propped by my mother into the gut skins she had washed and boiled over and over. This meant two days of intensive work, but the fleshpots were filled for the season. Slaughtering, that is, killing for one's own satisfaction, was not at odds with love for an animal. On the contrary, it was an integral part of life on our farm, of the network of respectful, loving human-animal relationships. Thus, of our economy of care.

Conclusions and discussion

What can we conclude from this small phenomenology of human-animal relationships on a Dutch farm in the 1950s and 1960s – from this *auto-bio-ethno-graphy*?

Allow me to begin with a more methodological remark. As is the case with every historical reconstruction, the narrative of our farm contains an intermingling of all sorts of levels, inasmuch as they can be distinguished from one another at all: *Die Geschichte, wie sie wirklich gewesen ist* (indeed, in itself a historistic/positivistic absurdity), the way in which I experienced that past at that time, my (selective) recollections nowadays, as well as the philosophically prestructured way in which I address this history in this contribution – in terms of care and economy, with all kinds of animal-ethical discussions in the background. Particularly this last issue is important. After all, to be honest, many of the above-raised issues concerning our interaction with animals were not a part of our attitudes at that time, not in that way. The fact that we never reflected on the moral dimensions of the agonising deaths of flies, as mentioned, is a typical observation of the present day, framed as it is by contemporary animal-ethical discussions on what is acceptable and what isn't and for which species. At the time, we never hesitated for a moment: not because we thought it was justified, but because we did not have a vocabulary at our disposal that enabled us to even pose such a question. We had no animal ethics, of any kind. We had no explicit rules for the interaction with animals.

As we have seen, this did not form an obstacle to genuine, sincere care of those animals. A mixture of diverse factors shaped the various human-animal relationships on our farm. Besides economic considerations, (moral) intuitions and probably also sentiment played an important role. But they were not romantic intuitions divorced from real-life practice, that is, false sentiments. On the contrary, as various examples have shown (the embarrassment about kicking the cow, sympathy with an animal in pain, the ruthless hunt for vermin), the diverse human-animal relationships were firmly entrenched in routines and customs. They were inspired by strong feelings and passed down from one generation to the next: i.e. by moral traditions. They were solidified in habits and therefore always implicit and unarticulated, as opposed to explicit ethical principles. This leads to a first conclusion: arguments in favour of animal rights and welfare may have the advantage of transparency and thus play a significant role in policy-oriented and legal contexts, but dedicated care about and for animals is evidently not, or at least not only, dependent on these. And vice versa, although sentiments originating in completely different contexts, such as the domain of domestic pets for example, may have a content that makes a strong moral appeal and, as such, fulfil a signalling, critical role with regard to our interaction with production animals, they will only have a durable effect if they are translated into the other practice; that is, if they are anchored in the routines and habits of farming life. Between the rationalist, universal ethics of rules and rights on the one hand, and local emotions and sentiments on the other, another field of research is to be won. We must display, clarify and articulate the various human-animal relationships, also in their moral dimensions: their institutional practices, the norms and values embedded in these practices, their consolidated moralities, implicit intuitions, and complex deliberation mechanisms.

The second conclusion is directly linked to this: care comes in various sorts and sizes. Consequently, if people wish to formulate an animal ethics of care, let alone an ethics of animal rights, then it cannot be one that is universally applicable. The notions of care, of what good or bad care is and the distinction between positive and negative care require differentiation between various animals and kinds of animals (the care for cows is completely different from the care about mice and rats), between the individual animal and a category of animals (the care given to an individual horse is completely different from the care given to a brood of hens) and between the practices within which the animals function (the care for porkers requires a different commitment than the care for a breeding pig, let alone wild boar, which is something completely different again). Following the same logic, there can sometimes be good reasons for making a distinction between humans and animals. A general condemnation of speciesism presupposes a much too abstract ideal of equality – as if universal human rights, i.e. the rights of the *human animal*, as the anti-specists say, can and should be regarded as a subgroup of even more universal animal rights. In this way, we drift further and further away from comprehending the diversity of human-animal relationships, both *de facto and de juris*. Whereas the notion of human rights is based on the principle of the equality of people, this type of equality cannot be seriously upheld in the case of animal rights, including the human animal – on pain of eroding the whole idea of equality. There is a price to be paid here.[13]

My third and final conclusion: economy and care are not mutually exclusive. On the contrary, they presuppose one another. Our farm was a classic example of an economy of care. Instrumentality and morality are not categories that supplant one another. Animals are not either an object/thing or a subject/living being – property or person. What an animal actually is – its significance, its status – is only expressed in the contextual, historical environment-based relationship between humans and animals. And that also applies *mutatis mutandis* to humans. Humans and animals are products of their pragmatic – that is, practice-specific – interactions rather than being predefined inputs. In the context of our farm, this meant that good farming demanded good care. There was no primacy of economy in the sense that the laws of the market gave us a licence to do what we liked with the animals. But it also meant that care was tightly interwoven with economic survival. There was no scope for 'soft' care. It was a farm, not a middle-class home or a seal sanctuary, zoo, or safari park.

What are the possible implications of these conclusions? I shall mention two, beginning with the final conclusion – that economy and care, instrumentality and morality are not mutually exclusive. Why shouldn't this conclusion apply to present-day farmers of the bio-industry? The adage of 'good farming demands good care' also applies to a factory farmer. One of my cousins, the owner of a hyper-modern dairy cattle company with over 200 cows and its own yoghurt factory, recently switched from milking three times a day back to the standard twice a day. Of course, it was primarily an economic question: milking three times a day demanded so much of his animals that the bills from the vet were higher than the additional money raised from an extra milking round. But it wasn't only that. His cows were ill so often and became so emaciated that he no longer enjoyed his work. It was not only economically irresponsible but 'difficult to take', as he said himself, thus expressing both an aesthetic and ethical feeling. So here, too, we have the combination of economy and care – even if the economic context and thus the preconditions of care have altered radically. After all, this is exactly the difference between our farm in the 1950s and 1960s and the modern, much more advanced bio-industry: more than in our times, the economic game is now played with daggers drawn. The margins have become smaller. Every economy generates its own care regime. Anyone wishing to combat the bio-industry would do better to take this into account, rather than typify the factory farmer as a criminal and murderer on the basis of abstract notions like animal rights – by broadening the margins for care, for example. It is not a matter of condemning the individual farmer but more a matter of altering the conditions under which he has to do his job.

As for the second implication of my narrative, it also applies to the animal-ethical side of the issue. Nowadays the issue goes right to the wire, economically as well as morally. As I already mentioned: at that time, we did not have explicit ethical rules. Nevertheless, we provided good care, at least according to our erstwhile moral intuitions. Perhaps animal ethics could be a bit more modest: don't judge too fast, first take account of contextual circumstances. Conversely, I have also observed that the questions that I posed with reference to our past were partly shaped by this more pronounced and exposed animal ethical context. There is nothing wrong with this. The historicisation and contextualisation of human-animal relationships that I applied and advocated here do not imply that animal ethics has become superfluous. On the contrary, the same arguments could be used to historicise and contextualise animal ethics, which would imply a strengthening, not a weakening of its normative authority. In the same way as environmental ethics became popular at the moment we realised that we were spoiling our natural environment, animal ethics has made its entrance in the era of the bio-industry and the technological manipulation of animals. Besides being a reason for a healthy portion of irony, this is also a sign of increasing moral sensitivity. Regarded in this way, animal ethics as an expression of genuine concern about animals' fate is a sign of civilisation and decency.[14] Economy and care, instrumentality and morality are not mutually exclusive. On the contrary, if the economic situation becomes harder, the animal-ethical, normative input will also become harder. More instrumentality demands more morality. And for every new practice, for every new context, the words have to be rediscovered – time and again. Explication and articulation of the implicit morality of previous or other practices, such as our farmers' intuitions half a century ago, can help in such situations. The erstwhile inner perspective can be applied as a critical external perspective to contemporary practices – and vice versa.[15] No ahistorical, universal animal ethics need be evoked here.

My father killed the dog with a stick. If necessary, I have my dog put down by the vet. In the context of those times and circumstances, my father's actions were understandable. Now, in another context and under other circumstances, we would do things differently, I guess. Probably, we would first anaesthetise the piglets – or perhaps not even castrate them at all if it turned out that there were other means to reach the same objective. Different times, different practices, different customs, different forms of care – different *animal farm love*.

Notes

1 This example was borrowed from Gaita's confessions regarding his own German shepherd dog, Gypsy. In his splendid *The Philosopher's Dog*, Gaita wonders why we are so foolish and where our (his) limits concerning care and sympathy actually lie. See Gaita (2002).

2 The same kind of sentimentalism underlies more organized, political representations of these reactions, as articulated by various animal (liberation and welfare) organizations and, in the Netherlands, the *Partij voor de Dieren* (Party for the Animals) – which has held 2 seats in Parliament since the last elections in 2006. Even these political reactions play heavily on the sentiment of our relationship with domestic pets.

3 For a discussion of the usefulness of this type of moral cross-fertilization between diverse practices of human-animal relationships, see Korthals (2002), who refers to the notion of practice-bound morality as expressed in MacIntyre (1985). See also Walzer (1983). For a radicalization of Korthals's *multi-practices approach*, see Harbers (2002). My contribution to this book elaborates on this last-mentioned publication – although it is more comprehensive now and set in the context of a slightly different issue.

4 For an overview, see Armstrong & Botzler (2003). Singer (1975) and Regan (1983) have become classics in this field. Subsequently, DeGrazia (1996), Francione (2000) and Franklin (2005) ought to be obligatory reading. In the same tradition, but paying more attention to differences in the capabilities between sorts, see Nussbaum (2006).

5 See particularly Wise (2000).

6 For similar criticism, see the ecofeminists who compare this allegedly masculine style of 'animal liberation' with women's liberation based on traditional notions of equality. Whereas the latter would only lead to emancipation on men's terms, the animal rights movement would only entail emancipation on humans' terms. These feminist theorists, often brandishing concepts of care ethics, argue in favour of *emancipation-on-their-own-terms* – of women and animals, respectively. See MacKinnon (2004). Regardless of how interesting this criticism may be, it occasionally leads, in my opinion, to very questionable alternatives. With regard to women, this quest for 'emancipation-on-their-own-terms' gives rise to all kinds of sensible ideas, but what does this actually mean in the case of animals? I believe little more than a romantic notion of noble savagery, a glorification of Mother Nature. It is not without reason that Merchant (1980) is mentioned here as the most important source of inspiration.

7 For a recent review of the latest in the animal-rights discussion, see Sunstein & Nussbaum (2004).

8 See, for example, the geographical studies by Wolch & Emel (1998) and Philo & Wilbert (2000), diverse cultural studies of Rothfels (2002), the more philosophical essays by Gaita (2002) and Haraway (2003), as well as the work of literators such as Coetzee (1999), not forgetting the dog-trainer Hearne (1986).

9 This does not mean that scientific research does not play a role here. On the contrary: see the much-quoted work by the ethologist Frans de Waal, or that of the primatologist, later sheep-researcher, Thelma Rowell, who studied the responses of animals to human treatment. Relationality between humans and animals has even been embedded in the methodical structure of ethological research. See Despret (2005) on this topic.

10 Thelma Rowell's sheep are also hobby animals – not animals essential for her survival.

11 This characterisation intentionally refers to actor-network theory – a way of thinking that is continuously present in this article, albeit implicitly, with its notions of relationism, anti-reductionism and complexity, among others. For a further elucidation of this theory as a theory of co-existence, see Latour (2005). For the notion of complexity, see also Law & Mol (2002).

12 This also applies to the narrators of relational stories about human-animal relationships – those historians, phenomenologists and ethnographers. In general, they have less difficulty with not all-too-gentle interactions with animals, or even with killing animals, than the much more rational, apparently less sensitive and less sentimental animal ethicists. For example, Hearne received severe criticism for the way in which she trains dogs. On closer inspection, animal ethicists tend to display a huge amount of sentiment to legitimise their otherwise strictly rational discourses. Evidently, an ethically 'soft', relational attitude can accompany a rather tough approach to animals, whereas an ethically 'hard', rationalistic style does not guarantee the exclusion of emotion and sentiment. See, for example, Thompson (2002) on the various philosophies concerning the treatment of elephants in Amboseli National Park, Kenya. From an animal-rights perspective an elephant should never be shot dead; from a relational standpoint, the issue is somewhat more complex. See also Klaver et al. (2002) on the problem of large herbivores in nature areas. From the standpoint of individual animal rights, these animals should be given food supplements in periods of food shortages; from a relational standpoint (not in terms of human-animal relationships this time, but in terms of relationships within the ecosystem), it is ethically justified to let nature run its course and let them starve.

13 See also Brom (1997).

14 This does not mean that the degree of moral sensitivity necessarily runs parallel to economic growth and welfare, as is shown by the way in which animals are (better) treated in numerous less prosperous countries and cultures than in our Western culture. Evidently, even the historicity of morality is not a linear path.

15 In methodical terms, historical narratives with a, rather nostalgic, backward looking character are thus assigned a positive, normative, forward-looking function; they demonstrate that other (moral) realities are possible. Cf. Berger (1992) and Mak (1996) on the decline of rural village culture.

References

Armstrong, Susan J. & Richard G. Botzler (eds), *The Animal Ethics Reader*. Routledge: London & New York 2003.

Berger, John, *Pig Earth*. Vintage International: New York 1992 [1979].

Brom, F.W.A., *Onherstelbaar verbeterd. Biotechnologie bij dieren als een moreel probleem*. Van Gorcum: Assen 1997.

Coetzee, J.M., *The Lives of Animals*. Princeton UP: New Jersey 1999.

DeGrazia, David, *Taking Animals Seriously*: Mental Life and Moral Status. Cambridge UP: Cambridge 1996.

Despret, Vinciane, 'Sheep Do Have Opinions', in Bruno Latour & Peter Weibel (eds), *Making Things Public: atmospheres of democracy*. MIT Press: Cambridge 2005, 360-368.

Francione, Gary L., *Introduction to Animal Rights. Your Child or the Dog?* Temple UP: Philadelphia 2000.

Franklin, Julian H., *Animal Rights and Moral Philosophy*. Columbia UP: New York 2005.

Gaita, Raimond, *The Philosopher's Dog*. Routledge: London & New York 2002.

Haraway, Donna, *The Companion Species Manifesto. Dogs, People and Significant Otherness*. Prickley Paradigm Press: Chicago 2003.

Harbers, Hans, 'Weak Ethics, Strong Feelings. Comments on Korthals', in Jozef Keultartz, Michiel Korthals, Maartje Schermer & Tsjalling Swiersra (eds), *Pragmatist Ethics for a Technological Culture*. Kluwer Ac. Publ.: Dordrecht 2002, 143-149.

Hearne, Vicky, *Adam's Task. Calling Animals by Name*. Alfred A. Knopf: New York 1986.

Klaver, Irene, Jozef Keulartz, Henk van den Belt & Bart Gremmen, 'Born to be wild: A pluralist ethics concerning introduced large herbivores in the Netherlands', *Environmental Ethics*, 24(2002)1, 3-21.

Korthals, Michiel, 'A Multi-Practice Ethics of Domesticated and "Wild" Animals', in Jozef Keultartz, Michiel Korthals, Maartje Schermer & Tsjalling Swierstra (eds), *Pragmatist Ethics for a Technological Culture*. Kluwer Ac. Publ.: Dordrecht 2002, 127-134.

Latour, Bruno, *Reassembling the Social. An Introduction to Actor-Network-Theory*. Oxford UP: Oxford 2005.

Law, John & Annemarie Mol, *Complexities. Social Studies of Knowledge Practices*. Duke UP: Durham & London 2002.

MacIntyre, Alasdair, *After Virtue*. Duckworth: London 1985².

MacKinnon, Catherina A., 'Of Mice and Men. A Feminist Fragment on Animal Rights', in Cass R. Sunstein & Martha C. Nussbaum, *Animal Rights. Current Debates and New Directions*. Oxford UP: Oxford 2004, 263-276.

Mak, Geert, *Hoe God verdween uit Jorwerd. Een Nederlands dorp in de twintigste eeuw*. Atlas: Amsterdam 1996.

Merchant, Carolyn, *The Death of Nature: Women, Ecology and the Scientific Revolution*. Harper & Row: San Francisco 1980.

Nussbaum, Martha, 'Beyond "Compassion and Humanity"', in idem, *Frontiers of Justice*. Harvard UP: Cambridge Mass. 2006.

Philo, Chris & Chris Wilbert (eds), *Animal Spaces, Beastly Practices. New Geographies of Human-Animal Relations*. Routledge: London & New York 2000.

Regan, Tom, *The Case for Animal Rights*. University of California Press: Berkeley 1983.

Rhothfels, Nigel (ed.), *Representing Animals*. Indiana UP: Bloomington & Indianapolis 2002.

Singer, Peter, *Animal Liberation*: A New Ethics for Our Treatment of Animals. Avon Books: New York 1990 [1975].

Sunstein, Cass R. & Martha C. Nussbaum, *Animal Rights. Current Debates and New Directions*. Oxford UP: Oxford 2004.

Thompson, Charis, 'When Elephants Stand for Competing Philosophies of Nature: Amboseli National Park. Kenya', in Law & Mol (2002), 166-190.

Walzer, Michael, *Spheres of Justice*. Basic Books: New York 1983.

Wise, Stephan, *Rattling the Cage: Towards Legal Rights for Animals*. Perseus Books: Cambridge Mass. 2000.

Wolch, Jennifer & Jody Emel (eds), *Animal Geographies. Place, Politics and Identity in the Nature-Culture Borderlands*. Verso: London & New York 1998.

Telecare
What patients care about

Jeannette Pols

Telecare and other IT applications in health care are 'hot topics' in the Netherlands. Telecare is being developed as a new way of shaping care for patients with chronic diseases. It can be described as 'direct patient care, in which the recipient is at home and spatially remote from the clinician, nurse or informal carer, and in which communication media are used'. It is unclear how telecare will change health care, as is the question of whether it will bring improvements.[1] To look for some answers, I will analyse the workings of three telecare practices. I will start, however, by briefly looking into the public debates on telecare: why is it so hot?

The debates about telecare are characterised by their oppositional nature: the positions are either pro or con. In this polarisation, there is not much analysis to back up the claims of either camp. In the Netherlands, the promise most commonly heard about telecare is that it will bring *efficiency*.[2] To this effect, it is first argued that by organising care practices better, telecare promises to solve the problem of an ageing society, with a growing number of patients and fewer professionals to care for them. Second, telecare is said to reduce costs by preventing diseases from turning into crises needing potentially expensive hospitalisation. The third way telecare is said to lead to efficiency goes together with the first promise: by delegating tasks from professionals to patients, the former will be relieved.

The counter-promises are similarly far-reaching.[3] There are complaints about the 'technology push' in telecare developments, in which producers are trying to sell devices nobody in their right mind would want to use, or that still have to prove their value or 'evidence base'.[4] Professionals worry about their relationships with patients when devices are put 'in between' them, turning care into a cold, risky affair See also: Pols & Moser, 2009; Pols 209. Others point to the organisation of Dutch health care as a marketplace, portraying it as a 'Wild West' populated by technology cowboys, where more muscle means more sales and nothing is regulated to assure quality.

Regarding telecare, stakes are high and the grandest of solutions are juxtaposed with the blackest of nightmares. But what happens to these ideals and these worries when one looks at the care practices where these devices are used? Perhaps not surprisingly, the practices differ from these predictions. The unpredictability of exactly how a new device will work when it is introduced to practice can be examined in roughly three ways.

First, there are the different patient groups at which the telecare devices are targeted, often one of the 'big three' chronic diseases: heart failure, chronic obstructive pulmonary disease (COPD) and diabetes. However, the actual patients within each diagnosis group are very different from one another. The disease may be mild or severe, medications may or may not be easily adjusted, the patients may be grieving and in denial, they may be very active with large social networks or lonely, inactive and isolated. They might count the calories of curries or cauliflower, cook without salt -or not. It is unclear how the telecare devices relate to these differences, and how the different patients relate to the devices.

The second way to understand the unpredictable workings of these new technologies is that there is not one but many types of telecare devices, each containing different 'scripts'.[5] Just like movies and plays, technologies can be seen as containing scripts that indicate to users/players which characters they are, what they should do and when they should do this. Interesting here is what kind of care activities the devices allow for or invite users to engage in, or exactly the opposite: what kind of questions or solutions the device does *not* allow for or discourages when compared to other care practices and devices. Technologies are not passive, even if they do not act on their own. They can be seen as normative actors. And these directives may turn out to be different than intended, particularly when one realises that the users have their own 'care scripts' as well.

This brings us then to the third reason for unpredictable outcomes: devices and scripts function in an environment of actual users, other technologies and within specific care settings with their own particular notions of what constitutes good care.[6] These different actors need to be aligned. This can be done by adapting scripts or expectations, or by adapting and accommodating goals and ideals in order to make the devices become recognisable and 'interesting' for all concerned.[7] Apart from the device and its producer, there need to be doctors, nurses and patients who are willing to use it, technicians and technological infrastructure, money, research, and so on. The establishment of what is called *the network*, which is needed to make a technology work, is a complicated process that involves many changes and translations. The resulting practice in which the device is finally used may be very different from what was visualised on the drawing board.

So there are different patients, different devices and different practices. The devices and their users solve particular problems by cooperating with each other, but in enacting these solutions together, *they also shape what these problems are*.[8] While shaping care practices, the lives of patients, the jobs of their formal and informal carers and the function of the devices is also shaped. This paper aims to explore the problems and solutions enacted in care practices using three types of telecare devices.[9] The first device monitors vital signs for heart failure patients, the second is a device for patient education and monitoring, also for heart failure patients, and the third device is used for videoconferencing in the care of patients with COPD. Which of the patients' problems do these telecare practices address -and therefore which practices do the devices help shape? What kind of self-care are the patients invited to engage in -what do the patients do and what are they required to do?

Coding devices

As a consequence of the unstable and evolving identities of the devices within their practices of use, it is not possible to make definite statements about the workings of a particular *device*. One can only pinpoint particular workings at a particular point in time within particular practices. To signify this, I will use code names to refer to the devices. The story, then, is about three possible care practices with a certain degree of flexibility for organising the networks differently. Even so, by focusing on particular functions at a particular moment in the evolution of these care practices, my aim is to make the reader sensitive to the possible ways in which telecare may help to shape concerns in patient care. A second reason for using code names is that the analysis is restricted to the enacted problems and self-care of the *patients*. It is not a complete picture.

'Heartline' and the problem of objective disease

Let us first look at a device that monitors vital signs for people suffering from heart failure, which I have given the codename Heartline. Until now, Heartline has only been used in hospital settings in the

Netherlands. Heartline is a device that provides a blood pressure meter and scale so that people can measure their blood pressure and weight on a daily basis. These measuring devices have wireless connections to a set-up box that uses the Internet to collect and forward the numbers to a central server. Here, the numbers are encoded with alarms if they deviate from the threshold values set by the patient's cardiologist. One concern is that patients will gain weight: for heart failure patients this could mean they are retaining fluid, which is potentially lethal if the fluid reaches the lungs. Another concern is that blood pressure might be too low as a consequence of medication use.

The encoded numbers are sent on to a call centre, where the nurse on duty has a sophisticated triage programme and an extensive software programme at his or her disposal. Every day, the nurse receives the alarms that signify deviant values via the screen, and she must follow these up by calling the patient and writing a note that makes the alarm message disappear. The call centre nurse has to discuss any changes in medication with the patient's cardiologist or their heart failure nurse.

Deviant values, objective diseases and subjective complaints

Which patient problems are enacted in this telecare practice? There is a problem when the patients have *blood pressure or weight values that deviate from their individually defined standards*. When one of the values crosses the threshold value set by the cardiologist, the computer protocol detects this and an alarm is sent to the nurse, who will call the patient.

> *Mrs. Floyd*: Well, they [the nurses from the call centre] were really kind and friendly people, honestly. It's just, well, to me, personally, see: if my weight is between 62 and 63 kilos and one day it is 63.1... This kilo or this 100 grams might be gone the next day, but you would get a call straight away. I think this is over the top.

Although 100 grams does not seem like much to Mrs. Floyd, to the logic of the device the threshold value has been crossed. This is what thresholds are for: to signal when they are crossed, whether by a little or a lot.

A representative from the company that recently launched this device says it is crucial to assemble 'objective parameters' that make these deviances visible. Because, or so says my informant, *patients lie*.

> *Industry representative*: It's the objective measurements you need. People lie, but they can't lie about their blood pressure. This is why Companion [to be discussed later in this

paper, and which does not use measuring devices] doesn't work. People can just report whatever they want. Heartline works with objective measurements.

Although one could formulate this in a milder fashion, the statement points out the nature of the problem: one needs to know the objective symptoms in order to trap the 'real disease'. 'Objective parameters' prevent 'cheating' by the patients, who tend to politely answer the question 'How are you today?' with an 'I'm fine, thanks!' This is why measuring vital signs is even better than face-to-face contacts, says my informant. By using the device, patients cannot pretend to be better than they are. Hard figures don't lie.

So the problem the device counteracts is that patients are not the best reporters of their own disease. They may underreport their own suffering. But this underreporting may also stem from the fact that the disease as it is diagnosed by the measurement devices is different from what people experience inside their own bodies. This is a perennial issue in medicine: laboratory diagnosis and complaints do not always coincide. Heartline is not attuned to what complaints the patients might have, but rather to the 'objective' state of their bodies. Objective disease and subjective complaints are separated.

The assumed unreliability of complaints explains why it is a problem that patients present themselves as 'better than they are'. It is not assumed that patients lie to show they are worse than they are, while their objective measures are good.[10] This would not be a problem from the logic of objective diseases. People who feel 'worse than they are' either go to the doctor or suffer in silence. This means they either come in and are reassured by the doctor, who might show them their numbers are okay or tackle other problems. Or they stay home feeling miserable, while *actually* nothing is wrong with them, that is to say: nothing is wrong with them that can be related to their failing heart. Even though they might be suffering, their bodies are fine because the measured values are fine.

However, the separation of subjective complaints and objective measurements does not completely eliminate the former. One could say that the other technologies connected to the measuring device – the call centre and the telephone – take care of the subjective complaints.

> Meeting with call centre staff: 'Time and attention are very important for these patients', says the project coordinator,

> 'What is heart failure? You go to the hospital, there is always a limited amount of time, and if you manage to solve one problem there, the next problem will pop up the following day. Information isn't absorbed all at once, or patients forget to ask the questions they wanted to ask. Here we have time for them'.

The call centre creates a space for whatever patients may experience as troublesome. Patients can call the nurses, who have time to talk to them. And indeed, some very good relationships have developed between patients and nurses over the telephone.

Daily measurements and compliance.
What kind of self-care does this monitoring care practice invite patients to take part in? Patients are invited to put on a cuff and inflate it to measure their blood pressure, and to get on the scale to measure their weight. *Patients have to measure this on a daily basis* so they can provide numbers to the nurses. This has to be done every day because of the nature of the measurements. A single measurement is meaningless. It is unreliable. Blood pressure can vary from one day to the next, even from one hour to the next.

To make the numbers meaningful, they need to be measured *frequently* so the individual measurements can be related to the preceding ones. Measuring failures can be filtered out in this way. So although the patients are unreliable in reporting on their disease, they still have to correct the unreliability of the devices monitoring them. Furthermore, patients continuously take measurements *over long periods of time*. Because their numbers may shift at any time, my industry informant intended the patients to use Heartline as long as they lived with their chronic condition.

Taking such measurements serves another self-care aim, which is that patients should *comply* with the therapy the professionals set out for them. Compliance is enforced in two ways. First, the monitoring device allows the professionals who interpret the numbers to ask the patients to come in when there is cause for concern. The numbers deteriorate when patients do not stick to their therapy or when a change in therapy is needed. Second, if a patient does not produce numbers every day, the call centre nurse will notice this and follow up on the patient.

In this way, complying with the treatment is not merely the patient's responsibility, but also that of the professional who interprets the numbers and makes decisions to change the treatment, whether these have to do with medication or lifestyle. The responsibility of the health care professional becomes very clear when the trajectory of the objective numbers is traced. These are encoded with risk levels determined by the cardiologist, to be interpreted by the call centre nurse and possibly discussed with the responsible caregivers. So although there are many translations and interpretations, this work is done by *professionals* and according to the protocols they define, not by the patients. In other words, in this care practice, patients care for themselves by *following their caregivers' instructions*.

Because they have access to their own graphs and are aware of their blood pressure and weight on a daily basis, patients can learn to interpret the numbers themselves. However, the patients we talked to were not very active in this regard, because they knew the nurse would look after them.

> Patient answering a phone call from the call centre: Ah, I thought it would be you, that you would call. My weight isn't right today.

Patients know when something is wrong. But their concerns are immediately taken up by the nurse. Within this care practice, patients are active in their own care. This activity is mainly within the realm of 'taking measurements' every day and following instructions. When it comes to interpreting symptoms and treatment decisions, Heartline intensifies professional care rather than delegating it to the patient. And patients like this: they feel safe, because they are being monitored and taken care of.

> *Mr. Johnson*: Of course you know a lot, because you have a lot of experience with your heart and with your body. But this takes it a step further, so to speak. It feels safer. The idea that there are people out there who are checking on you puts you at ease.

What patients can initiate is phoning the call centre nurse if they are worried, even though the numbers are not out of range. However, they rarely do. Although the nurse may also contact the patient, this is usually set in motion in response to deviant measurements. So although there is space for discussing subjective complaints, the main problem targeted in this care practice is the objective disease.

'Companion' and the problem of poor lifestyle and lack of knowledge

I will give the second device the code name Companion. Patients receive a white box for home use; every day questions appear on the display, and these can be answered using four buttons. It is used in three projects in the Netherlands: one for COPD, one for type 2 diabetes, and one (the one being analysed here) for heart failure.

How does it work? The questions the patient must answer daily are presented in written form on the display of the white box. The questions are derived from a general protocol of questions typical for patients with heart failure. The series usually starts with the question 'How are you today?' which can be answered using a 10-point scale.

The questions and answers are categorised into three areas. There are questions about the symptoms the patients observe in or on their bodies, the behaviour they engage in, and their knowledge of their disease and lifestyle. 'Symptom questions' involve observations on weight, shortness of breath and swollen ankles. The questions about behaviour ask if patients took their medications and stuck to their salt-free diet and fluid intake quota. The questions about knowledge involve multiple-choice questions: Does being physically active help relieve stress? How much fruit should you eat each day? The patients get immediate electronic feedback on their answers: the right answer is repeated and good answers are complimented. The session ends with a 'Thank you and see you tomorrow' message.

Once a day, after being encoded by a computer protocol that assigns alarm labels, the questions and answers are sent over the telephone line to the responsible heart failure nurses in the hospital. In contrast to Heartline, the warning signals involve general notions on healthy behaviour for heart failure patients. Companion is made for patients with a specific diagnosis to which the questions are matched.

Lack of awareness of fluctuating symptoms and poor routines

Which problems for patients are enacted in this care practice? One of the problems for the heart failure patients here is that their *symptoms may fluctuate* from one day to the next. On top of this *the patients should be aware of this*. There is some ambivalence here. When symptoms fluctuate, the nurses decide if something needs to be done. However, to become aware of these fluctuations the patients are taught to routinely observe their bodies. In this way, a lack of routine observation is targeted, rather than trouble inside their bodies per se. Instead of an objective disease (which is left to the nurses), in this practice *lifestyle* and *routines* are turned into the object of intervention for the patients.

In contrast to Heartline, observations are made not by using accompanying measuring devices but by using devices the patients have at home (mainly a scale) or their own observations. This takes the interrelatedness of the monitored symptoms more seriously: for heart failure patients, if there is a sudden increase in weight or ankle contour this could indicate fluid retention, and this is more important than their absolute weight or precise ankle perimeter. Unlike Heartline, various complaints are not turned into subjective particularities unrelated to disease, but are to be observed as symptoms themselves.

What about the reliability of these numbers and observations? Do the patients lie? The patients we asked were adamant that they reported the truth. The device would be useless, they said, if you did not give sincere answers, both about observations and complaints.[11] The heart failure nurse confirmed that Companion induces truth-telling better than face-to-face contacts. Beyond what can be done during face-to-face contacts, patients are taught to routinely measure their weight and check their bodies -and continue to do this.

So the main problem Companion addresses for the patients is that *they have poor lifestyle routines*. Although some of these routines are about observing symptoms and relating these observations, a link to other lifestyle routines is also made. When patients eat too much salt or are not careful with their fluid intake, this will affect their condition in a negative way. Hence, the device tries to enforce the right lifestyle, either by reminding patients or by explaining again why all of this is necessary. Thus, the problems enacted for the patients are the lack of proper routines and the right knowledge to help them deal with the disease.

Improving lifestyles, developing routines and being taken care of

What kind of self-care is enacted in this care practice? Foremost, this is about *improving patients' lifestyles*. The device makes the patients do this in two ways: by turning lifestyle into routines and by increasing their knowledge.

By making them answer questions on the white box every day, patients are invited to turn the observation of their bodies and behaviour into a daily routine. The use of the device is turned into a routine in itself, as is checking weight and fluid intake, which is requested every day.

> *Mr. Danick*: It's part of what you do, your life. How shall I put it. I get up in the morning, I go to the loo and step on the scale and write down the number. And then we go for breakfast. And after breakfast I measure my blood pressure and everything. It's all part of the routines, just like the box. And once all of this is done, I can get on with my day.

The device reminds patients and explains to them why they should continually act in certain ways. The materiality of the device addresses this routinisation. Answering questions by pushing buttons is very easy, is included in the morning rituals and takes just a few minutes to complete.

It is also made possible for patients to improve their lifestyle by *increasing their knowledge* about their condition and lifestyle. They can do this by filling out the questions on the telecare device: the 'health quiz'. This is the part the patients particularly like. They turn it into a game, competing with other members of the household, like on TV shows. An example:

> *What are two signs of fluid retention?*
> a. Weight loss and swollen feet.
> b. Shortness of breath and dry mouth.
> c. Weight gain and swollen feet.

Note that the question and possible answers contain hidden directives that are oriented towards a change in behaviour: look out for weight gain and swollen feet. Patients should learn more facts in order to get their lifestyles right. The device provides these facts: don't use salt, use alcohol in moderation, exercise and don't smoke. The patients should learn these 'directives disguised as facts' by adding them to the body of knowledge they have already acquired and practice them. The facts/directives are timeless and are the same for every individual with heart failure.

But there is something amiss with the universality of these facts/directives (apart from them being a universality phrased in Dutch). For example, 'reasonable deviations' do not exist for the programme, and there is no way to skip questions that do not fit a person's individual situation. The reasons for not complying are not scripted as meaningful or potentially meaningful, but as wrong, and in need of an alarm to report it to the nurse. There is only one best way to live your disease.[12]

In this practice it is the nurses who make space for individual variations. The nurses following up the alarms may decide whether to allow the patient to disturb the logic of the device. For instance, when patients are stable and do not want to exercise or say they can only manage a salt-free diet three days a week, the nurses will not nag them about this. The nurses solve the problem of the device's non-universal universality by ignoring alarms about these matters for such patients.

Another problem with the general protocol is that not every patient needs the same information. If patients are not using a specific kind of medication but still have to answer questions about it, this is confusing, and the answers will be random. So although Companion helps patients learn to stick to their lifestyle, there are difficulties in dealing with individual differences and exceptions. Ironically, the general protocol makes the information less universally applicable. When there are individual exceptions, the patients wait to get a call and *discuss their considerations with the nurse*.

The individual exceptions and inappropriate questions make it difficult for the patients to interpret the evaluation the device gives about their answers. And they are happy to leave it to the nurse to decide whether something needs to be done, knowing the nurses will call if there is anything wrong. Even though the device sometimes urges them to call the nurse, most patients do not do this. They know the nurse will call them if it is really necessary. One patient has tested this out:

> When I got that box, I thought: what does this rubbish mean! You get a lot of questions, yes, no, 1, 2 or 3, or all of the above. And I gave the wrong answer on purpose. And half an hour later, the phone rang. So I tested it out to see if it worked. And I did it again a few weeks later, because maybe they would only check on the new patients. And the telephone rang again! So they really do something with it.

And this seems to be crucial to the patients' enthusiasm for the device. They report that the device makes them feel safe because the nurses look after them. Their self-care here means letting the nurses take the responsibility. Thus the device does not function as a temporary educational device. When the aim is to educate patients by way of gathering the facts to build a 'body of knowledge' and effectuating behavioural change, the need for the device would be finite. But the patients want to keep it. They are being monitored more often than if they just go to the clinic every three months. They are checked every day. The nurse sitting 'on the other end' is very important to them. Their part in their care is to routinely 'speak the truth' to the device and to take the health quizzes. But again, it is left to the professionals to judge what the truth they report might mean. In this practice, the patients and nurses enact the device as a way for the nurses to keep an eye on the patients.

Videoconferencing and the problems of daily life

A third type of telecare device are the videoconferencing systems that provide screen-to-screen contacts. I will look at a system used for follow-up care in a clinic once patients have been discharged from a three-month rehabilitation programme for living with severe COPD. Webcams are used to connect the patients to their main health care professional in the clinic for follow-up care, and also with fellow patients they spent time with in the clinic. The clinic loans them a computer for three months, and patients are trained in the clinic to use the video programme as well as the internet and email. The idea is that this will facilitate transferring the lessons they learned in the clinic to the home setting, will give patients something constructive to do, and will also allow patients to support each other.

Fuzzy problems and the necessity of talking

What kinds of problems are enacted with the webcams during follow-up care? The webcam does not script the content of particular *problems* in a structured manner, as is the case with the devices discussed before. Anything can be discussed over the webcam, from vital signs to leisure time, and this 'anything' is multiplied by the different communication partners connected in this way. However, what *is* scripted is that the problems addressed by webcam contact are to be *established interactively*.

Let us look at what kinds of problems are actually discussed over the webcam in the particular context of follow-up care for COPD rehabilitants. There is one particular problem the webcam helps to address. Patients say that the webcam, like an actual visit to their caregiver, helps them to overcome their embarrassment about discussing how they are doing, especially if they are doing badly. The caregiver can see if a polite answer to a 'How are you doing?' question makes sense or not. The patients explain that this is not a matter of being unreliable about reporting on their situation, but that they are embarrassed to acknowledge they are doing badly, even though they were looked after so well.

Although caregivers say they use the video image to 'check up on' their patients (according to them: to spot ash trays or an unkempt appearance), their unreliability is not corrected here by objectifying information, but by extending the *trust* and intimacy of a relationship that has already been established.

> *Mrs. Miranda*: It's just much more personal [than the telephone]. You can see one another and… Yes, I have the feeling that a conversation lasts much longer – you tell much more than you would over the telephone. You are much closer to one another. It's actually as if you are just visiting your caregiver, as if you are in the same room together. You have to really make time for it.

The carer knows the patients well and knows what they look like when they are not well. So here, the video system addresses the problem of patients *being embarrassed to talk about their problems*. The imperative in this care practice is that they do this anyway, hence creating the possibility of revealing whatever is beneath the feelings of embarrassment. Is medication needed or a supportive listener instead? The webcam thus allows unsolvable problems to be addressed.

> *Social worker*: Take the two ladies I chat with on the [webcam]. This is supposed to be follow-up care after leaving the clinic, but is it? No. They simply have a lot of problems. And I hear their stories and nod sympathetically. I'm more of a sounding board (*praatpaal*), which is quite a different effect than on the phone.

Apart from talking to carers, patients in follow-up care in the rehabilitation clinic can use the webcam to talk to fellow patients they befriended in the clinic.[13] In this case, a contact may start with the *patient's worries or wanting to talk*. Fellow patients do not judge you, and understand what you are talking about. Because of their shared history in the clinic, they know about each other's difficulties, and are very supportive. They know what it means to live with COPD. A problem thus addressed is that the patients often feel that they are *not understood very well* or are misjudged.

> *Mrs. Jaspers*: What I find really very difficult about this disease is that you can't see from the outside that one is ill. And one time I'm better than another. And people simply don't have a clue what it means. My neighbour, she said: 'Oh, my grandson has eczema too'. When I told her about emphysema [the term formerly used for COPD]. They have no idea.

This misunderstanding is also related to the way in which the patients understand their own illness. They told me that one of the hardest things is to accept that you have this disease and will have to live with it. The patients describe a continual process of accepting and rejecting the reality of their disease. All patients recognise this process of shifting and fluid ontological states. Patients point out and discuss this over the webcam by 'reminding' each other to take care of their sick bodies and by sympathising with the grief of the umpteenth realisation that one is not well. Hence, the patients discuss a kind of knowledge of 'living disease on a daily basis'. In contrast to the unreliable subjective experience in the Heartline care practice – where it is placed in opposition to objective symptoms – experience here points to a shared reality of living disease. Experience is not suspect and a hindrance, but can be productively shaped and shared with fellow patients.

Living disease not only prompted the patients to have serious webcam conversations, but also opened up avenues for diversion.

> *Mr. Best*: Let's say, when you were tired, and you were out of breath..., well, you would go and play with that thing [the computer and the webcam], just to fool around a bit. Make some jokes. That would make you forget about everything for a bit. It's just, it helped me tremendously. It's made all the difference. Just to chat with them [the fellow patients].

The problem here is that patients get too absorbed in their problems. 'Diversion' is a sensible goal here. Mr. Best told me he was treated for depression when he learned about the irreversibility of his illness. Thinking about more cheerful matters and talking nonsense with his fellow patients helped him deal with his situation. Thus, *emotional matters* such as sadness and despair may also be addressed via the webcam. Because problems are shaped within the webcam interaction, jointly articulating them is at the same time engaging in taking care of them.

Share experiences, find out what to do and get a life

Videoconferencing helps bring about a kind of self-care that interactively shapes what the problems are. What the care patients are invited to practise is *getting help, not being alone* and *sharing experiences* in order to shape and address problems at the same time. Jointly shaped problems are not individual problems.

> *Mr. Torrance*: I think the contact with fellow patients is really nice. Because there is always a night where you wake up, and you're short of breath, and things don't work out.

> And then you think: is this me, is this my illness, or what? But if you can talk to another patient, and he or she feels just as bad, then you think: well, I'm not the only one suffering today. And then it may turn out that there's bad weather on the way or something like that. And then you can see: it's not only me.

The shared experience may help patients identify what is the 'me', what is the 'illness' and what is something else. The exchanges help patients shape ways of living with their condition and anticipate how their bodies will react to the circumstances. The set-up with fellow patients also makes it possible to 'just have a chat', to prevent one from becoming lonely, even if there are no physical bodies present and one has to stay at home to use the webcam.

Once again, the *nature of the care* patients are invited to engage in is thus foremost *a matter of jointly shaping problems and solutions*. Video chats allow patients to discuss, compare and even reject lifestyles, thereby sorting out how to live their disease in the best way possible. Of course, COPD patients also have to pay attention to lifestyle. If heart failure patients were to use the device, they would still need to watch their weight and fluid intake. But these matters are not specifically targeted by the device, and only come up when the patients (or their sparring partners) bring them up during a video chat. The video system allows patients and carers to develop and turn to different types of knowledge and questions. Thus, for the video system described here and the particular connections it helps to establish, there is not just one possible way to live one's disease. The practice allows for a multitude of *individual variations* for defining and solving problems or matters worth discussing.

When one includes the use of the computer that comes with the webcam – as is done in the care practice of the clinic – another way of self-care is promoted as well: the patients' *'broadening of their horizon'* and their engagement with activities they like rather than with their illness. Although it takes effort and training to use the computer, it is this effort that allows for new problems to emerge and to be solved. The supposedly technophobic elderly patients helped each other get started with email and the Internet. John, a former rehabilitant from the clinic, organises training sessions:

> *John*: We teach them how to write emails. And there was one man, he had a son living in Japan. And in the meantime

> he had become a grandfather. But he had never heard of the Internet. So he got this Internet connection at home, and his son sent him his email address. And I helped him type the email address, and when he got an answer he got pictures and saw his grandchild for the first time. Really, if you could see this older man looking at a picture with tears in his eyes... Then I think: the world opened up for him, really. That he could see pictures that had been taken two days before in Japan. That was really – you work for hours with this man, but you do take some pride in your work there [laughs].

This type of care actually encourages patients to focus not only on the things that are wrong with them, but also on the positive things they might want to do with their lives by 'bringing the world into their home' and by caring for each other.

In contrast to the routine use of Heartline or Companion, learning to use the computer, booting it up every time, making the appointments for the consultations, taking the time to get it all set up and seeing the person on the other end engages patients in a clearly marked activity. It creates *events* rather than routines. It is new and unexpected every time it is set up. A fluid mixture of medical, social, emotional and practical problems and solutions are shaped and addressed, staging events in the midst of many routines of getting through the days.

There is an ironic twist to this care practice. The patients have to turn in the equipment after three months, in keeping with the idea that they should become independent of the clinic, but conflicting with the idea that support by fellow patients and the use of email and Internet demand a more permanent use. This tension came into being for various reasons, one of them being the lack of clarity about what the device actually *was*. Was it to be used as 'follow-up care', linking patients to the clinic for as long as was needed for them to translate the lessons learned there to the home setting? Or was it intended as permanent support? This lack of clarity, muddled by technical and cost issues was keeping this webcam practice in a bind.

Which problems to care for?

At the start of this paper, I stated that telecare technology does not solve problems that are already there, but helps to enact particular problems as the ones needing to be attended to. I demonstrated that it is the nature of the problem itself that changes with the particular practice in which a device is embedded. These are specific normativities that the telecare devices help to enforce. Indeed, it has become clear there is no 'naturalised' disease 'out there' for which the telecare devices provide the only logical solution. Heartline helps to enact an objective disease that is differentiated from subjective complaints. Another technology in the composite – the call centre – is supposed to create space for the latter. For the same patient group, Companion helps to enact a problem with patients' routines, and also addresses patients' fear of their disease. The webcam practice locates the problems of COPD patients in daily life and makes it difficult to keep these problems to oneself or turn them into an identity or sole activity. Each device thus helps enact a different set of problems.

In line with the different problems enacted, care – which here means self-care by the patients – becomes different things as well. In the Heartline practice, patients care for themselves by routinely measuring and complying with interpretations and solutions put forward by the nurses. The Companion practice makes patients care for themselves by teaching and making them practise different routines and by being monitored by the nurses. The webcam in the rehabilitation clinic turns self-care into a quest for different people to talk to and events to be shaped and set in motion.

The different enactments of problems and self-care imply a different appreciation of what patients experience. The more their experience is questioned, the less the patients are addressed as active participants in their care. The monitoring of objective symptoms turns out to be something that professionals and devices have to take care of. The patients have little access to these and lack the knowledge to find solutions. The Companion practice takes patients' experiences more seriously, turning these into possible symptoms of disease that patients can learn about by making them the object of routine observations. Again, problems uncovered in this way are interpreted and dealt with by professionals. The more socially or interactively enacted problems that come with the webcam care practice turned experience into expertise, bringing other potential carers into the picture, such as fellow patients, people with whom one shares specific interests and ways of living disease. Framing problems as the problems of daily life makes professional responsibility and expertise one among many sources of solutions. Patients, too, are actively engaged in identifying their worries and the best way to deal with them.

Interestingly, the 'utopias' and their opposites discussed in the introduction were not encountered. Instead of a more efficient use of nursing capacity, all practices implied a greater workload for the nurses. Their workload grew because patients did not 'manage' themselves completely on their own, but care was intensified, be it in a different form than before. The resulting practices shaped different problems, and turned living with a disease into a very different life. There were no relative differences (more or less good care), there were qualitatively different ways of relating to very different problems and lives.

Why is their no active debate on these differences? One reason is that care practices are difficult to study, particularly because of the way most of these studies are designed and organised. Current telecare research consists mainly of individual project evaluations, not comparisons. Although many such evaluations exist, they focus on quantitative evaluations of predefined effects to be produced by the devices, or draw these together in meta-analyses.[14] This makes it very hard, if not impossible, to learn about shifting goals and different use practices, particularly when the goals and problems targeted are the *result* of innovative practices rather than their starting point. Although these studies into telecare effects may continue to accumulate, they will not show how these devices work.[15] If one wants to learn about the nature of these fluid innovative care practices, methods sensitive to this fluidity are needed. Qualitative methods are better suited to this, and allow for descriptions of very different effects, rather than measuring changes of just a few predefined ones (see also: Finch *et al.* 2003).

The ethnographic analysis in this paper *did* allow reflection on the question of what problems are determined to be worth taking care of. And indeed, one could think about whether one wants to live with routines rather than events, with more or fewer professionals looking over one's shoulder, about the time one wants to invest in self-care, the preferred nature and status of one's problems or experience, and the responsibilities one deems acceptable. These are not just medical questions, but ethical and political ones as well. But here is the irony: these questions cannot be asked in a politically meaningful way in The Netherlands. Telecare is outside the scope of ethical and political deliberations and decision-making. There is no place where debates about telecare actually take place and where decisions can be made. The space where telecare takes shape is in 'the marketplace' rather than in parliament.

What kind of telecare device, and therefore what kind of life one can live with one's chronic disease, depends on where one lives, what organisation is active there and what devices they bought, rather than on what one chooses or prefers, what fits one's situation best, or what defines good care or a good life. When, as in the Netherlands, health care is turned more and more into a marketplace, competing health care organisations and insurance companies will each organise their own projects without sharing their experiences with each other. Developing telecare, then, will be about having the best company and being ahead of the competition, rather than being about jointly discovering what the best possible care is for whom. Research data become business secrets.

The patient is the weakest partner in these market processes. Telecare projects are usually developed by starting a pilot project with a producer, financing and some related evaluation research. Only when all of this is arranged is the 'field' of professionals approached. This may cause delays, because the professionals might want to change parts of the device or need to negotiate within their organisation; key doctors need to attach their name to the project, and so on. A complex network must be in place before the devices are able to function at all and before the first patients are invited to use them.[16] In the practices of building these networks, the patients are the last ones notified. They have to live with the devices and what comes along with them, but are only involved when the network is already largely in place. Their option is to say either 'yes' or 'no'.

There is no political space for discussions about which telecare practices would be good ones. Instead of deliberations, there are these experimental practices in which the goals of these care practices are shifted and tinkered with by those involved. People and devices jointly invent possible forms of living with and caring for disease. Treating these experiments as proper experiments by opening them up for analysis about how they work may indeed be the type of politics that is better suited to telecare developments.

Acknowledgments

This paper was written as part of the project 'Care at a distance. A normative investigation into telecare' on which I am working together with Dick Willems (AMC) and Maartje Schermer (Erasmus MC, Rotterdam). I would like to thank them both for their collaboration and comments on earlier versions of this chapter. Thanks also to the Netherlands Organisation for Scientific Research (NWO) programme 'Ethics, Research and Government' (in Dutch: 'Ethiek, Onderzoek en Bestuur') for financing the research, and to the European Union for financing its continuation (EFFORT). I am grateful to Annemarie Mol and Ingunn Moser for their comments and our continued work together, and to Amâde M'charek for helping me grasp how this story should end.

Notes

1. See Willems (2004) for an exploration of ethical questions relating to telecare innovations.
2. The promise for using telecare devices in this small country is not that patients should have *access* to health care services, as was the case with the first developments in telemedicine in countries like Canada and the US (see Mort, May & Williams 2003). Cartwright (2000) gives a fascinating and critical analysis of the politics of telemedicine, where poor and vulnerable populations are used to test technologies for the army and space travel.
3. See Brown 2003 for the dynamics of hopes, hypes and their shadow sides.
4. See www.euractiv.com/en/health/doctors-unconvinced-ehealth-policy/article-170213, published 8 February 2008, last accessed 8 May 2008.
5. This term was introduced and developed by Akrich (1992) and Latour (1992).
6. All of these actors co-produce a particular care practice. For an analysis on what an actor is (featuring sheep as actors), see Law & Mol (2007). For more about the analysis of 'enacting good care', see Pols (2004).
7. This is a free translation of the French term 'interessement'; see e.g. Latour (1987) and Callon (1985). The term 'translation' is also used.
8. Dick Willems (1995) gives a beautiful analysis of how different types of drugs create different kinds of lungs.
9. The notion of 'enactment' was coined by Annemarie Mol and developed in Mol 2002. It signifies that the identity of objects may be learned from the way in which they are 'done' in relationships between activities, events, routines, things and talk in particular practices.
10. Thanks to Dick Willems for pointing this out to me.
11. There are different, more complex styles of answering where patients consider the effect of their answers on the activities of the nurse.
12. I have chosen not to use 'living *with* a disease' in order to stress that diseases do not precede practices and activities, but are in fact shaped by them.
13. Patients only talked to fellow patients over the webcam when they had established a friendly relationship before; they did not want to make webcam contact with 'strangers' (see Pols, 2010).
14. For examples of the multitude of these studies, see the *Journal of Telemedicine and E-health*. Eminovic et al. (2007) complain about the complexity of this kind of research and the haphazard way in which these studies are usually designed.
15. Moreover, it is a public secret that although devices may make it during the project phase, they tend to fall apart when the research infrastructure is gone. This is pointed out by Langstrup-Nielsen (2005) and Finch et al. (2003).
16. See also Nicolini (2006), who gives an account of the difficulties of matching telecare with actual work processes. Lehoux et al. (2002) describe the types of knowledge seen as favourable to telemedicine, and May et al. (2001) describe where professionals' constructs about the nature and practice of therapeutic relationships come into conflict with the use of telecare technologies.

References

Akrich, M. (1992) The De-Scription of technical objects. In: W.E. Bijker & J. Law, Shaping technology/ building society. Studies in sociotechnical change. Cambridge (MS), London (GB): The MIT Press, p. 205-224.

Brown, N. (2003). Hope against hype – accountability in biopasts, presents and futures. Science Studies, 16(2), 3-21.

Callon, M. (1985) Some elements of a sociology of translation: domestication of the scallops and the fishermen of St. Brieu Bay, In Law, J. (ed) Power, Action and Belief. Sociological Review Monograph. London: Routledge and Kegan Paul.

Cartwright, L. 2000. Reach out and heal someone: telemedicine and the globalization of health care. Health 4 (3): 347-77.

Eminovic, N., De Keizer, N.F., Bindels, P.J.E. & Hasman, A. (2007) Maturity of teledermatology evaluation research: a systematic literature review. British Journal of Dermatology, 156, 412-9.

Finch, T., May, C., Mair, F., Mort, M. & Gask, L. (2003) Integrating service development with evaluation in telehealthcare: an ethnographic study. British Medical Journal, 327, 1205-9.

Langstrup-Nielsen, H.L. (2005): Linking Healthcare – An inquiry into the changing performances of web-based technology for asthma monitoring. PhD. thesis, Copenhagen Business School.

Latour, B. (1983) 'Give me a laboratory and I will raise the world.' in: Knorr-Cetina, K. & Mulkay, M. (eds) Science observed. Perspectives on the social studies of Science. London, Sage: 141-170.

Latour, B. (1987) The Pasteurization of French Society. Cambridge MA: MIT Press.

Law J. & Mol A. (2007). The Actor-Enacted: Cumbrian Sheep in 2001. *Material Agency: Towards a Non-Anthropocentric Approach*. L. Malafouris and C. Knappett. New York, Springer.

Lehoux, P. Sicotte, C. Denis, J.L., Berg, M. & Lacroix, A. (2002) The theory of use behind telemedicine: how compatible with physicians' clinical routines? Social Science & Medicine, 54, 889-904.

May, C., Gask, L., Atkinson, T., Ellis, N., Mair, F. & Esmail, A. (2001) Resisting and promoting new technologies in clinical practice: the case of telepsychiatry. Social Science and Medicine, 52, 12, pp. 1889-1901(13).

Mol, A. (2002) The body multiple. An ontology of medical practice. Durham: Duke University Press.

Mort M, May C & Williams T. (2003). Remote doctors and absent patients: Acting at a distance in telemedicine? Science, Technology and Human Values, 28(2), pp. 274-295.

Nicolini, D. (2006) The work to make telemedicine work: a social and articulative view. Social Science & Medicine, 62, 2754-67.

Pols, J. (2004) 'Good care. Enacting a complex ideal in long-term psychiatry.' Utrecht: Trimbos-reeks, 2004. *http://www.trimbos.nl/default211.html?productId=575&back=1*

Pols, J. & Moser, I. (2009) Cold technologies versus warm care? On affective andsocial relations with and through care technologies, ALTER, European Journal of Disability Research 3 159-178.

Pols, J. (2009) The heart of the matter. About good nursing and telecare. Health Care Analysis, DOI 10.1007/s 10728-009-0140-1.

Pols, J. (2010b) Wonderful webcams About active gazes and invisible technologies. Science Technology & Human Values, forthcoming.

Willems, D. (1995) Tools of Care? Explorations into the Semiotics of Medical Technology. PhD thesis Maastricht.

Willems, D. (2004) Geavanceerde thuiszorgtechnologie: morele vragen bij een ethisch ideaal. Den Haag: Gezondheidsraad. Publicatienummer 2004/12/4. In: Signalering Ethiek en Gezondheid 2004. Gezondheidsraad. Publicatienummer 2004/12.

When patients care (too much) for information

Brit Ross Winthereik & Henriette Langstrup

Introduction

A particular, almost ritual, kind of problematisation has in recent years been used to introduce scientific papers, political discussions and policy documents addressing the application of information technology (IT) in health care. This introduction addresses the ever-increasing demand for care made by an ageing population, a growing number of persons with chronic diseases and patients who wish to be treated like consumers. Quality care and the money required to provide it are scarce resources in these accounts, and the challenge for Western health care systems is thus to find ways of preventing, meeting, curtailing or transforming demands for care. Within this context, IT-systems are mobilised that target patients as self-caring agents. IT-mediated self-care is often promoted as initiatives that simultaneously empower patients and free resources with which professionals can provide more and better care for groups of patients, who are unable to care for themselves. According to this rationale, if a group of relatively well-functioning patients can receive care through (access to) information and tools, more resources can be spent on more frequent encounters between health care professionals and so-called 'weak' patients.

The following chapter questions this assumption through analysing the pilot test of an online maternity record programme meant to prove the potential of a 'web portal', i.e. an Internet-based service for information sharing among patients and professionals in Denmark. It is a story about how the organisation behind the service, Sundhed.dk, sought to 'activate' pregnant women as patients and about how Sundhed.dk got both more and less than it had hoped for. On the one hand, they got less, since they did not succeed in making their targeted group of 'patients' active in the manner they had hoped, as only a few of the women involved in the project were using the on-line record on a regular basis. On the other hand, they also got more, as some of the few women using the record became active in ways that exceeded what had been imagined. These women did more than just keep themselves updated on information in their record; they also took responsibility for ensuring that the health care professionals used the internet service 'correctly'. This involved making active reviews of the health care professionals' record notes. In relation to the overall theme of this anthology, this chapter shows how the pilot project and the availability of the online record reconfigured relations between pregnant women and health care professionals in a way that was likely to change the meaning of care, but unlikely to free resources that could be delegated elsewhere in the system.

In the following we will show how the pregnant women in the pilot test started to care for information-sharing and for the care provider. This was a consequence of the specific framing introduced by the pilot project. Out of this attempt to frame the participants and their relations, as well as the socio-materially embedded responses from the involved professionals to this framing, an active, responsible, self-caring patient emerged. However, the woman that emerged did not much resemble the active patient inscribed into the visions of the online record. She was not active in the sense that she sat in front of her computer at home, using the information made available to her online to care for herself and thereby limiting the strain on the professionals' resources. Rather, the emerging 'patient' insisted on a specific kind of face-to-face interaction with health care professionals that involved discussing the content of the record. This was a kind of care, or *care for the care provider* that differed from the ideas of a patient performing *self-care* by directly engaging with IT-tools.

We use the notions of framing and overflow developed by Michel Callon and colleagues (Callon 1998, Callon *et al.* 2002) to describe how the configuration of IT-system, care setting and pregnant women together created a position for the woman from which she could monitor the professionals' behaviour. Framing, as described by Callon, is the act of disentangling entities from the networks in which they exist in order to treat them as bounded and separable from other entities, at least temporarily (Callon, 1998 Callon *et al.*, 2002). Frames should be thought of as sociotechnical constructs – or temporarily stabilised networks – that encompass discursive, human and material/technical entities. Because they are able to make the actors' entanglements with other networks invisible, such frames can generate certain paths or sociotechnical lock-ins, which progressively privilege some options while neglecting and progressively hindering others (Callon & Rabeharisoa, 2008). However, such framing is always incomplete in that the entities pushed into the bounded frame of the project do not necessarily conform to the identities ascribed to them. In addition, as the entities within the frame form a new network, new identities come into being and overflows are produced. This calls for new framings (Callon *et al.*, 2002).

The situation in which the pregnant women began to monitor the health care professionals is something that overflowed the frame that was initially set around the project.[1] Overflow, if connected too tightly with the visual image of a cup overflowing the boundaries of its china sides, may be misleading in that it suggests that what flows over was inside the cup from the start. In contrast, in our study an unexpected transformation happened as the pregnant woman emerged as active and responsible *during the clinical encounter*. That the woman would be active this way in this place was not part of the project's framing of the patient. Indeed, Sundhed.dk had imagined that the responsible patient would be a positive outcome of the project. But rather than being enacted in the clinical encounter, it expected that this would take place in the home of the pregnant women. A specific way of being active and responsible thus overflowed the frame of the project.

Shared care as a common frame

In 2004 a pilot project – the maternity care project – was initiated to test the ability of web technology to improve the communication among health care professionals internally and between health care professionals and patients. The pilot project was an initiative by Sundhed.dk, the organization responsible for the web service www.sundhed.dk, financially supported by major actors in the Danish health care scene. 'Sundhed' means health in Danish and one of the reasons to build and launch this web service, was to grant all citizens, whether patients or not, easier access to information about the health care system. The web page, which both patients and health care professionals can log onto, contains encyclopedic information, information about hospital waiting times, information about health-related services offered in Danish regions, a list of all the medications that has been issued to patients by pharmacies over the past five years, etc. Despite its obvious success as a web-based source of health information – the web service has won a number of national and international awards for its design and technical functionality – www.sundhed.dk is routinely used neither by health care professionals nor by patients. Thus, the organization behind the web service has not succeeded in turning the portal into a communication tool for health care professionals and patients, which was part of its commission. This poses a problem to the organization Sundhed.dk and its external partners as the overall goal for the portal was to be the shared platform that linked – and thus activated, but in a new way – all relevant actors involved in a care trajectory.

One of the very first things that happened in the attempt to build IT-support for maternity care was that Sundhed.dk started to look for an IT-vendor. The vendor was to design an IT-solution that would enable web-based communication about individual pregnant women among midwives, GPs, hospitals and the woman in question. Various IT-companies bid on how to build such a solution, and in the end a company was found. In their description of the new system, the company specified that they wanted to design a *'shared care solution'* (unpublished project description) that would enable care to be shared seamlessly across various boundaries; for example, among health care organizations and among health care professionals and patients.

The company pointed to diabetes and maternity care as offering good 'cases' for a testing of their design. In collaboration with Sundhed.dk, maternity care was selected as the case for a pilot test of Sundhed.dk's ability to work as a technology connecting diverse, distributed actors in health care.[2] The project participants at Sundhed.dk as well as the local midwives and doctors in the region where the new design – an online record for maternity care – was to be tested found it easy to relate to the conceptualisation of support of maternity care as essentially being a matter of establishing shared care. The participants also agreed that reorganising care delivery along the lines of shared care would ultimately benefit maternity care. However, a common definition of *what* shared care implied and subsequently *how* pregnant women would benefit was never made explicit.

Shared care was the trademark for the project. The notion thus produced a particular frame that kept together a number of disparate and distributed entities. We use the notions of frame and overflows to show that what constitutes 'the patient', 'the health care professional', 'pregnancy' or 'care' are, is not given. Because these identities are transformed as the relations among them are mediated in new ways, a project like the one analysed below generates a number of overflows, some of which change the foundation of the project. Before we go into detail about the overflows and their consequences, we would like to show in what way shared care formed a successful framing of the project.

In the vendor's initial description of the IT-design, the company used a famous definition of shared care introduced by Pritchard and

Hughes (1995) in which care is shared between organisations. A distinction is made between organisations located in the primary care sector and in the secondary sector. The patient is largely absent, or at least in a receiving role.

> Shared care applies when the responsibility for the healthcare of the patient is shared between individuals or teams, who are part of separate organisations, or where substantial organisational boundaries exist (Pritchard & Hughes 1995: 8).

In the definition that could later be found on the vendor's website, shared care refers to the sharing of information. No health care organisations are mentioned; instead, individual health care professionals and patients are the actors that are imagined to share. They do not share responsibility for care, but for information. A much more active role is thus ascribed to the patient than in the above definition. This second definition reads:

> The shared care concept covers IT solutions that make it possible to gather and exchange relevant information among health care professionals involved in the treatment of a patient in order to create continuity of care (...) At the same time, the IT solutions create a possibility for well-functioning chronic patients to actively participate in their own treatment. This can happen through information, self-monitoring, mobile solutions and online consultations. The participation has a preventive effect and may provide more freedom and better quality of life for the patient (www.acure.dk – authors' translation).

According to this definition, shared care applies when patients use IT-tools to monitor themselves and exchange information with health care professionals. Shared care here is defined as a means to freedom for patients through access to information; it means that the responsibility for care is partly in the patient's own hands and thus makes him or her free (to act, choose, and remain independent from paternalistic health care providers). A former Sundhed.dk project manager in his definition of shared care qualifies the meaning of freedom as a question of having access to electronic data about oneself.

> To me, shared care means that one starts with the patient and the relevant indications, i.e. data. That one always has access to the most recent and up-to-date data. And then it is about making a patient active in relation to his/her own case. Supporting the treatment by letting the patient play an active role (Interview with former project manager, 4/10 2004).

In the project manager's and in the vendor's second definition of shared care, the patient plays an active role. Freedom and agency are closely connected. But like the project manager says: *'it is about making a patient active'*. Thus, the patient is not active already, but can be *made* so. And having access to data through an online IT-system facilitates this articulation of the patient. Being active and free, thus, does not refer to making autonomous decisions about how to handle one's own care. Rather, it refers to the freedom established within the shared care frame. It refers to the possibility of accessing electronic and standardised data, i.e. knowing oneself as a medical case.

Charis Cussins (1998), Dick Willems (2000) and Annemarie Mol (2000) have all demonstrated how patients are made into agents through the use of medical technology. Presented with specific tasks and tools for diagnosis or self-monitoring, infertile couples in Cussins' case, people with asthma in Willems's case and people with diabetes in Mol's case are delegated knowledge and competences traditionally associated with the doctor. The analyses all show that this imagined autonomy has certain costs. For example, Mol shows how a device for blood sugar measurement that measures at specific points in time requires the patient to act like a health care professional. This, she argues, implies that the imagined freedom may better be understood more modestly as a question of particular liberties gained.

In our case, the online record system was hoped to be able to delegate new competences to pregnant women. It was thus the online system – rather than the doctor or the midwife – that was supposed to turn the pregnant woman into an agent. And perhaps for this reason, different health care professionals expressed an interest in the system that they imagined would do the work of 'activating' pregnant women in a way that saved them work.[3] A GP, for example, explained how he hoped that the system would stimulate the women to fill in information about previous births onto the record prior to the clinical encounter (interview with GP 27/10 2005). Another GP explained how, when she first heard about the project, thought that 'this shared care concept' would be very hard to put into practice. 'But then I discovered that it was simply about information exchange', she said, and explained that this made it somewhat easier to deal with for her (interview with GP 27/10 2005). The notoriously busy GPs were particularly intrigued by a system that could be used to delegate work to patients. But the midwives also saw potential in the system, given it kept 'strong' pregnant women at home, thus freeing time for the women with complicated pregnancies.

Among the health care professionals, information sharing became the framed stage onto which the project participants all agreed to stand. They agreed that shared care – seen as a matter of IT-mediated information sharing – was a good idea. As such the concept was a powerful tool for connecting the different stakeholders of the project. The stakeholders were also tied together by a shared normative understanding of who would benefit from this project. All agreed that one of the reasons why shared care was appealing was that it would be putting the woman at the centre of the care process. But when the woman was actually put in this position, a different version of the active patient was enacted. This patient turned out to be a means to more than one end, as we will show below.

To sum up, the project participants all joined forces to make www.sundhed.dk the vehicle for shared care, and part of this endeavour was to put the information-managing patient at the center of attention. There was no discussion about what shared care should mean, nor how it would affect pregnant women in different ways. This, however, turned out not to be a problem, it became one of the things that helped the project to progress. One of the reasons why the diversity among midwives, GPs, hospital staff, and pregnant women was not considered a problem was that everybody agreed that *real* shared care was not about care, but about information sharing.

The framing of pregnancy as a chronic illness

In the definitions of shared care used by the vendor and the project manager, the possibility of accessing information created active and responsible patients. Information thus served as a tool to enable health care professionals to empower pregnant women and pregnant women to empower themselves. Sundhed.dk thus wanted to make information about the maternity care trajectory readily available and turn pregnant women into agents this way. But why was the pregnant woman deemed a good place to start when building this future of shared care? For one, the pregnant woman was already seen as more of an agent than a patient in relation to constructing a trajectory through the health care system. Pregnant women were *already* (made) active and responsible.

Three examples of this: First, the pregnant woman was responsible for carrying a client-held record, which was used for information exchange among GPs, hospital, midwife and social authorities *prior* to the introduction of the online record. The woman was involved as an active participant in the process of information exchange; she existed as a holder of information related to her own case. Second, the woman was (and is) made responsible for the pregnancy through risk communication in the public sphere. For example, public poster campaigns with phrases like 'give your child the best start' suggest to pregnant women that they must not drink alcohol or that they must eat folic acid. Pregnant women also receive individual information on risk behaviour at consultations with health professionals. Deciding whether to smoke or not or whether to exercise or not inscribes her as somebody making active choices in relation to her pregnancy. Third, deciding what risk assessments, e.g. ultra sound screening, to choose (or not choosing an assessment at all), also inscribes her as an agent who makes active choices on behalf of her future child.[4] The pregnant woman as an image of a 'good patient' in terms of the pilot project relates to the way in which she takes care of her body. Not just for her own good, but as a delegate for the patient within the body, for the foetus. The pregnant woman was a good patient to test the technology precisely because she was not ill, but an active manager of risks.

In every research project the project-owners hope for success and this hope is often indirectly expressed in the inclusion and exclusion criteria that define and delimit the test group, e.g. by excluding 'complicated' research subjects (Epstein, 2007, p. 65) or by making sure the patient population fits the requirements of the tool (Berg, 1995, p. 87-88). Thought of in terms of framing, the continuous success of the framing depends on expanding the numbers of actors entering the frame, while limiting the possibilities of negative overflows or externalities that might come with the inclusion of such new actors. This explains why it is pertinent to choose a test group whose members resemble that which one seeks to create. It also explains why not all kinds of pregnant women, but only women with 'uncomplicated' pregnancies were part of the 100 pregnant women that made up the test group. 'Complicated' pregnancies might have allowed other and more difficult entities into the frame (other professional groups, other social services, other kinds of medication and treatment regimes), making it harder to achieve a successful framing of the project from the beginning. Clearly, for Sundhed.dk it was important that the project would work as a 'good example' so that it could form the basis for similar projects. The pregnant woman was a particularly good representative of the active and responsible patient who, all the stakeholders agreed, would be a precondition for realising shared care. They even agreed upon the term chronic disease management to describe the kind of practice the IT-system would be part of. They thus compared pregnant women's behaviour to that of chronic patients' behaviour, but in a highly specific version (i.e. active, responsible, well-functioning, proactive etc.). It was not an elderly chronic patient with constant pain and a complicated set of illnesses.

When pregnant women are compared to 'well-functioning' patients with chronic illnesses, the similarities between the two groups are emphasized. Pregnant women are turned into persons resembling (chronic) patients in certain aspects. In this framing both have a condition that to a large extent structures their lives. Both have many encounters with the health care system and both can and *should* be approached through various forms of measurement. Thus a certain aspect of the pregnancy is focused on: the condition that can be managed, measured, controlled, monitored, documented etc. Pregnancy becomes a medical case concerned with the management of health risks. But through this comparison, the person with a chronic illness is also portrayed in a particular way. Here, as in many other places and situations where the demand for care as a resource is sought to be managed more effectively, people with a chronic illness are being performed as responsible and active in their contact with the health care system. The overall effect is that both pregnant women and people with a chronic illness are seen as persons who benefit from relating to their condition as managers of risks and for whom the central device for doing so is information.

Challenging the frame

We will now turn to what happened when the system was implemented and met daily practice. The project participants – employees at Sundhed.dk, local project managers, doctors, midwives – needed to learn how to practice maternity care through this system. To be able to do so, they had to have pregnant women use the system as well. Thus, the pregnant women had to learn how to use the online maternity record in *their* daily practice. Both of these demands produced overflows.

The online record, which was supposed to provide support for shared maternity care, was a virtual transcript of two paper-based records previously used in maternity care. The record could be accessed by health care professionals involved in the care for a particular pregnant woman, as well as by the pregnant woman herself from home. Different health care professionals in maternity care usually use different kinds of documentation tools, and a client-held record usually serves as the main coordination mechanism among health care professionals located in different physical and organisational settings. The new record worked in a very different way, as all the health care professionals now had to write in the same (online) record without any use of paper-based records, including the client-held record. When the health care professionals realised that this new record-keeping system demanded that they structure information about pregnant women to a higher degree that previously and that they would need to change their work routines (i.e. not use paper records during consultations and read all entries in the online record to get an overview), as well as store patient information at a server located at the Sundhed.dk main office, they tried to negotiate the framing of the project. This was done in order to maintain a practice based on specialisation, in which each specialty provides care according to a certain expertise and knowledge regime and only subsequently informs other professionals about relevant issues and changes in relation to the pregnant woman's condition.[5]

Their negotiation began with a discussion about a button for printing the record. The designers of the system had reasoned that, since this was an online record, it would not be necessary to print the full record. Thus, to save money they did not include this function. After a period of discussion, the health care professionals and the local project manager both advocated the ability to print the entire record. As mentioned, one of the ambitions of the online record was that information about pregnant women produced in different locations would be structured in similar ways. Printing would create a number of local copies of the record; which one would then be considered the original? But the health care professionals, who argued that they could not use the record without a print option, negotiated this aim. If they had 'their own' prints, they could keep a selective overview of their particular interventions and of information relating to their area of expertise, thus also having "their own" version of the patient. The conclusion was that Sundhed.dk requested the designers add a print-button.

The resistance that the professionals expressed through their wish to maintain previously existing socio-materially embedded work practices can be seen as resistance to comply with the singular patient inscribed in the online record. It produced an overflow of the frame set around the project. The addition of the print-button worked to maintain stability by containing this particular overflow and reframe the project. Now the health care professionals could use the record as an online tool, as a paper record, or as both. And so they did. But because handwritten notes were often made on prints of the online record, the electronic record made it harder for the health care professionals to find the information they needed during clinical consultations with pregnant women. Did this mean that the online record prevented health care professionals from keeping a record complete with information? Yes and no. On the one hand, paper scattered the record and electronic sources were far from complete. On the other hand, to the health care professionals a complete record meant a record that contained *relevant* information (and this varied). Completeness to them was thus not a universal feature of a record. Instead what mattered was that the record could support the establishment of completeness, meaning that the record would allow a health care professional to trace the author of a piece of information and request new information when needed.

Pregnant women care for information

During the project the participating women developed an interest in 'a complete record' quite similar to the version of a complete record that the IT-designers had. When a woman discovered that a piece of information that, from her point of view, would make the record complete was missing, she would make sure that the doctor or midwife added this information. Interestingly, in some of the cases this happened at a time when the women experienced complications in the pregnancy and thus no longer fulfilled the inclusion criteria of the experiment (which was only for women with uncomplicated pregnancies). Few of the pregnant women demonstrated interest in reading their record at home. One of them said: 'If all is well with the baby, I see no reason to access their record from home' (Interview with pregnant woman 31/5 2006). By referring to 'their record', this woman suggested that the record was not hers, but belonged to the health care professionals.

Two of the women who were followed as part of our research experienced complications during their pregnancies. One had premature contractions, was hospitalised and later had to keep to bed for three weeks. The other developed a metabolic disease and had to be closely monitored during the last trimester of the pregnancy. As they experienced complications, they also experienced an increased need to communicate with health care professionals to communicate about the pregnancy. These two women – we will call them Sandra and Louise – began taking an interest in their records and started wondering why information was missing from the record that they could access from home. They also started wondering whether the health care professionals would at all be able to provide proper care during the birth when information was scattered around in so many different locations and media. That information is located in different settings is, of course, not a new situation. Before the online record was introduced, doctors, midwives and others involved in the care, would keep information stored in their own records, and would use the client-held record for communicative purposes only. The newness of the situation is that the partial nature of the information used by health care professional and the processes through which the information is gathered and managed was made visible to the pregnant women.

The introduction of the online record thus, for some women, created the need for accessible and complete information, and they now started considering the implications of giving birth assisted by somebody that they had never met before, and who did not have access to a complete set of information. How documentation is organised and the means by which information is shared is something that is usually not given much attention by pregnant women. But through the online record and the possibility of access, the pregnant women experienced this as very important. The notion that good care was based on the availability of complete information, as framed by the project, became a matter of urgency to them. Whereas it was assumed that shared care would only be realisable with the pregnant women as an active manager of electronic information, it turned out that the record's lack of performance as a tool for information sharing *among the health care professionals* was what activated the women. They were, however, not activated in the sense that they became active managers of information as hoped for in the project's frame. Instead they began monitoring the health care professionals' production and use of information. Their agency was thus linked to what the women saw as the health care professionals' lack of care for obtaining complete information in the way they imagined would be possible through use of an online record. This is interesting, as it is precisely because the health care professional cared for (relevant) information that he/she did not use the online record extensively. Since the online record did not allow for information to have a clear sender and receiver to the same extent as a client-held record, sharing work around the pregnant woman became harder as the online record was the only tool for documentation. And for this reason, pregnant women and midwives began experiencing how pieces of information that could not easily be requested elsewhere was also missing in the online record.

In the following observation from a consultation with a midwife, Louise was activated by a situation in which she found information to be missing (she was backed up by the midwife, who entered the information on Louise's request):

> Louise, during a midwife consultation, tells that she was admitted to the hospital before Easter because she had contractions. She was told that the cervix has shortened and that she would give birth prematurely. She tells the midwife what medication they gave her. The midwife checks the online record. There is no account in the record about her admission to hospital.
>
> Louise expresses a deep dissatisfaction with the lack of information in the record. Later in the consultation the midwife asks Louise to repeat what happened at the hospital. Louise mentions the date for hospital admittance and the name of the medication and the midwife types all this information into the record (observation midwife consultation, June 2006).

This observation shows how Louise became engaged in disciplining the midwife in her desire to turn the record into a complete representation of her case. Disciplining was, to begin with, delegated to the technology (among other things through the absence of the possibility of printing the full record), but when health care professionals began using prints, and when the modes of communication among health care professionals became increasingly opaque, other disciplining practices emerged. Thus, Louise took upon her the responsibility of reviewing the record's content during the encounter with the midwife.

Prior to implementation, the online record was imagined to work as a device that would turn pregnant women into agents through the possibility of accessing information online from home. It was not part of the framing that a transformation of the health care professionals' practices would occur. But as the online tool was implemented without the option that pregnant women could write in the record themselves, it changed the dynamics of the consultation. Whereas it was imagined that the women would increasingly do administrative work for the doctors and midwives, it was the doctors and midwives who now filled in information on request.

Consequently, the notion of care changed its meaning as different expectations and practices unfolded. When Louise discovered that the online record was not used by midwives, nurses and doctors to share all information, she interpreted this as a matter of non-sharing and of non-caring. Through the project, a substantial difference between what the pregnant women and the health care professionals saw as a complete record developed. This fed into a substantial difference between Louise's understanding of care and the understanding implied in the framing of the project. When she discovered that the health care professionals did not share *all* information it made her wonder: 'If they don't share, how do I know they care?' The framing of the project implied that *she* would care better for *herself* by reading information that had been entered by health care professionals. Yet, it had not at all been imagined by Sundhed.dk that the pregnant women would engage in monitoring who shared what, when and why.

This version of the active patient provided another illustration of overflow. And like the first, this overflow was contained by another reframing. An example of this is provided in the following field note.

> *The obstetrician browses through prints of the online record, which is all she has as there is no computer in her office.*
>
> *Obstetrician*: When I glance through the record [she lifts up the prints of the online record] it seems difficult to get an overview of your case. The only thing written here is that someone has seen you in December.
>
> *Sandra* [pregnant]: I don't have anything with me about my visits here either.
>
> [I, the observer, ask what the obstetrician is looking for and she answers that she is looking for a short statement of why Sandra must be monitored so closely as well as the results of the examinations she has already gone through].
>
> *Sandra*: I don't have anything on that in the papers [printouts] that I have here.
>
> *Obstetrician*: It is not recorded in ESTERIA [database where ultrasound scans are stored] why you are being followed. It is frustrating that I cannot see that it is the fourth time you are here. [She browses through all the printouts in front of her once more]. When were you here the last time?
>
> *Sandra*: The 28th of March.

> *Obstetrician*: I don't have anything on that. Have you got a print? [Sandra shows her a printout that she got when she was scanned the last time].
>
> *Obstetrician*: It is not good that your midwife does not know what we are doing out here.
>
> She takes one of the paper records that were previously used in the maternity care and fills in the results from all the scans. She asks the woman to hand the paper record to her midwife and says, full of regret: 'It is not fair that you are the one who must remember all this'. *Observation outpatient clinic, April 2006).*

At this meeting, some obvious gaps in communication between hospital and midwife were made visible, or rather, produced. Communication among obstetricians is apparently not made easier by the possibility of using an online record. The notes exemplify how the woman became part the solution to the problem of missing information. She took upon her the responsibility for ensuring completeness, while the obstetrician produced a way of containing the destabilisation of the frame by filling in one of the paper forms that are usually used in maternity care (the client-held record). She then asked Sandra to give the information to her midwife. This course of action resembles an almost complete return to former practice, where pregnant women were responsible for carrying information back and forth among health care providers. The difference is that this time the client-held record is mobilised, *not* as a means for communication where entries have a clear sender and in some cases also a well-defined recipient. Instead, the client-held record was introduced as a means for adding information to the online record in the hope that this information would complete it.

While the two pregnant women challenged the version of the patient as someone who is able to perform self-care through access to an online health record, they supported the assumption that the presence of complete information is crucial for good care to be given. What is at stake here is a tension between different versions of what role information plays for good care. We are not arguing that health care professionals do not care for information; they need information, too, but they resist working with a record that forces them to carefully read through each and every entry made by other health care professionals. Their view on the role of information in relation to care thus differs from the belief that it is possible to design a record that contains complete information.

Conclusion

In this paper we have traced some transformations in how care is understood and enacted in a health care system that is undergoing major changes. The scarcity of resources is a main concern in the Danish health care system. From this follows an occupation with how to limit access to health care resources by particular groups, especially those labelled as strong patients. We have analysed how it was hoped that an online maternity record would create a platform for information sharing among health care professionals and pregnant women, leading to less need for costly encounters. The online record was seen as a tool that would support the strong, while those labelled as weak would then ideally be able to see professionals more frequently. We have shown how the project was framed as an attempt to activate well-functioning patients to engage in a specific kind of IT-mediated self-care. The project failed in this regard, but succeeded in turning pregnant women into active patients, even though this version of an active patient was somewhat different than the one imagined by the project makers.

What characterises this version of an active patient? At first glance, the active patient emerging resembled the one imagined by Sundhed.dk, in that she wished for complete and electronically available information. But this patient differs in that she engaged in monitoring what the health care professionals wrote in her record. In contrast to the women's wish to view (and supplement) what was written about them was the health care professionals' view on the role of information in relation to care. For the health care professionals, caring was possible without access to a patient's information from one single information source. Not that they thought information is superfluous for good care; but to them information was only relevant if it had a context; for example in the format of a clear sender. To them, overly standardised or context-free information blocked good care. There is a tension between these two versions of a complete record and in their view on the role of information for good care.

Sundhed.dk did not detect the difference between the image of an active patient inscribed into the system and the various images held by project participants. *Shared care* as a multiple and dynamic object thus never made its way into the Sundhed.dk organisation. Instead, the framing that shared care was *good* was kept intact while other stories were mobilised in the project to explain (away) the online record's failure to perform. These included the lack of technical infrastructure at the hospital, GPs' and obstetricians' unwillingness to collaborate, the trouble for the pregnant women to ensure the right level of data security on their personal computer, etc. Our research group also failed to destabilise the frame despite attempts to make Sundhed.dk focus on unintended effects produced by the pilot project. Our evaluation of the pilot project focused on the lack of good project management (e.g. the failure to establish a shared expectation about whether the health care professionals would continue using the online record in their work after the pilot, or whether the end of the pilot was also the end of working with the record). We have tried to make up for this lack in later work, like the present analysis (and Winthereik 2008), but these analyses appear in journals that are unlikely to be read by Sundhed.dk employees and stakeholders. They also provide types of results that are hard to translate directly into implications applicable to IT-design or guidelines.

Where to go from here? Assuming that individuals in need of care can be made active only in certain ways and certain locations is problematic. Believing that it can be predicted how they will be activated is also problematic. When the pregnant women became controllers of the health care professionals' writing, they emerged as active patients who tried to influence what was written in the record. Rather than wanting to be kept updated through online access, they wanted to add information. They wanted to deliver, not just receive information. Our analysis has indicated that when pregnant women are activated this way, they start negotiating what good care is and how to get it. Introducing online access to health records from home, therefore, is not likely to keep the strong women out of the clinic and thus does not free resources for weaker ones. Reflecting on these experiences, what seems often to be missing in attempts to create health care systems that are patient-centred is the acknowledgement of the unexpected ways in which patients emerge. This happens in the encounters with devices made to activate them. Our analysis has shown how maternity care is shaped in collectives of health care professionals, project-makers, vendors, and IT-systems. Attending to how care for pregnant women is intertwined with their care for information sharing may extend our understanding of technologically mediated care practices. This, however, depends on our willingness to be surprised by and learn from the encounters these heterogeneous collectives produce.

Notes

1. Frame and overflow are notions developed in relation to a discussion of the behavior of economic markets and their externalities. Callon has used the terms in analyses of concerned social groups to describe the co-production of political engagement and scientific knowledge about congenial diseases (Callon and Rabeharisoa 2008).

2. Shared care is not a standard model for organising health care, as the concept is rather loosely defined and much variation exists in the way shared care has been used. The shared care concept has been used in the medical literature since at least the 1950s and tends to be a way of conceptually including the home situation in the care network. In the wake of the increased use of information technologies within health care, the notion has had a revival as a way of describing how health care should ideally be provided (see for example Branger, van't Hooft *et al.* 1999).

3. See Langstrup & Winthereik (2008) for a discussion of some of the difficulties and hard work involved in 'crafting' patients who can participate in a testing of an online self-monitoring tool for asthma patients.

4. For more reflection and discussion on the agency and autonomy of pregnant women, not least to new medical technologies, see e.g. Weir, 1996; Rapp, 1995; Cussins, 1998; or Akrich & Pasveer, 2004.

5. The experience of a situationally bound practice that differs across settings but is successfully coordinated by various means corresponds to the description made by Annemarie Mol (2002) in her analysis of how atherosclerosis is 'done' differently in different settings (the clinic, the laboratory), while simultaneously the different 'versions' of atherosclerosis are coordinated across sites.

References

Berg, Marc (1997) *Rationalizing Medical Work. Decision-Support Techniques and Medical Practice*. Cambridge: MIT Press.

Branger, Peter, A. van't Hooft, van der Wouden, J.C., Moorman P.W., van Bemmel, J.H. (1999). Shared care for diabetes: supporting communication between primary and secondary care, *International Journal of Medical Informatics* 53 (2-3), pp. 133-142.

Callon, Michel (1998) An essay on framing and overflowing: Economic externalities-revisited by sociology. In Callon, M. (ed.): *The laws of the markets*. Oxford and Keele: Blackwell and the Sociological Review.

Callon, Michel, C. Méadel & V. Rabeharisoa (2002) The economy of qualities. *Economy and Society* 31 (2): 194–217.

Callon, Michel & V. Rabeharisoa (2008) The Growing Engagement of Emergent Concerned Groups in Political and Economic Life: Lessons from the French Association of Neuromuscular Disease Patients, *Science, Technology and Human Values* 33 (2), pp. 230-261.

Cussins, Charis (1998) 'Ontological Coreography. Agency for women in an infertility clinic.' In Berg, M., Mol, A., eds. *Differences in Medicine*. Durham: Duke University Press.

Epstein, Steven (2007) *Inclusion. The Politics of Difference in Medical Research*. Chicago: The University of Chicago Press.

Langstrup, Henriette & Brit Ross Winthereik (2008) 'The Making of Self-Monitoring Asthma Patients: Mending a Split Reality with Comparative Ethnography', *Comparative Sociology* 7, pp. 362–386.

Mol, Annemarie (2000) What Diagnostic Devices Do: The Case of Blood Sugar Measurement. *Theoretical Medicine and Bioethics* 21, pp. 9-22.

Mol, Annemarie (2002) *The body multiple: Ontology in medical practice*. Durham, Duke University Press.

Pasveer, Bernike & Madeleine Akrich (2001) 'Obstetrical trajectories: On training women/bodies for (home) birth', in: R. Devries, C. Benoit, E. R. van Teijlingen, and S. Wrede (eds.) *Birth by Design: Pregnancy, Maternity Care, and Midwifery in North America and Europe*. New York, Routledge, pp. 229-42.

Pritchard, Peter & Hughes, Jane (1995) *Shared care: The future imperative?* London: Royal Society of Medicine Press.

Rapp, Rayna (1995) 'Real Time Fetus: The Role of the Sonogram in the Age of Monitored Reproduction.' In *Cyborgs and Citadels*, ed. by G. Domit, and S. Traweek. Seattle: University of Washington Press.

Weir, Lorna (1996) 'Recent development in the government of pregnancy.' *Economy and Society* 25, pp. 372-392.

Willems, Dick (2000) 'Managing one's body using self-management techniques: Practicing autonomy.' *Theoretical medicine and Bioetics* 21, pp. 23-38.

Winthereik, B R. Shared Care and Boundaries: Lessons From an Online Maternity Record. *Journal of Health Organization and Management* 22 (4), pp. 416-427.

Care and its values
Good food in the nursing home

Annemarie Mol

It is five past nine when I arrive at nursing home Y, a home for people with dementia who, for one reason or another, need institutional care. The door can easily be opened from the outside, but from the inside only with a few clever tricks. I address a woman who is cleaning the floor, and she points me to ward Blue. There I find the small serving kitchen where Jessy, the food assistant of the day, is expecting me. She asks whether indeed I want to learn more about eating and drinking in the nursing home, as she has been told. As I confirm this, she starts to teach me. Just now, she explains, the last few people are having breakfast. Earlier, the table was set. There were plates and cutlery. There were slices of white and brown bread, ham, cheese and liver paste, chocolate sprinkles, peanut butter, coloured sugar sprinkles, jam and sugar. Bread with things savoury and things sweet: a typical Dutch breakfast. 'But some people are late. I've made their breakfast for them.' Jessy takes a plate out of the fridge. A plastic film covers two slices of light brown bread that have been spread with margarine. There is Gouda cheese on one and jam on the other. A sticker says 'Mrs. Tilstra'. 'You get to know people.' Jessy continues to explain, 'and this is what Mrs. Tilstra likes for breakfast'. She takes off the thin plastic film and carries the plate to the living room, to a frail woman who has just been wheeled to a table by the window. 'Good morning, Mrs. Tilstra, here's your breakfast. What would you like to drink with it? Can I get you some tea?' Mrs. Tilstra nods, tea, yes, that would be fine.

During the rest of that day I learned a lot more – just as I did in other places where I recently observed practices to do with eating and drinking. Two of these were houses where elderly people live individually or as a couple in their own room or apartment. In one of them, Riverview, I spent some time in the kitchen and some in the restaurant. In the other, that I call Highsight (as the view from its 12th floor was impressive), I followed Emma, the service assistant responsible for serving residents their food and for pouring them coffee, tea and juice. If this was needed she also helped people to move: from their room to a day time activity centre, the hairdresser, the in-house shop, the restaurant, or back again. At this point, I would like to thank all the residents in whose lives I peaked during those days of fieldwork. And even more, I would like to thank Jessy, Emma and the others (nurses, nurse assistants, food assistants, service assistants, restaurant helpers, cooks, kitchen personnel, trainees, volunteers) for being such good teachers. But what would it be to do so? Many of the residents no longer read or even speak. Some may be dead by now. And while the carers are sharp and articulate enough, they are unlikely to come across this text as it is in English, not in Dutch. I better be honest about it: rather than my informants, this text addresses distant audiences. Writing it, implies that I do not further immerse myself in the embodied presence of a care home. Instead, I draw events observed there out of their context to make them travel elsewhere. And yet writing is not just a way of moving away from daily care practices, but also one of taking (small parts of) these practices along to public settings. Articulating what care entails, or so I hope, might help to shift the simplified schemes that are currently used to govern it. While texts (in a foreign language at that) are alien to daily life on the ward or in the kitchen, they may still be a homage to care practices. And seek to strengthen these.

The practices that in this text I will write about have to do with a particular kind of care. *Nourishing care*. In nursing homes and care homes for the elderly a lot of energy is put into preparing, distributing and eating food. When and how might we say that the nourishing care that ensues is *good*? There is no quick and easy answer. For as soon as one starts to look into it, various *goods*, in the plural, appear to be relevant to practices to do with food. Food may be nutritious, plenty, or tasty; a meal may be cosy or provide lots of choice; and then there are cleanliness, variation, short waiting times and what not to appreciate. The relations between such *goods* are strikingly complex. For even if they all have to do with food, the various relevant values tend to predicate different objects: food stuff, a dish, a meal, a kitchen, an atmosphere, and what not. And while values sometimes go together, on other occasions they clash – giving rise to ongoing tensions or a victory of one alternative over the other. Where, finally, to locate a value/evaluation: in the object of appreciation or in the appreciating subject? This is neither obvious nor a constant when it comes to appreciating food. Given all this complexity, it makes little sense to try to squeeze all the values to do with food into the one-dimensional scales of *quality assessments* or *accountability schemes*. The 'overall' quality of nourishing care does not depend on the addition of bits of good along a single scale, but on tinkering with *different goods* that map onto different dimensions. In what follows, I will try to unpack these rather condensed sentences. Seeking to elucidate care, I will tell you some stories to do with food and its values.

Nutritional value and cosiness

A first crucial value when it comes to food is its *nutritional value*. How many proteins, carbohydrates and fats are contained in the food that Mrs. Tilstra gets to eat on an average day? Does she absorb enough carbohydrates not to have to burn up her own body, enough vitamins and minerals to allow her to make new enzymes and to grow new skin? Attending to the nutritional value of food is important in institutional care for the elderly. All too often the residents of care institutions suffer from nutritional deficiencies. They lose weight and become weak; their resistance against infections diminishes; and they become more forgetful than they would be without, say, vitamin B12. To prevent nutritional deficiencies, then, it is important that the food that people get to eat contains the nutrients they need. Regular meals have to be nutrients-rich and varied. And as many elderly people in care institutions are not all that eager to eat, there are also additional products on the market that pack lots of nutrients into small quantities of food. Fortified yoghurts for instance, which, while tasting of banana, chocolate or strawberry, may hold as much as a fifth of a person's daily needs in a tiny bottle.

But nutritional value is not the only relevant good when it comes to providing nourishing care. Over the last decade many have insisted that not only the *substance*, food, deserves attention, but that the *practice*, eating, is at least as important. Meals are events. They are good events if they are *sociable* and *cosy*. From a text called *Ambiance scenario* I learn how (Dutch) cosiness may be configured. (The term used in Dutch is *gezellig*, a word that combines sociability and cosiness and famously cannot be translated in neighbouring languages. Even the German *gemütlich* doesn't quite do.) The *Ambiance scenario*, while concerned with as immaterial a value as 'cosy', insists on materialities. There should be a proper table cloth on the table, or (if this is asking too much) the paper place mats used should be nice and colourful, not dull and white. Rather than eating alone, it is better that people do so together. Putting serving dishes on every table is more homely and inviting than dishing up plates in the kitchen. During the meal, the room that is used to dine in should be quiet instead of buzzing with strangers walking around, in and out. There should be enough light. Maybe some easy listening music will cheer things up. Cosiness depends on ever so many elements of the dinner table and its surroundings.

Nutritional value and *cosiness* relate to different objects. The first is an attribute of a substance, food, the second of a practice, eating. Thus they do not fit on the same scale. And yet neither are they independent variables. In research settings there appeared to be a positive correlation between them: 'The results [of this research] indicate that creating a cosy, pleasant atmosphere during the meals in a nursing home, improves the nutrition related condition and the quality of life of the residents'.[1] If the ambiance of their meals is improved, the residents of nursing homes tend to eat more. And as they are often inclined not to eat enough, this implies that the nutritional value of the food they end up absorbing also improves.[2] Thus, even if they belong to different dimensions, in this case attending to one good (cosiness) is a way of serving the other good (nutritional value). It follows that feeding the residents of a nursing home ward with expensive fortified yoghurts is not the only way of improving their 'nutrition related condition'.[3] It is also possible to target the ambiance of the meals. The physicalities of the body, then, do not just underpin, or allow for, what people may do in daily life. The converse is also true: daily life practices, rather than just being more or less pleasant on their own terms, are also immediately relevant to people's physical condition. Eating bodies and the practices of eating make each other be.[4]

The *ambiance scenario* that I just quoted from, lays out suggestions for improving the practices around eating and drinking in care institutions for the elderly. These have been experimented with in a few exemplary wards and the scenario is meant to spread them out to other institutions. On ward Blue the *ambiance scenario* has been taken on board.[5] Serious efforts have been put into turning meals into pleasant experiences. There they are: the tables set for joint meals, the colourful place mats and the serving dishes that the scenario talks about. But alas. The *nutritional* value and the *cosiness* that fitted together so easily in the research setting, turn out to clash in daily life on ward Blue. The point is not that here, somehow, cosiness would fail to improve people's nutritional condition. The point is that cosiness entails more than (given the specificities of Blue) can be achieved. Ironically, this has to do with the need to attend to 'nutritional value' first. What is going on? According to the *ambiance scenario* cosiness demands that nurses, nurse assistants and volunteers sit with the people under their care at the dinner table. Nobody in Blue would disagree. 'You see that table, in the corner?' Tessa (one of the nurses) asks me, 'a while ago the ladies who sit there, were still able to talk amongst themselves. Now they no longer can. You can get them to talk alright. If one of us sits with them we can get them to talk. But in practice we rarely manage to do so'. This is because Tessa and the others spend most mealtimes at the tables of the people who need to be fed.

The ladies at the table in the corner would have enjoyed a conversation. Tessa might have talked with them about the plants on the window sill, the weather outdoors, or the activity they engaged in that morning with the physical therapist, whether or not they still remember it.[6] But such cosiness is not available to them. This is because they are physically capable of eating by themselves. It takes Mrs. Sanders some effort to hold her knife in one hand and her fork in the other, but she can do it. She cuts up her food attentively, shovels some onto her fork, and carries this up to her mouth. The other women at her table, with varying degrees of ease or awkwardness, do likewise. At the next table, by contrast, most people would starve if they were left alone with their plate. Take Mr. Hendriks. Half the time he even forgets that Lenneke is sitting next to him and she has to remind him that he is eating. 'Please, open your mouth now, Mr. Hendriks, I have another mouthful for you.' As chewing is difficult for Mr. Hendriks, his food is mashed. Lenneke gently touches his lips with the spoon. Then he opens his mouth, gulps up the food, and swallows.

That *nutritional value* takes precedence over *cosiness* here, does not imply that the care provided is bad. In any case, making judgements from the side line is not the task that I have set myself. Instead, I would like to understand how goods and the relations between them are handled in practices like ward Blue. And this much is obvious: in the particular circumstances of that ward there is an irreducible tension between the *cosiness* that would be good for some and the *nutritional value* needed by others. These goods just cannot both be served at the same time. It is not that the people working on the ward do not try hard. Just as the ambiance scenario suggests, some have had their own lunch before the residents and others will have it afterwards. When the residents eat, everyone on duty is available to help. In addition to paid personnel there is a daughter who feeds her mother and a volunteer who has taken Mrs. Stuiveling elsewhere. And yet there are not enough hands to go round. At the time that I visit, there happen to be so many residents who need to be fed, that those who are able to eat by themselves are left to their own devices. *Nutritional value* wins over *cosiness* since life depends on it.

Is this a general lesson, then, that when it comes to it the necessities of the physical body overrule anything else? Is *survival* always given priority over values to do with *daily life*? Not quite. If, in a few months from now, Mr. Hansen will keep his mouth shut when Lenneke touches his lips with a spoon, he will not be forced to eat. If he will turn his head away, his refusal to eat will be respected. Lenneke and her colleagues will try to reach out to him. They will experiment with soup, fruit, fortified yoghurts, what have you. 'A while ago we had this old man who only wanted pancakes', Jessy tells me, 'So we made him pancakes. Three times a day. There, you see, on the small heater we have in the serving kitchen. Pancakes with syrup. Until he no longer wanted those either. And then, after a couple of days, he died'. The care staff in Blue seek to attune the food for people who are no longer eager to eat to their residual desires. But they do not force feed. Nasal tubes that end up in people's stomachs to carry food there against people's own inclination, are not used. Thus, while nutritional value 'wins' over cosiness when they clash because life itself is at stake, physical survival is not a supreme good in nursing home Y. When it comes to it, living one's daily life with *dignity* and being allowed to die a *good death*, are even more important.[7]

The taste of the eater and the taste of food

Nutritional value and *cosiness* are not the only goods relevant to food and eating. There is dignity too – and there are many more. Interesting among these is *choice*. In the Netherlands care institutions have taken to heart the criticism that they are patronising total institutions with little room for individual specificity. Trying to respond to this criticism, they sought to grant their residents more 'choice'. But choice about *what*? It does not fit the institutional logic to allow residents to choose which specific nurse or care assistant will attend to them. Neither do people get to choose every morning between the swimming pool and a long outdoor walk, whether on their own legs or in a wheelchair. There is not enough personnel for that. *Choice about food* can, however, be organised. And as eating is a recurrent, important daily event, introducing food choice seems an ideal (real as well as symbolic) way to attune institutional care to the wishes of the people being cared for. How to go about it?

The most widespread way of introducing food choice in Dutch care institutions, is to provide residents with a menu.[8] This is a sheet of paper on which a list of food items has been printed. For every item that makes up a meal, there are two or three alternatives to choose between: just put a cross in the little box in front of them. In the High-site coffee room a trainee (who is taking her break) tells Mrs. Veenstra (who doesn't stop talking) that in half an hour from now, Emma will come to fetch her menu. 'I'd better hurry up, then', Mrs. Veenstra says. At which point I ask her if she would want to explain me how it works. Mrs. Veenstra immediately invites me into her room. There, she first shows me the photos of her son, who, or so I learn, is just wonderful. Then she tells me that she is 93 years old. And then she sits down behind her table with the form in front of her. 'Half the time', she says, 'you don't get what you ask for'. However, she does not seem all that sure about what she is asking for. 'So you don't order meat every day?' I comment when I see that she skips both meat boxes of the Wednesday. 'Oh, but I do', she says. 'Usually I hardly eat any, but sometimes it is good.' At that point she notices her omission and puts a cross in one of the meat boxes for the Wednesday. I look at the date. It is three weeks from now. That must be convenient when it comes to buying supplies, three weeks. But how is Mrs. Veenstra supposed to know *now* what she would like to eat *then*, and to *then* remember what she preferred *now* over its less attractive alternative? All in all, however shiny the ideal, this particular form of 'food choice' does not provide Mrs. Veenstra with a lot of *pleasure*. 'Done!' she says when her form is filled, with a mixture of pride and relief on her face. Demanding task accomplished.

In ward Blue none of the residents would be able to fill out a form. So instead of handing out menus, the central kitchen provides ward Blue with a choice of serving dishes. For every hot meal (for every lunch that is) there are two kinds of filling stuff (potato, pasta or rice), two kinds of meat and two kinds of vegetables. Even among the residents who have hardly any words left, many are perfectly capable of making a choice when they get to see and smell what they might eat. Without hesitation, Mrs. Verhagen points at the beans, she doesn't want broccoli. Organising things in this way, turns 'food choice' into a far more pleasurable experience. And yet in Blue it comes at a cost: *cosiness* suffers. The *ambiance scenario* suggested that serving dishes be put on every table. A carer who joins them at their table might then help residents who need help with the serving. However, since there are two serving dishes of broccoli and two serving dishes of beans for *five* tables, putting these dishes on tables would deprive the residents of choice. To cope with this the carers on ward Blue put the dishes on trolleys. Jessy and Linda (a care assistant) push the trolleys around and present people with the options of the day. 'So, beans for you then, Mrs. Verhagen, there you go!' Thus (under these particular circumstances) realising one good, *choice*, comes at the cost of another, *cosiness*. Other values suffer even more. Notable among these is the meal's *culinary* value. In restaurants one tends to have a single option for each course. As your main course you may chose between composites, say, 'grandmother's chicken', 'lasagne with fish' or 'pumpkin with chick peas and cashew nuts'. In institutional menus, by contrast, the main dish is divided into pieces. Mashed potatoes or boiled potatoes. Mince or stew. Broccoli or beans. Eaters have to compose their main course from such components. The *nutritional value* of the food has been taken into account: the mashed and the boiled potatoes offer carbohydrates, the minced meat and the stew are counted on for proteins and fats and the broccoli and the beans are supposed to supply eaters with vitamins and minerals. The conventions of Dutch home cooking are also respected: 'potatoes, meat and vegetables' form a so-called *proper* meal. However, the fragmentation that ensues does not fit in with the culinary tradition, where a meal should hang together as a whole. In the culinary tradition, the various tastes, forms and colours that come together on a plate should be in *harmony* with each other. This is hard to realise if menus are fragmented.[9]

Organising food choice is a way to respect the fact that people have different preferences. It takes into account that when it comes to food, we all have our own *taste*. What it disregards, however, is that taste is not only an attribute of those who eat, but also of food itself.[10] Many of the professional carers whom I get to talk to, deplore the fact that in the institution where they work, the taste of the food itself is not sufficiently attended to. When we are having coffee, Tessa says: 'I don't think the food here in Blue tastes very nice. But, listen, we will be serving lunch soon. You may taste some for yourself. We sometimes do so, too'. The shift strikes me. While in the choice scenario *taste* is located in people (who base their choice on it), Tessa's advice suggests that *taste* is an attribute of food that everyone is able to recognise (just taste it for yourself).[11] A few weeks later I am in the kitchen that provides Blue with food. Remembering Tessa's suggestion I ask the cook: 'Do you get to taste what you prepare?' His answer is immediate: 'Not if I can avoid it'. This is a cook who tries to keep the spirits in his kitchen up by making jokes. He makes jokes all the time. And yet this particular joke speaks of a particular disappointment. All in all, or so I learn, circumstances bring along that the cook prepares food that does not meet his own criteria for *tasty* food.

The kitchen, once designed for a single home, is now being used for *five* such homes. In the home where the kitchen is situated, people eat what has been cooked the very same day.[12] The food for the other four homes is put into serving dishes, chilled quickly, and then put into trolleys that are stored in a cold room. The trolleys are delivered to their destination the following morning. There, someone unloads them and puts all the dishes in need of reheating into a large micro-wave oven. (In Blue this is among Jessy's tasks and she takes me along to see her do it.) It is all very *efficient*. But the implication of this system, called 'split cooking', is that the kitchen is too small. The potatoes overflow the pan. Frying meat is impossible, as the hot plate is too small. Putting all the pieces of meat one by one on that small plate and turning them over takes too much time. And then there is the cooling and reheating. 'Reheating doesn't suit food, does it', says the cook 'it makes a mash of it'. And then, more carefully, he adds that for some dishes like potatoes it doesn't make much difference. But for vegetables it does: they lose their *colour* and their *crispiness* when they are reheated.

And then there are the ingredients. That day's carrots come deep frozen in large, plastic bags. 'Why do you have this brand of carrots rather than another?' I ask while inspecting one of the bags, its obligatory 'information' printed in thirty languages. The cook casts me a look that says: 'Can't you guess *that*?' Then he shrugs and tells that they are the *cheapest* brand. The residents are granted a choice between carrots and peas, but they never get to choose between various kinds of carrots or various kinds of peas. Nor does the cook. This is a task of the kitchen manager, who also decides about the menus. Somehow the kitchen manager balances off price, taste, nutritional value and other goods. But how? What makes him opt for the cheapest carrots? Does he ever taste them? He is not on duty when I am around and nobody working lower down in the hierarchy seems to know. At some point I interview someone higher up: the member of a board of governors of a large care institution. 'Do you ever talk about the taste of food in a board meeting?' I ask. The short answer is: no. The slightly longer answer is that food *safety* is crucial to governing boards: it is not to be compromised, accidents and scandals are unwelcome. But apart from safety, the only aspect of food that ever reaches board meetings are figures to do with the costs.

What to conclude? Has *cheapness* become an all but overriding good in institutional care management in the Netherlands? Not quite. Safety is actually very expensive and attempts to provide people with food choice have not been cheap either. But *survival* is a publicly sensitive good, while tastiness is not. And *choice* is a widely celebrated ideal, that resonates with freedom, which is much more respectable than pleasure.[13] Thus, while the *taste of eaters* came to be a focal point of Dutch health care management, the *taste of food* itself, as material as it is ephemeral, does not quite fit the agenda. Most of my informants (nurses, care assistants, kitchen personal) deplore this. They invest their soul in their work and would much rather prepare, serve and feed *delicious* food.

Measuring and tinkering

So far, I have demonstrated that the various goods to do with food and eating may add up or be in tension and that the *qualification* 'good' may be made to depend on the appreciating subject, the object appreciated, or the interplay between them. The next issue I would like to address, is how to best *serve* the goods to do with food. In the Netherlands, as in many other places, the quality of care has become tied up with measurement. In the words of a recent Dutch report (written in English): 'Over the past few years, Government policy has come to increasingly focus on making the quality of healthcare visible and measurable by means of 'performance indicators'. The aim of this is twofold: 'To set up a transparent form of public accountability, and to encourage healthcare professionals to improve the quality of their service'.[14] Rather than engaging in what they call a 'principled discussion', the authors of the report have done some meta-counting: does the use of performance indicators indeed lead to *transparency* and to the hoped for *improvement* of the quality of professional service? The answer turns out to be disappointing. The authors suggest some technical adjustments. But they also warn policy makers to not exaggerate their desire to govern. Health care professionals might well lose their *intrinsic* motivation as a result of the harsh *extrinsic* pressure that measuring 'performance indicators' imposes on them.

Here, I would also like to address the question whether or not measuring is likely to lead on to improvement. However, I use no numbers and neither have I investigated the motivation of care personnel. Instead, I will present you with a few more stories. They exemplify what 'measuring' might entail in practice and what the practice of separating out 'indicators' so as to measure them, implies for the quality of care. First, then, what it is to measure. In line with the idea that the residents in nursing homes are its customers, has come the marketing strategy to assess 'client satisfaction'. Does the 'product' provided to the 'customers' of residential care, live up to their expectations, or not? In the context of eating and drinking this leads on to the question if residents if are satisfied with their meals. But what is it to ask people if they like their food?

Let me to take you to the restaurant of Highsite. Many of the residents as well as of the elderly people who live in the semi-independent apartments built next to it, are having lunch there. They have just finished the soup. Like the other women around (Emma and a few other service assistants, restaurant assistants and volunteers) I walk around clearing crockery and, again like them, each time someone leans to the side so that I can take their cup and saucer, I ask 'Was it good?'. A women in a flowery dress looks at me and answers: 'Yes, dear'. Her tone is soothing. She sounds as if she wants to reassure me. She must presume that I am a new volunteer or maybe work here. Well, she is grateful for that. Oh, yes, dear. Thus, her answer to my question has nothing to do with the taste of the soup. Instead it is about care: this person wants to care back for the people who take care of her. At the next table I get a polite 'Yes, thank you', of another woman who then adds, in a conspirational tone: 'It is as well to make the best of it, isn't it? I'm not complaining'. Complaining, so much is clear, won't improve anything. Again, then, this answer does not provide 'information' about the quality of the soup. It rather signals a posture. This is a person who realises only too well that she cannot leave Highsite. She has nowhere else to go till the end of her days. In those circumstances, praising the soup is a sensible way to make life tolerable.

It is a quite specific, but therefore no less enlightening example. What, at first sight, may seem to be a mode of gathering information, turns out, in practice, to be part of an interaction. Questionnaires would work in a similar way. But if 'measuring' does not necessarily create transparency, then what about improvement? Do measurements help to improve care? They may do. If Jessy measures the temperature of the ward's butter and notes down the result in a notebook, this may warn those who read the numbers about a faltering fridge before bacteria have a field day there. In this way, the good *safety* is quite probably served better than if Jessy had no thermometer and no notebook. But it is not always that easy. Take breakfast in Blue. The *ambiance scenario* recommends a joint breakfast with set tables rather than pre-prepared sandwiches. Joint breakfasts are defined as good care. It would be easy to measure how often this particular *good* is achieved. I haven't done this, but I learned from Jessy that the answer would be: *never*. However, to conclude from there that care in Blue deserves to be improved on this particular point, would be to disentangle the 'joint breakfast' from the context of daily life on the ward. As it happens, days on a ward for people with dementia do not start with breakfast. They start with getting up, washed and dressed.

None of these activities are obvious. In some cases a nurse assistant may just say 'Good morning, Mrs. Sanders!' and point out where to find a wash cloth and a clean enough dress. But Mrs. Verhagen would put her cardigan inside out if nobody were to help her. And Mr. Hendriks isn't able to do anything much at all. As he is incontinent, being showered in the morning is nicer for him (and better for his skin) than just getting a 'down below' with a wash cloth.[15] But that takes time. And what with all the residents in need of help, the morning ritual takes a lot of time. That is why a *compromise* has been crafted. Those who arrive in the living room early get to eat jointly at a breakfast table that has been set. Those who are late (because they like, or don't mind, staying in bed longer, and are thus washed and dressed later) get a personalised breakfast on a plate.

If a 'joint breakfast' were to become a 'performance indicator' this creative compromise would not only go unnoticed: it might well be undermined. For if high scores on performance indicators would come to matter (for being officially approved of, for receiving a 'high quality' mark, or for getting money), this one might yet be achieved. Getting everyone out of bed, washed and dressed could be seriously speeded up. Mrs. Verhagen might appear at the breakfast table with her cardigan inside out and Mr. Hendriks would no longer get his morning shower, but 'performance' would substantially increase. Alternatively, the morning ritual might still be carefully attended to (there is, after all, not all that much to do after breakfast for people who have trouble washing and dressing themselves and in Blue the possibilities for 'activation' are not endless). But in that scenario the early risers would have a long wait for their morning food. It is quite likely that they would get restless and agitated, while again the 'performance' measured would increase. Thus, in one way or another, increasing the score of ward Blue on the performance indicator 'joint breakfast', would imply a deterioration of the overall quality of its care.

The potential undermining effect of performance indicators, then, is not only that their *extrinsic* character risks to undermine the *intrinsic* motivation of professionals. Something else is going on as well. For it is not only relevant *who* carries 'the' norms, but also *which* norms are put into play. And here, the one-dimensional character of 'performance indicators' clashes with the *multiplicity* of goods relevant to care in practice. Setting performance indicators frustrates compromises because goods that are not counted, can no longer be appropriately attended to. Thus, performance indicators may have *perverse effects*. Instead of helping to serve the quality of care, they may as well undermine it. Maybe this need not surprise us. For when you look at it, the entire setup is strange: accountability systems invite those whom they call to account, to *boast* about their work. After a certain amount of adjustment time, during which they work hard to improve their 'performance indicators', professionals and institutions should be pleased with themselves. Look, our indicators are fine, our work is good, they are invited to say. But improving the practice in which one is engaged, calls for the opposite attitude. Modesty, self doubt. Attentiveness to what does *not* work. Those who want to improve the practices in which they work, should be on the lookout for tensions, frictions, problems. For sites and situations where different *goods* do not easily go together. For clashes and places where it hurts.

When I ask Tessa and Mark about *problems* to do with eating and drinking, they promptly mention *smell* or rather the lack thereof. Since the kitchen in Y is no longer operational, there are no food smells in the corridors before meals. That is a pity: food smells increase people's appetite. It is at this point that Tessa also tells me that the food in Blue does not taste as good as it should do, and that she recommends me to taste it for myself. As it happens, Tessa and Mark are impressively articulate about 'clashes and places where it hurts'. But they do not leave it at that. They also try to accommodate the clashes and alleviate the hurt. If bread is too tough for people to swallow, they organise porridge for them. If joint breakfasts are introduced as an ideal, they still feel responsible for washing and dressing, and they invent a compromise. They tinker. Adapt, attune, or compensate. 'Tomorrow we have chips', Tessa tells. And Mark adds: 'Have you ever had chips from a microwave? Don't even try, they aren't crisp. So tomorrow we have cancelled lunch from the central kitchen for a day, except for the people who need their food mashed. And we have ordered chips from the local carry out. We have done it before. People love it. You can see them enjoying chips'. Even if people rarely give straight answers to questions such as 'was it good?' or 'did you like it?', it is not all that difficult to *sense* whether or not their food accords with them. Tomorrow the residents of Blue will eat voraciously and radiate their pleasure. Mark is looking forward to it already.

In practice, then, improving care is a matter of *tinkering*.[16] In line with this, asking residents if they like their food, should not be glossed as a measurement technique at all. Rather than a way to gather information, it is a mode of caring. If the women who assemble the crockery in the restaurant ask the diners: 'Was it good?' they pass on the message: 'I care about you'. Or maybe theirs is a performative question, one that is meant to *make* people appreciate the food they eat. Chatting and being sociable, after all, improves the ambiance, and, as the ambiance scenario puts it: 'Identical food tastes better in surroundings that are pleasant than in those that are not'. (p.7) Asking people if their food is good, may also evoke an old repertoire: one of confirmation. If a host asks 'Was it good?', the appropriate answer is: 'Yes it was, thank you'. And while people nod, or say yes in so many words, as a long time ago they have learned to do, they may yet start to appreciate their food. Thus, if Lenneke keeps on asking Mr. Hendriks 'Is it good?' while she feeds him, she never expects an answer. Rather than wanting to *know* whether or not he takes his food to taste good, she tries to *improve* this taste. Carers asking questions do not necessarily seek to establish a fact, they may as well try to serve a good. They tinker.

Yelling

As soon as one starts to look into it, various *goods*, in the plural, appear to be relevant in relation to food. They have complex relations between them. The *cosiness* of eating may serve the *nutritious value* of the food that people eat, while some people's cosiness clashes with other people's need for nutrients. Thus, while *here* 'cosiness' and 'nutritional value' are interdependent, *somewhere else*, they are in tension. And just as fascinating is the question of where to locate a qualification. Take taste: is that a characteristic of food 'itself' or is it in the eye, or rather the mouth, of the beholder, that is to say, the taster? As taste interestingly moves between these sites, improving taste, too, may move between attending to food itself and attending to its appreciation. And how, finally, to best attend to the quality of care, how to serve its various goods? *Measuring*, or so I argued, however much it is put forward as crucial part of improvement strategies, may not be all that suitable to this aim. Once we attend to the fact that all measuring is an intervention, it may turn out not to be the most appropriate intervention. It may not provide the information that is hoped for, or it may have perverse effects. More generally, drawing a *single* good out of its complex settings all too often fails to serve the *overall* quality of care. The quality of care rather depends on compromises between goods. On a persistent willingness to tinker. Crucial for good care, then, are those who *feel* the tensions between different goods as these cause frictions in their daily practice.

That is my conclusion. But how to end? When we say good bye, as her working day is over, Jessy asks: 'Will you write all of this down?' Yes, I will. 'And do you get paid for that?' Her tone is incredulous. But no,

I don't plead guilty because I get a salary for writing while in Blue another pair of hands would be ever so welcome. It is important for care practices to be put into words and get more presence, be represented, in the sites from where they are governed. Obviously, the work of words is not straightforward or direct. Those who decide about the budgets, rules and regulations of (Dutch) health care, are as unlikely to read this text as the people who figure in it. But neither is working *in situ* in one setting (hospital, care home, home care service) or the next (be it as a hands-on carer, a manager, a consultant or a researcher) the only viable way to contribute to good care. The theoretical repertoires, the very languages, in which we talk about care also deserve to be enriched, fine tuned and tinkered with. Doing so in English (that travels far more widely than Dutch) brings along the possibility of comparing and contrasting the specificities of ever so many sites and situations. This is a great good when it comes to making words and crafting languages.

So, no, I am not ashamed to be theorist. There is something else that bothers me. It is that somehow writing about the *goods* of care is just too *nice*. Too cosy. There are also *bads* to address, but how to do so? In the present context, engaging in criticism would be gratuitous. I would risk nothing by passing moral judgements. So what I seek instead, but cannot quite find, is a good *tone* for writing about care practices that do not live up to the ideals of those who do the care work. How, while telling stories, to address the ever pressing scarcity of time to care, or the just not good enough taste of the food? Compared with most of the rest of the world, the luxury of care homes in the Netherlands is impressive. And, girl, do we get old. But somehow there are nagging lacks to face. What is lacking? Resources, managerial wisdom, space to improvise, fantasy? Maybe there are also irreducible lacks, like the ones staged in tragedies, where there is no good option. And then there is the misery that tends to come with 'disease itself' – even if disease is never 'itself alone' as it cannot be separated out from the varied ways we care, and live with it, in practice.

The evening meal in Blue resembles breakfast. By the late afternoon, the table is set once again with slices of bread, ham, cheese and liver paste, chocolate sprinkles, peanut butter, coloured sugar sprinkles, jam and sugar. Tanja (now on duty) has quickly helped someone who needs feeding and manages to join the table in the corner, that of Mrs. Sanders and the other women who might enjoy a conversation. Immediately it becomes clear that they do. First, talk is about liver paste. Mrs. Gremmen silently points at the liver paste when Tanja asks her what she would like. 'Would you like liver paste, Mrs. Gremmen?' Tanja repeats in so many words, just to make sure. Mrs. Gremmen nods and gets a slice of bread that has been spread with it. By then, Tanja has shifted the topic to holidays. Mrs. Sanders used to go to France. 'Did you go camping, Mrs. Sanders, or did you stay in a cottage?' They took a tent along. Camping was great. 'And what about you, Mrs. Gremmen?' Tanja asks. The look on Mrs. Gremmen's face suggests that she works on remembering. Tanja lists countries not too far from the Netherlands, but she doesn't hit on the right one. Then Mrs. Gremmen, whose voice I haven't heard all day, suddenly says: '*Austria*'. She smiles, deeply pleased. 'Austria!' Says Tanja: 'Ah, that must have been nice. Did you go for walks then?'

It is obvious that the great good of *cosiness* is admirably being served here. And yet it never gets cosy in the living room. There is too much noise for that. Mrs. Stuiveling doesn't stop yelling. While yelling, she pushes her chair aside and gets up. She claps her hands uncomfortably close to other people's faces. It is loud. And it is heartbreaking. 'On and on it goes', Tanja tells me a bit later, as she goes to have a coffee and takes me to the door, 'whatever we try to do. Sometimes she hits us. She is agitated and unhappy. We've suggested to give her medication, but her son is against that. And he is on the clients' council'. What to make of this? The cosiness of everyone else in the living room clashes with something to do with Mrs. Stuiveling. But with what exactly? Maybe Mrs. Stuiveling's right to yell and to not be drugged even if she is difficult to live with; maybe the sums of money that would be required to give her individual care. Maybe her son's right to be autonomous in her name; or maybe the desire of the management team to avoid problems with the clients' council. Whichever way, the nursing staff keeps trying to have cosy meals even when Mrs. Stuiveling is present. But in practice, stories about trying to tinker towards good care do not necessarily have happy endings.

Acknowledgments

A thank you note does make sense in relating to my colleagues. Over the last few years I have worked on care in various forms collaboratively with Jeannette Pols, Ingunn Moser, Rita Struhkamp, Dick Willems, Tsjalling Swierstra, Mirjam Kohinor, Can Karayalcin, Hans Harbers and Alice Stollmeijer. Thanks. More authors than I can footnote, as well as those who wrote the various other chapters in the present book, also provided valuable inspiration. With John Law I not only discussed health care, but also worked on care in other sites and situations, and, invaluably, once again he corrected my English. For inspiration and discussion while working on this text I would like to also thank: Peter van Lieshout, Mieke Aerts, Amâde M'Charek, David Healy, Nick Bingham, Ingunn Moser and Jeannette Pols (a second time). Thanks, too, to the Paul Cremers Stichting for inviting me to give a talk to managers of care homes and for putting me into contact with the homes where I did my field work; and to the person who arranged all this field work for me. (I do not mention her name to grant anonymity, not just to her, but also to everyone whom I observed. As the ethnographic convention has it, all names in this text are invented.) Finally I would like to thank the Netherlands Organization for Scientific Research, notably its section Ethics, Research and Policy, for the grant that allows me to study: 'Good Food, Good Information'.

Notes

1 For this research see: Nijs e.a. 2006. The quote is from the *Ambiance draaiboek*, p 7, my translation.

2 As a part of my larger research project on food, I also did field work with dieticians. There the overwhelming concern is with eating *too much*. The contrast with the concern in elderly care with eating *too little* is filled with interesting lessons. But that is another story.

3 Nutritional science has topicalised and researched 'nutritional value' by splitting up foodstuffs into biochemical components that one may list on a package. The *ambiance scenario* accepts that but wants to add something social (sociability, cosiness) to it. However, as beautifully argued in Pollan 2008, we do not need to accept the terms of nutritional science to begin with. In the present text I want to note this, but do not to further develop it.

4 The eating body, is not a body we *have* and/or a body we *are* (the two sides of a coin that the tradition of phenomenology presents us with) but can be understood far better when theorised as a body we *do*. See for a further exploration of the 'body we do', Mol & Law 2004.

5 This not a coincidence: a copy of the scenario was sent to me by the person who works on improving the care around eating and drinking in the larger institutional conglomerate of which nursing home Y is a part, the same person who also organised my field access. Later I came across this text various times on the internet. It is an important document in the Dutch nursing home landscape.

6 See about such talking practices Pols 1992 as well as Taylor, present volume.

7 For a more extensive analysis of food refusal in Dutch nursing homes, see Harbers e.a. 2002. There we show that while for doctors food refusal is a symptom of dementia, and ethicists tend to take it as a non-verbal expression of the will, those engaging in nursing care caringly tinker with textures and tastes (food in its materiality) to figure out what might still appeal to people. Note that in the Dutch context there is a remarkable general agreement about the undesirability of tube feeding for people with dementia who no longer wish to eat.

8 For another, similarly practically oriented, shift from the ideal of food choice in the abstract, to practices to do with realising food choices, see Struhkamp, 2005.

9 Actually, in most menus the dishes are presented as two lists. Each of these lists is designed to be a coherent meal. On the Friday that I observed in the kitchen, for instance, fish was being served (in accordance with the Roman Catholic tradition.) There were carrots to go with this as 'fish and carrots' form a traditional combination in the Dutch kitchen. At the same time, nothing stops the eaters from having their fish with peas (the alternative vegetable of that day). This is precisely *at the same time* what provides eaters with freedom (they don't have to eat carrots if they don't happen to like carrots) and what undermines the meal's harmony (if we'd accord the 'fish carrot' combination with such culinary credit to begin with).

10 And what is in the food, and what in the eater, is not easy to separate out. For the way the taste of food and the taste of eaters co-constitute each other, see Teil & Hennion, 2004.

11 I did not taste the food in Blue. For between subjective and objective taste, there are (sub)cultural specificities to do with eating. The proper Dutch 'potatoes, meat, vegetable' meal, happens to not remotely resemble what I eat at home, and in a restaurant I would go for the 'pumpkin, chick peas and cashew nut' option. What about deviant or culturally marginal diets in the care homes? Yes, they cater for vegetarians, too, I was told. Vegetarians could eat the same potatoes and vegetables 'of course'. Instead of meat, they would get something like an omelette, a vegetable burger or a cheese wrap. Once a week the kitchen would cook (the Dutch version of) an Indonesian meal. They would make more than the required amounts for that day, and freeze the extra portions in individualised plastic dishes, for people with a preference for Indonesian food. As it happens, the day I was in Blue, one woman indeed got her personal plate of *bami*. With great gusto she ate every last bit of it. See on all this A. Mol, *Bami goreng for Mrs. Klerks. And other stories on food and culture*, in preparation.

12 Not just the residents: for a few Euro, personnel can buy a hot lunch, too. Volunteers sometimes do so to avoid eating at home, alone. One of the restaurant assistants told me that she always eats lunch at work when there is bami, even if at home she will still have to cook for her husband and children in the evening. The cook, she explained, has a hand of cooking bami: it is very good. Thus, there are not only complaints about the taste of the food in the care homes where I observed. It is also gratefully appreciated.

13 For the fascinating history of the entanglement of nutritional science with the protestant ethos of thriftiness, and its total negligence of anything to do with taste or pleasure, see Conveney 2006.

14 Wollersheim e.a. 2006 p. 13. English is in the original.

15 Washing is as complex a practice as eating. And like eating it does not fit dreams about accountability. See for this: Pols 2006.

16 This proposition is more extensively presented and argued for (with the case of the care for and of people with diabetes) in Mol 2008.

References

Coveney, John (2006 2ᵉ druk) *Food, Morals and Meaning*. The pleasure and anxiety of eating, London: Routledge.

Harbers, Hans, Annemarie Mol & Alice Stollmeijer (2002) Food Matters. Arguments for an Ethnography of Daily Care, in *Theory, Culture and Society* vol 19 (5/6) 207-226.

Mol, Annemarie (2008) *The Logic of Care. Health and the problem of patient choice*, Routledge.

Mol, A. & J. Law, (2004) Embodied Action, Enacted Bodies. The Example of Hypoglycaemia, in: *Body & Society* Vol. 10 (2-3): 43-62.

Moser, Ingunn (2008) Making Alzheimer Matter. Enacting, interfering and doing politics of nature, *Geoforum* Vol 39 (1), 98-110.

Kristel Nijs, http://www.zorgvoorbeter.nl/docs/Draaiboek_Ambiance.pdf

Kristel Nijs, Cees de Graaf, Els Siebelink, Ybel Blauw, Vincent Vanneste, Frans Kok and Wija van Staveren (2006) Effect of Family-Style Meals on Energy Intake and Risk of Malnutrition in Dutch Nursing Home Residents: A Randomized Controlled Trial *The Journals of Gerontology Series A: Biological Sciences and Medical Sciences* 61:935-942.

Pollan, Michael (2008) In *Defence of Food*, London/New York: Allen Lane.

Pols, Jeannette (2006) Accounting and Washing: Good Care in Long-Term Psychiatry, *Science, Technology & Human Values*, Vol. 31, No. 4, 409-430.

Teil, Geneviève & Antoine Hennion (2004) 'Discovering quality or performing taste?', in M. Harvey, e.a. (eds.), *Qualities of food*, Manchester and New York, Manchester University Press, p.19-37.

Rita Struhkamp, (2005) Patient autonomy: A view from the kitchen, *Medicine, Health Care and Philosophy*, vol 8, 105-11.

Good farming
Control or care?

Vicky Singleton

I am with Jack, a semi-retired farmer of a small family farm, on his routine morning check of his herd of cattle. He repeats the check every evening. It is mid winter and the cattle are inside a huge modern steel farm building that reminds me more of an aircraft hanger than a cattle byre. The building is known on the farm as 'the big building'. It is relatively new, built by Jack and his sons. It is very warm inside and it smells sweet, of hay and cow manure. The 62 cows and calves are separated into several groups by metal partitions. Some of the cattle are tearing mouthfuls of hay from the big bales that Jack has just placed in the central aisle, using his tractor with metal lifting spike attachment. The cattle stand on a deep litter of layered manure and straw; fresh straw has recently been laid on top. The cattle are calm and clean. They look healthy and content.

Jack leans on one of the partitions and surveys his herd. He seeks any ailing animals, unusual behavior or body changes that require closer inspection, for example indicating that a cow is about to calf. He admires the cattle. His gaze appreciates their health, breeding and beauty. His positioning on the other side of the partition, the dog by his side ready to protect and the stick in his hand, respect the size and weight of the cattle and their tolerance of one another and of us. Occasionally he talks to me or to a cow. Pointing at a black faced cow and her calf he says: 'That one can be aggressive when she has a calf, she's a good mother. You have to keep your distance but I know she cares well for the calf'.[1] To her he says: 'Come on old girl, how's that calf doing?' He searches for a specific animal and asks me if I can see 'one that's walking badly'. I can't see any that I think may be injured. He sees the one he is looking for, identified because of the particular arrangement of black and white patches on its body. He moves towards it and prods its hind quarters gently with his stick to make it walk, so he can assess its movement. It reluctantly moves a couple of steps. Jack is injecting it every day and is satisfied that it is improving.

Chapter 11

We walk back towards the farmhouse. Jack looks at the hedges and comments that he knew this would be a hard winter because the hawthorn trees had been laden with berries in the autumn. He reflects that he is pleased with the year's harvest; he has enough hay to feed his herd for the whole time they are cared for inside. Last year he had to buy some feed in late spring to supplement the previous year's poor harvest and in the face of a lengthy, wet winter that soaked the fields, slowed the grass growth and delayed the cattle being put out to graze.

We sit at the wooden table in the kitchen. Jack is 76 and Mary is 67. Farming is in their blood. They have farmed their current farm for 32 years and worked on family farms prior to that. They were both born into farming families and they don't know a life without livestock to care for. Jack picks up an official looking A4 envelope and takes out a thick wad of papers. He pushes it in front of me and asks, 'What is this about? What do they want now?' The front sheet is a letter headed with the logo DEFRA, the British Government Department of Environment, Food and Rural Affairs. Jack says he receives lots of letters and leaflets about the farm and that this is what he currently finds most anxiety promoting about farming. He tries to carefully read all the letters and leaflets to find out what he must attend to and what can be safely ignored or simply noted. He worries about missing something important that could mean he loses money or his beloved livestock. I quickly scan the letter and tell Jack that this is an invitation to attend a non-compulsory information-giving event about environmental schemes related to farming. He does not have to attend to this letter now but I suggest that he could benefit from returning to it. I explain that Jack and Mary may be able to claim government support for environmentally sensitive farm practices. Jack carefully puts the paper back in the envelope and gets a pencil out of a leather folder. Slowly he writes on the envelope, 'Farm' and then he pauses, trying to decide what to write next. The pencil hovers over the word for a moment and then he puts the pencil down. He doesn't know what to label this paperwork, where to file it or how to respond to it. He places the envelope in a plastic box next to the table. Mary says: 'We get so many letters. It's a full time job just keeping up with the paperwork'. Later she says:

> Keeping the livestock alive is one thing. Keeping on the right side of DEFRA, the Environment Agency and the taxman, that's another. (Mary, Jan 07.)

I reflect that caring for cattle on the farm is a demanding series of daily routines accompanied by considerable knowledge specific to this farm, its land and these cattle. This includes regularly checking the cattle, responding to their immediate needs, predicting and planning their food supply and developing knowledge of the temperaments and health of individual cattle over time. Cutting across this care work is legislation. Indeed, as Mary suggests in the quote above, the activities that constitute the legislation often seem 'other' to the daily on-going care of the cattle. The recently introduced UK Cattle Tracing System is an example of such legislation. Drawing on fieldwork on small family farms in North West UK and attendance on a taught course at a local agricultural college (January to March 2006) this paper considers the work involved in the implementation of the Cattle Tracing System on farms and draws out tensions between the legislation and the work of caring for the cattle on the farm.[2]

The Cattle Tracing System: The control dream

The British Cattle Movement Service computerized Cattle Tracing System (CTS) is a set of practices that have at their core a dream of control. Lucy, one of the tutors at the local agricultural college who, for 30 years, worked for UK Government organizations legislating on farming, most recently for the Rural Payments Agency, part of DEFRA, introduces the System in the following way:

> It holds every bit of information. It was difficult to get this up and running. Now it works incredibly well. We have full traceability of animals. It is a super system. (Lucy, 6.2.07, Ex DEFRA employer; Agricultural College.)

The Service is based in Workington, Cumbria, North United Kingdom and it aims to hold details of the birth, death and movement of every bovine animal in the UK (not Ireland). European Union legislation required all Member States to introduce a computerized tracing system by the end of 1999. The UK Cattle Tracing System was introduced on the 28th September 1998 and has been developed and expanded since then.

It is claimed that the System provides more comprehensive and accessible records of animal movement than previously available. For example, Lucy said:

> We have had to clean up our farm systems, to become pure as pure. Now it's extremely clean. It's all about traceability

> and now we have full traceability of animals. We have excellent systems. (Lucy, 6.2.07, Ex DEFRA employee; Agricultural College.)

Excellent records of cattle movement are associated with 'purity and cleanliness' by Lucy because they aim to provide comprehensive knowledge of cattle movement and increased accountability of farmers, animal movers and sellers. Thereby, the System aims to prevent the spread of cattle disease. The Cattle Tracing System is a key part of the response to the relatively recent outbreaks of animal diseases in the UK. Lucy explains:

> With BSE, Foot and Mouth, Bird Flu, the legislation has been heaped on, and it's still coming. (Lucy, 6.2.07, Ex DEFRA employee; Agricultural College.)

That is, the Cattle Tracing System, through its aim to hold knowledge of all cattle movement, dreams of being able to control all cattle movement. Hence it is both a response to and an attempt to prevent the reoccurrence of horrors previously experienced, for example the 2001 UK Foot and Mouth Disease outbreak. This outbreak is associated with funeral pyres of piles of slaughtered animals, a high emotional, social and financial cost to farming families, limited public access to the countryside, damage to rural economies through detrimental effect on tourism and debates and confusion about cause and treatment. (Convery *et al*, 2008; Mort *et al*. 2005; Law, 2006) The extent of the outbreak was worsened by lack of knowledge of and control of animal movement. The media images traveled widely and portrayed the stench of rotting carcasses and inefficient, 'impure' records contaminated by 'bad' farming practices of record keeping and care of animals. The Cattle Tracing System promises more effective management of disease. And many farmers recognize this as one of the goods of the System, not least because it may improve sales of beef. Beef consumption has reduced in recent years due to consumer concerns about human health and cattle welfare. The System aims to ensure that beef is fully traceable in terms of where it comes from, where it has been, where and how it is slaughtered. Food miles can be recorded, places of slaughter and conditions of transport can be monitored, and farm practices can be inspected. DEFRA claim: 'Cattle tracing is now an integral part of the Government's commitment to improve consumer confidence in British Beef' (Rural Payments Agency web site). Lucy states:

> I would eat anything now if it is produced in the UK; the systems are very good for the consumer. (Lucy, 6.2.07, Ex DEFRA employee; Agricultural College.)

Lucy's claim is problematic because there are various consumers for whom the System may not be good. For example, what of a consumer such as a rambler who enjoys walking the fields but is distressed by the sight of tags in the ears of cattle, finding them ugly. Moreover, I am wondering if the systems are wholly good for the farmers. In fact, Lucy suggests that there are tensions between the System and farm practices of care when she says:

> It is good legislation in that it is there to protect the consumer. But, unfortunately, it has placed a huge burden on the farmer. Whether you farm 3 acres or 3000, the paperwork is exactly the same. (Lucy, 6.2.07, Ex DEFRA employee; Agricultural College.)

It will become evident below that the burden placed upon the farmer is not only in relation to paperwork. The Cattle Tracing System presupposes various practices that must be carried out on the farm in order for the System to be implemented. However, these practices risk being forgotten *because* they take place on the farm. Moreover, many of the practices on which the Cattle Tracing System depends (and also interferes with) are primarily *care practices* rather than the control work of, for example, inputting bar codes into a centralized computer system. Hence, these care practices are frequently in tension with the control dream that underpins the Cattle Tracing System.

Making the control dream work on the farm

All cattle must have ear tags for the Cattle Tracing System to work. Tags are identification ear attachments. They are inserted into the calf's ear soon after birth by the farmer on the farm. Lucy said: 'A tag is for life; it cannot be changed or taken out. It is the identity of the animal' (Lucy, ex-DEFRA employee, Agricultural, Jan 07). In dairy herds the animal must be tagged within 36 hours of birth, for beef herds within 20 days from birth. Since 1st January 1998 all animals must wear 2 official tags (normally one in each ear). Each tag bears a crown logo, UK prefix (country code), herd number and the animal's unique lifetime identification number. The farmer allocates this number according to the herd register. There are regulations about the size and character of the tags. The primary ear tag is yellow, plastic and comes in two pieces. It is a minimum of 45mm high and 55mm wide with letters a minimum 5mm high. Farmers must ensure that regulation tags are inserted within deadlines, that they remain in place and that they correspond with written records. The tags are inserted via a hand held gun. The farmers must restrain the young calf (or the cow when replacing a lost tag), hold the gun to the ear and release the trigger to force the pin through the ear. The calf or cow usually resists the restraint and jumps when the pin is inserted. Some farmers have been injured during this process – either by the calf or cow moving and resisting or by a protective mother cow.

All cattle must have a passport. British Farmers must register their cattle and report all births, deaths and movement within the Cattle Tracing System. Within 27 days of birth (that is within 7 days from tagging) farmers must apply for a passport for a calf. The passport contains all the animals details, including the ear tag number, breed, sex, date of birth and genetic dam and the date the passport is issued (and re-issued). When a calf is born the farmer allocates it one of the passports he has been sent from DEFRA having inserted the ear tag with the matching number. The farmer signs it and attaches one of the farm's barcode labels. This barcode sticker is the key to how the Cattle Tracing System works. It is a computerized system. The bar code stickers supplied to the farmer include the name and address in English, but the system works by reading bar codes.

It is a statutory requirement that a herd register is kept, is up to date for each animal and has no missing information. It must include the following information to be completed within specific deadlines:

Information to be recorded	Deadline for completion
Date of birth or age of animal	Birth to be recorded in 7 days (Diary herd), 30 days (other herds)
Ear tag number	
Breed	
Sex	
Dams official identification number (if the calf is born on the holding)	
Date of movement on or off the holding and place from/to which the animal moved	Within 36 hours of movement, passport to CTS within 3 days
Date of Death	Within 7 days and passport returned to CTS, if animal under 24 months age. If over 24 months animal sent for BSE test.

Most farmers I have met keep a hand written record. Jack has a book, the size of an A4 pad, obtained from DEFRA. He reviews it and writes in it daily. He records more information than is deemed essential by the Cattle Tracing System. He makes notes about the individual animals including about their temperament, where they calf, if they have been unwell and any medication. He writes in pencil so that he can correct any mistakes. He keeps the book next to the table in the kitchen so it is easily accessible and so that he can sit down while writing it. Some farmers keep their register in their cattle housing.

Observing Jack it is evident that this formal written record is in addition to the wealth of information that he holds in his head and can retrieve as needed. I witnessed on numerous occasions Jack making a decision about an animal's health and needs based on knowledge gained from interacting with the animal over time. Furthermore, Jack holds and incorporates his experiential knowledge of and informal evaluation of the body shape, physical build and temperament of an animal within decisions about breeding and selling.

Farmers must keep accurate Movement Records. When an animal leaves a holding the farmer must fill in one of the tear out sections in the passport, tick the box for either on or off movement (onto the holding or off the holding), complete the date of movement, attach the sticky holding label, sign the card and then detach and post the movement card. The Cattle Tracing System reads the barcode sticker and updates the record for that particular animal. It is a statutory requirement to report all cattle movements through the Cattle Tracing System.

Movement includes moves to and from temporary holdings or between holdings in the same business. As detailed in the table above, there are deadlines to be met. Farm records of movement must be completed within 36 hours by both farmers (or by the farmer and the auction). The passport must be returned to British Cattle Movement Service within 3 days.

Implementing the System: Collisions between the control dream and care practices

The above account of the constituents of the Cattle Tracing System demonstrates that the System depends upon a whole series of practices being carried out on the farm. While the System dreams of control, its successful implementation depends upon farm based care practices which, I show below, are not about control but are responsive, flexible and unpredictable. Hence the control dream and the care practices frequently collide with one another.

Cattle Movement: Predictable vs. Unpredictable

> We had a call the other day, said that one of our cattle was out on the road. It wasn't one of ours; we thought it was probably one of Steve's. We put it into our field, called him and he collected it later… Turned out a car had come off the road the night before, knocked down his fence and drove off without telling him. The cow got out and went for a walk. (Laughs)… A good walk, down to back of beyond. Probably trying to get to the other cows. It was bellowing to get in with them so she (telephone caller) thought it was one of ours… Anyhow, we kept it off the road. (Jack, September, 2006.)

Any movement of cattle outside a five mile radius within a holding or onto another holding must be recorded in the farm movement record and via the Cattle Tracing System. It is claimed that this is because the cattle are likely to mix with livestock from another holding and could be a disease risk. As far as I am aware, the cattle movement described in the above story was not recorded in any formal way. This is something farmers are faced with on a fairly regular basis.

The Cattle Tracing System requires and claims knowledge of all cattle movement. However, full control of cattle movement on the farm is a precarious achievement. It is not possible all of the time. That good care includes knowledge of where one's cattle are is not in question. Indeed, all farmers that I have spoken with and observed spend considerable time counting and recounting their cattle and very carefully monitoring cattle movement and containment. Maintenance of fences and hedge boundaries, maintenance of buildings and movement of cattle to different grazing sites take up a great deal of farming time and are a major constituent of good care. Yet, farmers are often faced with the unexpected. For example, that which has been contained escapes. In the above example, the fence was no longer a fence, the car didn't stay on the road, and the cow did not stay in the field. A specific collision of events and materials led to movement of a cow from one holding to another in an unanticipated manner. This is, at the same time, a collision of control versus care modes of monitoring cattle movement. On the farm monitoring cattle movement is distributed and modest and appreciates that sometimes things 'go wild' and do their own thing. It accommodates the unpredictable.

Tagging: Timetabled versus flows

Mary: Well we have calves born dead sometimes. Not very often but sometimes.

> *Vicky*: What do you do then; do you have to ear tag?
> *Mary*: No, no you don't then, you just tell them and that's okay. But, y'know, well, (hesitates) well, you're supposed to get the ear tag in quickly and the passport sent off. Well, once, we couldn't do that. We were late. We'd been away on holiday and busy. We just said it was born 2 days later than it had been born. You couldn't do that if it was more than a few days. I mean we wouldn't do it for any longer. (Mary, February, 2007.)

The Cattle Tracing System demands adherence to a timetable for ear tagging and passports. The System cuts across the complexities of daily farm life, including care of the self through taking a holiday or responding to other aspects of life that demand attention and time. Care of cattle is embodied by an array of entities that can and do make unexpected demands that make it difficult to keep to a strict timetable.

Having said this, sometimes the located specificities of farm life dovetail with the requirements of the Cattle Tracing System. The same farmer says:

> He [her husband] puts the ear tags in as soon as they are born, usually. It's easier. You can actually sit on the calf. He gets one of the lads [his son] to do it, or someone else; he can't easily do it, especially not on his own. It gets harder if the calves are older and our sons go mad because it's more difficult. (Mary, February, 2007.)

So, accepting that tagging has to be done, carrying out the procedure as soon as possible after birth is seen as best practice by the Cattle Tracing System and by farmers but for different reasons. For the Cattle Tracing System it is primarily about control – so as not to miss a record of a birth. For the farmer it is about care – to tag when the calf is most easy to handle and hence risk of injury is low and it is less stressful for the calf than when they get older and larger. In Britain there has been public discussion about the risks of carrying out tagging to the farmers. For example, in March 2007 a case was reported of the death of a Scottish farmer when tagging a new born calf. The protective mother cow attacked the farmer leading to crush injuries and his death.[3]

In contrast to the control required by the Cattle Tracing System, as a care practice tagging must be flexibly implemented. Tagging can be a dangerous activity that requires considerable skill and knowledge. It can also require high levels of strength and physical fitness. For example, when a calf is born outside in the field rather than in the cattle housing they can quickly become able to move rapidly and catching the calf requires not only skill but running speed and physical stamina. Furthermore, not only does the farmer need to tag a lively, strong calf but often has to cope with a protective mother cow. A lone farmer may not be able to do this task alone, he or she must rely on neighboring farmers, relatives or friends. Placing the tag in the calf's ear and scheduling this procedure may not be straightforward. The Cattle Tracing System tagging timetable is linear, disembodied, and calculable. It is made of numbers on a piece of paper. It is tabled and made up of a series of discrete moments of accounting. Tagging on the farm is embodied and relational, embedded in a *flow* of events rather than a linear timetable. It involves an array of heterogeneous elements; it includes the requirements of the Cattle Tracing System and paperwork and also, for example, the size and aggression of the animal, the time and place of the birth of the calf, the needs of and demands upon the farming family, and the strength, health and physical fitness of the farmer.

Individuals versus Collectivities: Colliding styles of practice

In the above example of the cow escaping the field the farmer displays consideration for his neighboring farmer and for the cow, if hit by a car. He wanted to get the cow off the road; this would prevent accidental damage to the cow, or even to a motorist who could collide with the cow on the road, and loss of livelihood for his neighbor. Good care of cattle on the farm is located in relations of caring for fellow farmers, their livelihoods and their cows.

Another example of this 'collective caring' is offered by a farm practice of 'bull hire'. The Cattle Tracing System regulations state that movement to another holding, even for bull hire, must be recorded in the movement book and via the passports. Bull hire is when a bull is taken to another holding to service the cow(s). The alternative is to use Artificial Insemination and there is considerable support from DEFRA for this as best practice as it reduces risk in relation to biosecurity – spread of infection. Indeed, there is a strong argument that keeping a bull is risky on too many grounds – human health and safety (they are potentially dangerous animals), economic (they eat a lot for little gain) and biosecurity (they can cross contaminate infections).

On the other hand, one of the small farms that I have observed does keep a bull to run with their herd. Moreover, the bulls often do travel to other farms to run with another herd. Reasons for this are multiple. Some farmers said that they like having a bull. They like to see a bull in the field, 'a magnificent animal when they look their best'. They also talk about it making good sense in relation to greater chance of success of impregnating cows. The reproductive cycle of a cow is central to the success of a dairy or beef cattle farm. Cows must be in calf within a particular time frame following the birth of a previous calf. And cows are fertile for just one day. The signs of fertility can be ambiguous. To identify the day on which the Artificial Insemination staff must visit to inseminate the cow, the cow must be carefully monitored. If the herd runs with a bull there is less chance of missing the fertile day and less need for close surveillance.

So, some farmers do like a bull to run with their herd and one way to off-set the costs of keeping a bull is to share a bull between herds. That is, neighboring farmers borrow a bull for a short time. This alleviates the owner's costs of keeping a bull. As stated above, the Cattle Tracing System states that such 'bull hire' must be fully recorded and monitored. In practice this does not always happen. In one instance that I was told about the bull is walked along a bridleway next to the farm to 'go on his holiday' at the neighboring farm. Having observed this practice I also know that this presents an opportunity for the farmers to meet, to talk, to discuss their farming practices as well as to update on respective family activities. It is a social activity. It is a collective caring farming practice.

The Cattle Tracing System tends toward individualism – that of the farmer and each cow. Yet, when caring for cattle on the farms the cattle are part of a herd and moreover, the farmer and the farming family are part of a farming community. Good care is about caring for and appreciating the collectives – communities and herds.

Practices: Punctuated vs. continuities

Jack, the elderly semi-retired farmer that I mentioned at the start of this paper, spoke about how he learned many things from working on his grandparent's farm. His grandfather was a farmer and butcher in the 1930s.

> He would take my elbow and lead me across the field, without saying anything... he'd show me a nest with young birds in it... He knew where they all were around the farm... He wanted me to be careful when working around the nest. He would do the same if there was an unusual plant growing... he would keep the cattle off them. (Jack, February 2007.)

I have many examples of this kind of description of good farm practices as being passed along generations. Practices as learned through doing and as sets of continuities.[4] Farming practices may be *done* rather than known or told and they may be *silent and implicit* rather than explicit and verbal. And, they may not fit within the explicit, formal Cattle Tracing System.

I have previously mentioned the knowledge Jack 'held in his head' along side the information recorded in his formal written herd register. I witnessed numerous examples of Jack drawing upon knowledge learned through on-going interaction with an animal and coupled with information about cattle breeding and handling gained from years of *doing it*. All the farmers I have observed demonstrate similar knowledge practices. For example, when a cow is calving they will often refer to the individual history of the cow, how many times she has calved before, what the birth was like, if the cow was previously a 'good' mother, if she is very protective and hence there is a need to be wary and cautious around her. The cattle on these small family farms often have a local history that is included in what is best practice in relation to that particular animal at specific moments. A further example is an occasion when the farmer was anxious to delay tagging a particular calf because he knew, from previous experience of the mother, that she is aggressively protective and likely to become very distressed at the attempt to remove and tag her new born calf too soon. He knew that she would become calmer and tagging easier and safer given some time.

While the Cattle Tracing System creates continuities in terms of traces of the movements of individual animals, in other important ways the system punctuates continuities of care on the farm. It creates discrete moments of accountability that may displace or at least colonize embodied practices of 'care'. Care that is unarticulated and located in specific knowledge of a particular animal or is an embodiment of years of practice is displaced by some of the demands of the Cattle Tracing System that are explicit, formal and universal, for example, tagging a calf as soon as possible after birth.

Displacement and dependence: Record Keeping past versus present

I have suggested that the Cattle Tracing System is staged as progressive, for example by employees of DEFRA such as Lucy whose job it is to implement the System. Lucy stated that it is a change in farm record keeping that has cleaned up the ineffective systems that were there before it. The System claims a break with the past and a more controlled future for record keeping. However, while the Cattle Tracing System claims to displace farm practices, it rather depends upon them. It is necessary to the Cattle Tracing System that there is widespread agreement that keeping full records of animal management, including detailed records of movement, births and deaths, is an essential element of good care practice. If farmers did not keep records the System would break down. Furthermore, repeatedly I have come across examples of effective and efficient systems of monitoring animal movement that pre-existed the Cattle Tracing System. Mary a woman farmer, married to a semi-retired farmer, says:

> We've always kept records, this book since 1994, our son got it, it's not the DEFRA book but it's the same. It records the movement of animals... He (husband) does what he's always done, even if there is a better way to do things he carries on doing what he's always done... He's always recorded deaths, sales, where moved to, killing, breed, mother and ear tag number. It's funny DEFRA think this a big change, it is a pain at times, the inspections, and you don't have long to get the tags in, but he's always kept a good record, this book started in 1994 and he'll have the one before that somewhere, he never throws anything away. I suppose it's good practice. (Mary, February 2007.)

The Cattle Tracing System has imposed a 'new' system of record keeping on the cattle farm. It claims to have displaced and improved previous systems. However, effective farm systems of record keeping, linked to Government organizations, have existed for a long time. In addition, farmers very often keep their own records. For example, one of the farmers I spoke with keeps a small leather notebook with him at all times in which he writes an extensive record of births, deaths, movements, injuries and various other variables and specificities about individual animals. As Mary says in the quote above, record keeping is one aspect of good farming practice – good care of the livestock on the farm.

The implication of enacting the Cattle Tracing System as cleaning up previously inefficient and dirty systems is the relocation of best farming practice to the Cattle Tracing System and its version of record keeping and thereby the *dis/location* of this aspect of good care from the farm. However, the Cattle Tracing System grows out of established practices of keeping records present on the farm. There is a tension between past and present and between control and care. The Cattle Tracing System claims to clean up ineffective farm based practices and yet it must build upon them in order to work at all.

Farm inspection: Care displaces control

Further to the above, we shall see below in the practice of farm inspections that record keeping is most effective and efficient when it is responsive to the specificities and unpredictability of embodied farm-based cattle care – when it prioritizes care over control.

Farm inspections are a moment when the Cattle Tracing System and farmers and their constitutive practices, materials and people physically come together. I have become particularly interested in what happens on the farm at these moments. This is one account:

> *Mary*: They don't give you much notice. We've had two… the second visit, two people came, with a print out with all our numbers on. They were matching their paper with the ear tag numbers with our records… Then they found a problem… The inspector marked it, no ear tag. She said, I have to put it down, nothing will happen, there's only this one, I just have to mark it down.
> *Interviewer*: What happened?
> *Mary*: There was a discrepancy between my husband's book and their records and the ear tag… He'd marked it down wrong… he always writes in pencil, and it had smudged, it looked like a different number, not a naught. Now we always double check… We got a letter from DEFRA a few weeks after, telling us we had had a discrepancy and that others could affect our single payment. It frightened him, he said, we could have lost money couldn't we? You get penalties on your single payment, you lose percentages. We were alright, this one didn't matter, just a mistake. (Mary, February 07.)[5]

This is a moment when the complexity of daily farm practice is included in the Cattle Tracing System. The description above suggests that it is a problematic and discomforting moment for both the Inspectors and the farmers. The work of Helen Verran, a postcolonial technoscience scholar, suggests that we should consider such moments of disconcertment carefully. These are moments of practice when different ways of working collide. In this case the Cattle Tracing System dream of control collides with the situated care of the farmers. The moment of disconcertment, when the 'error' is at once recorded and dismissed, is a moment of practice when the different systems are respectfully engaged in 'generating new ways to go on, and re-generating old ways of going-on together'(142, 1999). The Inspectors record the discrepancy but note that nothing will happen. In this particular instance there are no other discrepancies and the Inspectors evaluate the farmers as having made a mistake rather than as trying to deceive. The discrepancy is classified as an understandable mistake and the tension between the control of the system and the care of the farmers is dispersed. The Inspectors mark the discrepancy while reassuring the farmers. This seems to be an example of care practices displacing the control dream of the Cattle Tracing System.

Conclusions: 'The care has gone'

I began this paper with the following quote:

> Keeping the livestock alive is one thing. Keeping on the right side of DEFRA, the Environment Agency, the taxman, that's another. (Mary, January, 2007.)

The words of this farmer enact a dualism between legislation and farm practices, between DEFRA and the farm. She suggests a fundamental difference between legislation and care of the livestock. For her caring for the animals is other to the activities that constitute the legislation. Hence, while there is agreement between farmers and DEFRA that effective, responsible practices of monitoring cattle movement are a crucial aspect of 'good cattle farming', the ways of working to achieve this are different for the System and for the farmers.

The Cattle Tracing System involves cattle identification numbers, holdings, keepers and computerized records. It draws together, combines and circulates information about cattle movement. It imposes a timetable for farm records and it demands tagging and individualization of cattle. If necessary the System will control cattle movement through monitoring imposed restrictions in the event of a disease outbreak. Farmers, people who run slaughterhouses and livestock markets and dealers can be called into account for their part in breeding, holding, selling and slaughtering cattle. Thereby, the System way of monitoring cattle movement is centralized, disembodied, formalized and standardized activities that can be monitored and regulated. That is, the System attempts to control farm practices and cattle movement.

However, farmers' practice is embodied, located, and responsive to their livestock, their land, their family and themselves. Their practice includes cattle that are part of a herd, named land, know-how that has been passed through generations, neighboring farmers, living in a community, pencil written notes, families, friends and personal health and capability. That is, farming practice is necessarily responsible for *and responsive to* a variety of heterogeneous entities and involves managing their varied, competing needs. The demands of the Cattle Tracing System compete with those of the cattle, neighboring farmers, family members, materials such as fences and gates and personal health / the doctor. Hence a crucial difference between the System and the farming practice is that the former *dreams of control* while the farmers *practice care*.[6]

Moreover, the System is demanding. The System adds to the work of managing the livestock but is not primarily about caring for the livestock. Rarely does the System respectfully sit along side of (or is displaced by) livestock care practices. The exception may be the example of the farm inspection that is detailed above – but this was related to me as an exception. The high demands made on the farmer and the livestock by the Cattle Tracing System demonstrate that the System affords limited recognition of the significance and the complexity of many embodied livestock care practices. Indeed, the time, anxiety and energy required to *do* the System on the farm is not visible in the passports, letters and required herd records.

That is, the effects of the System on the farm are not only demanding but they are also non-innocent. They include colonization, displacement, punctuation, disembodiment and invisibility of care practices. These effects are evident in relation to the livestock, the farmers and to government workers. Lucy closed her interview with the following moving statement:

> The increase in legislation is one of the reasons I don't work for DEFRA any longer. It felt like a policing bureaucracy. For 30 years I felt that I was helping the farmer. I would go onto farms and they'd offer me a cup of tea and sit down and chat. That stopped... Later, when I was training

Inspectors, they would tell me how badly they were treated by farmers. The farmers would be angry and aggressive. I told my Inspectors; put yourself in the farmer's position... We can give only 48 hours notice of Inspection. Many farmers will spend those 48 hours worrying, in a state, they could lose serious money if one cow hasn't got the right paperwork... *The care has gone.* (Lucy, 6.2.07, Ex DEFRA employee; Agricultural College.)

This erosion of care is experienced even though the System must be embodied in care practices on the farm to be workable at all.[7]

In addition, while the Cattle Tracing System is not inherently more efficient and effective than farm practices, it has been staged as such drawing upon its characteristics as a way of working. Because the System is formal, centralized, explicit and disembodied, its way of working is more easily transported and made visible than located care practices. The information and paperwork that constitutes the System is mobile and stable.[8] It is circulated between farms, the offices of the System, European Union and UK Government documents and offices, agricultural training colleges, slaughter houses, livestock markets and policy advisors. It is combined with other knowledge and legislation, such as other Government policy. This mobility and combinability enables the System to be staged as efficient and effective and to displace, colonize, and damage the farm care practices which are less formal and are located, embodied and decentralized. This is one important way in which the System, despite being difficult to live with, has achieved durability, it commenced in 1998. Nevertheless, as we have seen, another aspect of the durability of the System is that it is variably practiced on the farm.

In my attempt to articulate some of the work of living with the Cattle Tracing System on small family farms I have shown a series of tensions that emerge on the farm *between* attempts at control that are the effects of the System and practices of farming care. In some examples the tension is livable, perhaps even productive of a new way of working between the system and the care practices, as in the example of the farm inspection. In other examples, the effects of the System are loss and damage to crucial practices of care. Consider the examples of the tragic death of a farmer during tagging a calf, the sense of loss felt by the Government Inspector and the farmer having to defy the System when putting a neighbor's escaped cow into the nearest field. Nevertheless, the System depends upon the very practices of care that it is displacing, as in the example of keeping comprehensive records of cattle movement. Good farming emerges as embodied, located, collective, responsive practices that are crafted by care rather than control and that remain in tension with the effects of the System that dreams of control.[9]

Notes

1 Cudworth (2007) writes about gendering of cattle and of farm related occupations, on the farm and at slaughter houses. Birke, Bryld and Lykke (2004) propose considering the perfomativity of animality and argue that feminist science studies have given scant regard to nonhuman animals. They argue that it is important for feminist theory to address the complex relationships between humans and other animals, and the implications of these for feminism. See also Donna Haraway (2003, 2007).

2 Sally Hacker defines a family farm as, 'where people who live on the land also work it and make decisions about it'. (69, 1990)The family farms that I am coming to know are varied in their size, land type (upland, lowland and both), livestock, crops, family membership and also in their relationships to larger corporations. For example, one family farm has become a part of a consortium of local farms which enables localized decisions about food production, marketing and distribution. This farm occupies a position somewhere between agriculture and agribusiness, as defined by Hacker (1990). The definition of family farm seems to be under negotiation in 21st Century Britain, partly in relation to understandings of and national policies on agri-environmental issues such as food miles, organic production and landscape management. There is also a reported growth in hobby farming and small holders – the differences between these and family farms is ambiguous. (NFU, nfucountryside, Feb 2007) Hence, there is not a universal constitution of 'family farm'. Rather, each family farm is a specific arrangement of varied heterogeneous elements including: government and local directives and systems, land, practices, animals, people, plants, food, machinery, technologies and money.

3 Reported in various farming news journals. For example, see http://www.fwi.co.uk/Articles/2007/03/20/102420/scottish-farmer-killed-while-tagging-calf.html

4 John Gray's (2000) anthropological account of people living and working on hill sheep farms in the Borders region of the UK offers detailed examples of farming knowledges being passed on through practice.

5 The Single Payment Scheme (SPS) is the principal agricultural subsidy scheme in the European Union. The Rural Payments Agency, an Executive Agency of Defra, is the single paying agency responsible for the scheme in England.

6 See Annemarie Mol (2008) for a version of this argument with the example of diabetes care.

7 In this way, the Cattle Tracing System offers another example of the lesson that formal systems for managing daily practices must be tinkered with and adapted in practice in order to work at all. (Timmermans and Berg 1997; Morris 2006. Singleton 2005; Moser 2008.) Technological systems are perpetually in process, moved from one location to another and whether they work or not depends upon their being continually done and remade on location.(Singleton 2006, Moser 2007) Furthermore, the work of practice of technological systems is often made invisible if and when the system works smoothly. STS tells this as, technologies are black boxed. As is the case with the Cattle Tracing System, when 'working' and having achieved durability, we often no longer see what is needed to make them work unless controversy opens the black box or technoscience scholars prise it open. (Latour 1988b).

8 Latour (1988a) offers a detailed account of this argument with his case study of the pasteurization of France. In Laboratory Life Latour and Woolgar (1986) describe scientific texts as immutable mobiles and link these characteristics to the construction of scientific knowledges as facts that achieve durabiliy. More recent work, such as de Laet and Mol (2000) on the Zimbabwe bush pump and suggests that 'durability in practice' may be linked more to mutability or to an oscillation between stability and fluidity.(Singleton (2006) on public health policy.)

9 In Singleton (1998) I have written about the necessity of professional ambivalence to the durability of the systems in relation to public health policy in the UK.

References

Birke, Lynda, Bryld, Mette and Lykke, Nina (2004) Animal Performances: An Exploration of Intersections between Feminist Science Studies and Studies of Human/Animal Relationships Feminist Theory 2004; 5; 167.

Convery, Ian, Mort, Maggie, Baxter, Josephine and Bailey, Cathy (2008) Animal Disease and Human Trauma: Emotional Geographies of Disaster, Palgrave Macmillan: New York and Hampshire, UK.

Cudworth, E. (2008) 'Most farmers prefer Blondes': entanglements of gender and nature in animals' becoming-meat, Paper presented to the Annual Conference of the British Sociological Association, University of Warwick, March 28th-30th 2008.

de Laet, Marianne and Mol, Annemarie, (2000) The Zimbabwe Bush Pump Mechanics of a Fluid Technology, Social Studies of Science, Vol. 30, No. 2, 225-263 (2000).

Farmer's Weekly Interactive, *http://www.fwi.co.uk/Articles/2007/03/20/102420/scottish-farmer-killed-while-tagging-calf.html*

Gray, John N., (2000) At Home in the Hills: Sense of Place in the Scottish Borders, Berghahn Books: New York and Oxford.

Hacker, Sally (1990) Farming Out the Home: Women and Agribusiness pp69-88, in Sally Hacker, 'Doing It The Hard Way' Investigations of Gender and Technology, Unwin Hyman: Mass., and London.

Haraway, Donna (2003) The Companion Species Manifesto: Dogs, People and Significant Otherness, Prickly Paradigm Press: Chicago.

Haraway, Donna (2007) When Species Meet (Posthumanities) University of Minnesota Press.

Latour, Bruno and Woolgar, Steve (1986, reprint) Laboratory Life: The construction of scientific facts, Princeton University Press.

Latour, Bruno (1988a) The pasteurization of France, Harvard University Press: Cambridge, Mass.

Latour, Bruno (1988b) Science in Action: How to follow Scientists and Engineers Through Society, Harvard University Press: Cambridge, Mass.

Law, John (2006) Disaster in agriculture: or foot and mouth mobilities Environment and Planning A, 38(2) 227-239.

Mol, Annemarie (2008) The Logic of Care: Health and the problem of patient choice, Routledge.

Morris, Carol (2006) Negotiating the boundary between state-led and farmer approaches to knowing nature: An analysis of UK agri-environment schemes, Geoforum, Vol 37, Issue 1, January 2006, 113-127.

Moser, Ingunn (2008) Making Alzheimer's disease matter. Enacting, interfering and doing politics of nature, Geoforum, Vol 39, January, 98-110.

Mort, M., Convery, I., Baxter, J. & Bailey, C.(2005) Psychosocial effects of the 2001 UK foot and mouth disease epidemic in a rural population: qualitative diary based study, British Medical Journal, doi:10.1136/bmj.38603.375856.68. References and further reading may be available for this article. To view references and further reading you must purchase this article. Nfucountryside (2007) February, Associa Ltd., North Gate, Uppingham, Rutland, UK, LE15 9PL.

Singleton, Vicky (1998) Stabilising Instabilities: The role of the laboratory in the UK Cervical Screening Programme pp86-104 in Marc Berg and Annemarie Mol (eds.) Differences in Medicine: Unravelling Practices, Techniques and Bodies, Duke University Press: Durham, NCa.

Singleton, Vicky (2005) The promise of public health: Vulnerable policy and lazy citizens Environment and Planning : Society and Space, Vol 23 (5) October 771-786.

Timmermans, Stefan and Berg, Marc (1997) Standardization in Action: Achieving Local Universality through Medical Protocols Social Studies of Science, Vol. 27, No. 2, 273 – 305 (1997).

Verran, Helen (1999) Staying true to the laughter in Nigerian classrooms pp136 – 155, John Law and John Hassard, Actor Network Theory and After, Blackwell Publishers: Oxford.

Varieties of goodness in high-tech home care

Dick Willems

Good care, good technology

Healthcare care is a technology-intensive practice. Even the most mundane forms of care use technical objects such as thermometers, bandages or pain killers. Even so, technology has an unclear place in our thinking about good care – if anything, technology and care are often opposed. In this vision, technology, 'crowds out' real care, and as a result doctors, nurses and other caregivers do what is technically possible, not what is medically needed. Another point of view takes it for granted that technical objects will not do anything we humans do not want them to do. Any undesired consequence of the use of technology lies in the way we use it, not in the technology itself. Technology, in *this* view, is nothing but means to an end. I believe that these two positions expect either too much or too little from care technology. This paper investigates the idea that a vision of good care is part of every care technology in a way that does not *determine* healthcare, but also does not leave it completely open: an incorporated vision that makes it hard, but not impossible to act in other ways.

> The ventilator is sitting next to Mr. Van Dijk. A black rubber bellow moves quietly, making a gentle humming sound. It is connected to Mr. Van Dijk by a tube that goes to his neck and disappears behind an elegant brown scarf. On the other side, the ventilator connects to an electricity outlet.
> We sit down and have coffee and, most of the time, the ventilator quietly hums. I know that it pumps air through the tube going to Mr. Van Dijk's neck. Somehow the machine seems to be as modest as possible, especially when compared to its relatives in hospital: large machines full of displays that frequently make disquieting sounds. Most of the time, this quiet puffing is all the machine does. Every now and then, however, it starts making various alarming sounds. At such moments, the machine is trying to alert the people around so that they can prevent Mr. Van Dijk from choking.

This scene illustrates what I will be looking at in this paper: how visions of good care are incorporated into care machinery. However, this scene also shows that there is not just one description of good care in a technology, but quite a lot of them: for example the ventilator is at the same time very present but trying to be modest, quiet most of the time but alert to anything that might announce trouble, integrated into the environment but also, inevitably, springing to the eye of the visitor – in other words, the normativity of the machine is complex.

The assumption of this paper is thus that there is not just one version of good care, neither for human caregivers nor for care technology. There are varieties of good care, or, to use Von Wright's term, *varieties of goodness* in the machines used in technologically advanced home care, one of those areas where the goodness of the care provided and the lives people live is constantly uncertain. Technology plays an important role in this form of care.

The term 'varieties of goodness' was introduced by Georg Henrik von Wright, a Finnish analytical philosopher (Von Wright 1963). His idea was that the systematic study of the good can only become fruitful if the existence of various forms of goodness is acknowledged. Going back to Aristotle, he argues that the heterogeneous use of the term 'good' in everyday life does not simply reflect a careless and unsystematic use of the word, but that it parallels the ontological variety of 'goodnesses': a good sleep, a good conscience, a good blood pressure monitor or a good character. Von Wright distinguishes between the instrumental and technical good (being good at something), the medical good (being good for something or someone) and 'good' in the sense of virtue. Varieties of goodness, thus, are not different norms or values, but different moral registers or vocabularies.

The study of varieties of goodness can be relevant to caregivers and those involved in the development and use of technology, but it may also be relevant to the discipline of bioethics because it sheds new light on the normative role of technology. Thus, it may be possible for bioethics to increase its relevance to everyday technological healthcare practice.

As mentioned before, the focus of this paper is on varieties of good care as performed by the machinery involved in advanced home care. I will start by describing the technical objects in a strict sense and widen the perspective from there. I will take advanced pulmonary care as an example: oxygen provision to patients with chronic obstructive pulmonary disease (COPD), and artificial respiration for patients with severe neurological disease. I will discuss varieties of good care (and possible conflicts between them) in a gradually expanding way. I will first discuss the way in which these machines improve oxygen uptake by the body, either by enriching the air or by supporting the work of the lungs (section 2, 'Improving breath'). Next, I will speak about the way in which these technologies co-create a good environment for themselves and for the people using them, thereby expressing care-related versions of a good home. I will explore the ways in which advanced home care technologies create contexts in which they can work (section 3: 'Good environments'). Lastly, I will analyse the role of care technologies in undoing the situations they have created when the care stops, which, in these types of diseases, is invariably because the user dies (section 4: 'Good ends'). The question of this section is how advanced home care technology cares for a good death. I will end by describing what I think this type of study of varieties of goodness could mean for thinking about healthcare improvement.

Improving breath

This paper discusses two types of technical objects used by patients who have trouble breathing as a consequence of either lung disease or generalised neurological disease. The first technology provides oxygen and the second artificial ventilation.

Oxygen provision: enriching the air

> The Vivisol is an oxygen concentrator, a machine that provides oxygen to Mrs. Beek. It makes a slight sound that reminds one of a motorcycle at a distance. A thin, transparent tube runs from the machine to Mrs. Beek and bifurcates just under her nose. Mrs. Beek does not stay attached to this device the whole day; she puts it off to go to the bathroom and for dinner. In total, she tells me, the machine is on for about 10 hours a day. Vivisol can be set to deliver different quantities of oxygen, between 0.5 and 5 litres per minute. It enriches the air Mrs. Beek inhales through the tube so that, even with her diminished lung function, she will be able to take in enough oxygen to live her daily life. It enables Mrs. Beek, even though breathing remains a hard job for her, to walk around, make her meals and go into town on sunny afternoons.

Many patients with severe COPD need extra oxygen. They are then often put on Long Term Oxygen Therapy (LTOT), usually for the rest of their lives. LTOT involves the use of oxygen for at least 15 hours a day, but preferably continuously (NVALT, 2001). The problem for COPD patients is that they feel out of breath as soon as they stand up from their couch. Giving them oxygen does not restore their breath, but makes each breath transport more oxygen. For these patients, 'good air' is much richer in O_2 than for the rest of us. Mostly, an oxygen flow of 3 litres per minute is sufficient to maintain acceptable arterial oxygen pressures.

The primary activity of oxygen devices, then, is to add oxygen to the air the patient breathes so that oxygen reaches the body, even with insufficient breathing. Breathing itself is not improved (as with ventilators, as we will see later on), but the air is made richer in oxygen.

Oxygen-providing devices come in two varieties: the first are containers that store oxygen in an oxygen factory. There are two forms of containers: some contain up to 2000 litres of oxygen as a gas (so-called *cylinders*), others contain 20-40 litres of oxygen in a liquid state, which can be transformed into 850 litres of oxygen gas when it is provided to the patient. The second variety, fundamentally different, are the *concentrators* like Mrs. Beek's device that, by way of a system of sieves and chemical reactors, concentrates the oxygen from the ambient air.

Whereas containers merely store and distribute oxygen, concentrators do the entire job of concentrating, enriching and distributing: they are miniature oxygen factory. This may seem ideal; however, oxygen concentrators are less modest than the containers: they make a constant humming noise, often disliked by the users, and they are relatively big machines that need electricity.

The small, *portable* concentrators need a car battery as a power supply; they weigh about 10 kilograms and need to be transported using a wheeled trolley, which makes them quite cumbersome. Because of the risk of power supply disturbances, a 10-litre cylinder containing ready-to-use oxygen is provided as well, so that patients using oxygen concentrators need to be able to use both types of devices.

After having been stored in a container or extracted from the ambient air by a concentrator, the oxygen must be brought into the lungs of the patient. Three forms of access to the lungs have been developed: nasal masks, nasal cannulas and transtracheal cannulas. Masks have the inconvenience of covering up mouth and nose and are therefore only used at night, by patients who need large quantities of oxygen. Some users switch between modes of administration.

Cannulas, very thin transparent tubes through which oxygen-enriched air flows, come in two forms: transtracheal (through the air pipe) and nasal (into the nose). Both of these 'access routes' do something that is qualified as good care, and yet these are different: they incorporate varieties of goodness.

To start with the nasal cannula: it uses a normal, existing route of oxygen into the body: through the nose. No special access into the body needs to be made. A transtracheal cannula, on the other hand, demands an 'unnatural' access into the body. The patients have must undergo a small operation. But then again, this disadvantage is balanced by a different goodness: a transtracheal tube sends the oxygen straight into the lungs, bypassing the so-called 'dead space' going from the mouth or nose to the lungs. It is more *efficient* than a nasal cannula. Where a nasal cannula needs to deliver oxygen at a rate of 2l/min, a tracheal one can reach the same effect with 0.5l/min. Thus the transtracheal cannula is more efficient than the nasal tubes in that they spend as little effort as possible to reach a goal. This greater efficiency is the reason why transtracheal tubes are used more often for very severe patients, who need more oxygen per minute than can be reliably transported through a nasal tube.

There are other differences between nasal and transtracheal tubes, which are also related to versions of goodness. For instance, nasal cannulas are less easily infected or blocked than tracheal ones. The person who wears one can also take it off any moment – this is not as easy with a tracheal cannula. Mrs. Beek has no trouble removing her nasal tube, for instance, when she wants to drink her tea; this would be impossible if she had a transtracheal one. On the other hand, it would also be less necessary, because a transtracheal tube interferes less with drinking tea than a nasal one. Here we have another good of the transtracheal tube: it hardly interferes with eating and drinking.

Visibility and privacy

> Mr. Jansen tells about what he considers a real improvement in oxygen provision: the possibility of integrating the nasal cannula into the frame of his spectacles. The cannula that he used to have was very visible indeed, sometimes making it difficult for him to participate in social events.

Visibility in public space is a central theme related to oxygen provision. A transtracheal cannula can easily be made invisible. The person who uses it just wears a high collar or a scarf. A nasal tube, on the other hand, is visible to people – everybody knows that the person who is wearing it is on oxygen. Hence the many attempts to make nasal tubes as invisible as a tracheal one, for instance, by concealing them in the rim of a pair of glasses. Some oxygen users with perfect eyesight even wear spectacles just to be able to conceal their oxygen tube. Wearing spectacles, even unnecessarily, is considered less of a nuisance than visibly wearing an oxygen tube (but then again, wearing a tube is less of nuisance than oxygen shortage). On the other hand, visibility is not always regarded as a disadvantage: some patients told me the visible nasal cannula helps a lot while standing in line at the supermarket, because most people tend to let them cut in.

Not only the access routes, but also the oxygen machines themselves are visible to different extents. More than concentrator users, patients using oxygen cylinders or liquid oxygen go out with their miniature container on their backs or in their bags – in both cases, their oxygen provision remains visible. They can go virtually everywhere in the company of their oxygen containers. By doing so, they take healthcare technology into the public domain of shopping malls, airports and train stations. What used to be hidden in healthcare institutions or in the homes of people now comes into the open.

This is less true, however, for users of concentrators. Their technology is much harder to take out, because it is heavy and it needs electricity. This leads to many patients like Mrs. Beek going out for a brief stroll without their oxygen. Different versions of the good, especially effectiveness, seem to come in conflict here: encouraging the possibility to take a stroll is part of the goal of treatment of severe COPD, but the price concentrator users pay for that is an interruption of the oxygen provision, which lowers another form of effectiveness: providing sufficient oxygen to the patient's blood. Undisturbed strolls are incompatible with maximum oxygen enrichment. One of the doctors I interviewed explained how this incompatibility had led to a debate in his profession:

> One of the debates among physicians prescribing oxygen is whether patients should be using their oxygen while shopping or not. Some say that it is better if they do, because that gives them more oxygen when they need it, during exertion. Others say exactly the opposite: according to them the effect of oxygen lies in the numbers of hours it is administered – it doesn't directly enhance endurance.

> That's also my view: patients do not need to carry their oxygen device when it bothers them most, both because of the weight and the visibility: while they're shopping.

This quotation tells of two conflicting versions of what is good: the first one says that it is best to supply oxygen when a body needs it most, while walking instead of sitting; the other says that the important thing about oxygen is that it should be administered a certain amount of time each day. This second option leaves some space for people to choose when they want to use the oxygen.

Supporting the muscles: artificial ventilation

The second category of technical objects figuring in this paper supports patients with breathing difficulties in a totally different manner. These patients suffer from different diseases that cause insufficient breathing, namely neuromuscular diseases such as Amyotrophic Lateral Sclerosis, which eventually lead to a paralysis of the breathing muscles. Enriching the air with oxygen would be useless for these patients, since they are physically incapable of breathing at all. They need a device that, partially or entirely, takes over their breathing: a ventilator (also called a respirator).

Ventilators such as the one Mr. Van Dijk (see section 1) uses may measure up to 1 metre in height and 50 centimetres in width and depth. Some of these machines, however, are smaller and fit on a wheelchair. Their most conspicuous part is the bellow that is inflated and compressed about 15 times per minute; moreover, a ventilator contains various tubes, including a thin one used for suctioning. As mentioned in the sketch of Mr. Van Dijk's situation, the ventilator makes a continuous humming sound, sometimes interrupted by alarms.

> On one of my house visits with the artificial ventilation nurse, we drive up to the compound of a large farm in the middle of green pastures. The farm has a second home built next to it, and that's where we're going. The parents of the farmer live there. The nurse explains to me, while we are walking towards the home, that Mr. Van Dijk, who started the farm, has had ALS (amyotrophic lateral sclerosis, Lou Gehrig's disease) for a few years, and the disease is rapidly progressing. He has been on continuous artificial ventilation now for about a year. The nurse visits him every month to check if the couple are still managing, to change the tracheostomy tube if necessary and to support the family.

CHAPTER 12

> The patient's wife opens the door and while we walk to the room, she tells the nurse that he is not in good shape today: he is coughing a lot and he is ill-tempered. In the middle of the spacious living room with very little furniture, a man sits in a wheelchair. He has a visible tracheostomy, and on the back of the wheelchair is a machine of about half a metre high with a few indicators on it. It is connected by a wide tube to the tracheostomy.

Different forms of goodness can be found in home care ventilators, even though these display less outward variety than oxygen-technology. A home ventilator is conceived of as a relatively unobtrusive machine containing a smaller number of indicators and alarms than its equivalent in hospital. Non-intrusiveness and modesty are relevant varieties of goodness: the home should be as undisturbed by the technology as possible. However, there is also friction and compromise here: the alarm sounds given by the device are loud and disturbing, and they are meant to be so. In this case, good care obviously means freeing the patient's airway from mucus when needed, and as he cannot make this known himself, there has to be an audible form of alarm.

If one enters a room with a ventilator-dependent person, it is not only its visibility that is striking, but also its audibility. Ventilators have a strong presence in the homes where their users live. If the French aestheticist Mikel Dufrenne is right when he says that one of the characteristics of a good technology is that 'it is not ashamed of being a technical object', then the ventilator is a very good technology indeed (Dufrenne 1964). There is a constant, soft, regularly puffing, and somewhat soothing sound from the air bellow at the back of the machine. This could also be part of the definition of good care upheld by the ventilator: it makes a reassuring sound close to, even though it remains different from, the sound of breathing. It would have been quite different if the machine had been completely silent.

The wife of the farmer in the little story above tells us that her husband is ill-tempered, but that is hard to see for me, because he does not speak, let alone address his visitors in an unfriendly manner. For the ventilator to work optimally, it needs the most direct entrance to the lungs: a tracheostoma. However, this immediately makes patients unable to do what most of us can do with our breath almost at all times: speaking (ALS-patients remain able to speak for some time after their respiratory muscles have become paralysed). So there is a conflict here between the goods of being able to breathe and being able to speak. Most patients who cannot speak because of their disease or because of the artificial ventilation use their eyelids for 'speaking' (or maybe more exactly, writing.). Each letter corresponds to a number of blinks. The person they speak with starts guessing the words after two or three letters; the correct word is indicated by a long blink.

There is an obvious conflict of goods here, between optimal oxygenation of the blood and an optimal ability to speak. In eyelid speech, the conflict is solved outside the technology, but there could be solutions for this conflict *within* the technology. To explain the possible 'internal' solutions, I have to say something about a mundane part of the machinery: the inflatable cuff.

Tracheostomas are provided with an inflatable cuff that is used to close off the trachea around the tube in order to prevent the air from escaping by mouth. Goodness, here, is efficiency: no air will be wasted when the cuff is fully inflated. Patients who are not completely ventilator-dependent, however, have the option of leaving the cuff uninflated during the day as much as they wish, in order to be able to speak. The cuff is an example of how a conflict of goods related to the same device (efficacy versus communication) may be dealt with. The inflatable cuff allows the user to switch between two conflicting varieties of goodness; it performs its function exactly because it allows for inflation and for deflation.

There is another conflict of goods, between unobtrusiveness and the treatment of a sometimes life-threatening cough, where the machinery provides both the conflict and its solution:

> The machine hums in a quiet breathing rhythm. The man does not seem to notice our entering the room, but his wife starts talking to him and then this wonderful eye-lid conversation takes place. It makes one understand immediately why these machines have to have alarms: patients who are on permanent artificial ventilation have no way of asking for attention if things go wrong. Eye-lids cannot cry for help. In fact, in the middle of our conversation, the alarm goes off, and that is when the nurse says that he is really coughing, even though nothing like an ordinary cough can be heard. This is a clear sign of the extent to which the machine and the person have become one: coughing has become indistuingishably an activity of both the machine and the body.

There is a clear dilemma here: on the one hand, the patient needs continuous breath support, which not only makes speaking impossible but also makes coughing inaudible. The last thing one would want to happen is a patient choking because he cannot ask for suctioning (i.e. removing mucus from the windpipe). The solution to the dilemma, even if imperfect (the wife of one of my interviewees once did not hear the alarm, which almost lead to a fatal choking), is made part of the technical object: an alarm, reacting to even a tiny increase in pressure in the patient's airways, is built into every ventilator.

Good environments

We tend to take the term 'home' in home care technology for granted. However, homes change when advanced medical technology moves in. Home care machines not only contain and perform ideals about effectiveness, as shown in the previous paragraph, they also contain and perform a variety of goodness concerning the environment they work in. They do not operate in a ready-made context that is already fully there, they have to make their own environment.

What ideals concerning the home are packed into the technology? What norms and values do oxygen containers and concentrators hold about their 'terrain', to use Simondon's (1985) term? What does a good home consist of for these devices?

> I enter the home of the Jansen family in a small town in the east of the country. It is a long house, the front being a somewhat indefinite area that formerly served as a grocery shop. From there, I pass an unassuming little kitchen, which opens up into the living room. The first thing I notice is the puffing sound of the respirator next to Mrs. Jansen. She is entirely paralysed and propped up in a wheelchair, with the respirator attached to it. It is connected to an electricity outlet. Around her, a couch and several chairs have been grouped. We sit down and the nurse explains to Mrs. Jansen and her husband who I am. After some introductory talk, we move into the specially constructed ground floor bedroom, because the nurse must replace the transtracheal cannula. First we cross a small space that obviously serves as a medical storeroom. It contains a spare respirator and lots of bandages, spare tubes, etc.
>
> The husband explains that the room was built as an extension of the house after it became clear, about five years before, that his wife would remain dependent on the respirator and would therefore be unable to sleep on the

second floor. On my question of whether she had not seen the upper floor since coming home with her respirator, they answered that this was the case. She told me it had been hard for her to acknowledge that there was a large part of her house that she would never see again.

The new bedroom contains a hospital bed and another regular bed, several medical-looking cupboards and two small chairs. The bed is in the middle of the room, with enough space around it for a nurse to be able to circle it.

I ask whether they feel their house has changed since the introduction of the respirator. Well, obviously, they say. Not only has it been enlarged, just to accommodate the respirator and all that comes along with it, but it also has been necessary to widen up doors and corridors for Mrs. Jansen to be able to leave the house. Extra storing space also had to be found. 'We had been thinking of moving somewhere else but finally, adapting this house to the new needs proved cheaper and also more attractive – we know our neighbours, some of them are available for help, etcetera, so we didn't move, finally.'

The Jansens' example shows how the home that home care technology migrates to does not stay the same: the ventilator demands a specific type of home for it to function. It incorporates a version of the home as a spacious place, with an extensive ground floor or an elevator, and wide door openings.

Similar things can be said about oxygen technology. The old, classical oxygen cylinder asks a number of things from the home: that it be accessible for the almost daily exchange of these huge and heavy objects, that it be spacious enough to allow for their presence and their being moved about, that it not be crammed with stuff. The house needs to have at least one large bedroom, or else it has to be possible for the user to sleep in the main room, since the oxygen has to be taken at night. It is not hard to imagine that conflicts between the home and the oxygen cylinder occur quite often.

Most importantly, the cylinder asks for a house without fire: no smoking, no open heating. Any pulmonologist has horror stories about patients lighting a cigarette next to an open cannula from which oxygen freely flows – with severe burns or incinerated houses as the result. Many patients divide their homes into normal and no-fire zones – a clear example of how technology sets norms for its environment. Concentrators, on the other hand, are less prone to explosion danger than cylinders, so care does not depend on the willingness of those around them not to smoke. If we look at the wider environment, one might say that the dominant form of goodness in home care machinery is independence from hospitals. Patients using this form of technology no longer need to stay in heavily regulated environments such as hospitals, but may live where they feel most at home and where there are less rules imposed by the professional organisation – although those imposed by their family, their disease and the technology remain.

What does independence mean for oxygen concentrators? First, of course, that care does not depend on the firms distributing oxygen. The economic troubles these firms may go through, the potential breakdown of the machinery that isolates the oxygen and puts it into the containers, the workers that may go on strike are all relevant to O_2 provision in cylinders, but not to the concentrator (which, on the other hand, may have to deal with power outages).

Second, care by the concentrator does not depend on the intactness of the transport system. There is no worry about whether the delivery will be on time, whether the lorry will be hampered by snowstorms, roadblocks or engine breakdown. Your home may be anywhere that has electricity and you will still be able to use an oxygen concentrator. This may be what grants the concentrator its independence, but at the same time makes it more dependent on the reliability of its elements, which, in turn, can only be maintained if monitored. So the concentrator, even though independent by some measures, is still vulnerable: it depends on regular checks and maintenance to keep doing what it should. It may not need filling from an oxygen tank, but it does need regular visits by a technician. Technologies do not provide blank independence, but different mixtures of dependence and independence.

Even so, a good concentrator can still survive on, for instance, the thinly populated islands to the north of the Netherlands. Goodness also implies that the quality of care should not depend on where you live, and that it should not be necessary to move to an urban area because of the need for care. One variety of good care incorporated in the concentrator thus seems to be that it should be geographically universal, or at least as universal as electricity.

Good ends

The techniques I have discussed in this paper will usually remain in use until the patient's death, so the next way to investigate their normativity is to look for varieties of good dying inscribed in these machines. To put it differently: the previous sections described how devices contain versions of a 'good' situation for respiratorily disabled people, in this section I will look at how these devices 'undo' these situations in a good way.

Some of the professional caregivers I spoke with worry that mechanical ventilation in the home can, at least in principle, be continued indefinitely, and therefore almost inevitably will lead to the problem of when and how to stop it. As one of the home care technology nurses told me, 'The problem is that you can keep the body alive beyond the point where you could say that the person, in a sense, has already died. Then you would have the ventilator-dependent body and nothing else'. Apparently, the logic of the technology is to always continue, never to stop. The device contains no 'stopping rules' – the good death inscribed in the device would seem to be the endlessly reported death. But is it? Maybe technological objects contain other versions of the good death apart from this problematic one. The following quote is from an interview with the wife of a bedridden ALS patient on artificial ventilation.

> Oh yes, we have spoken a lot about how he will die, what he wants and what not. He has always said that as soon as he becomes unable to communicate with his eye-lids, he wants the doctor to end his life. We discussed it with our doctor, who agreed with it, but he asked us to formally make the request before my husband cannot communicate any more, because he needs to be able to talk with my husband, and a second doctor will need to do so, as well... You know, I think he has lost so much already of what he could do when he was healthy, that I feel he has been dying bit by bit the last four years...[crying]..., haven't you dear? But still, what is left is worthwhile to go on for. Sometimes I curse that machine for keeping him alive, but most often I am very happy that he is still with me. You know, he's still the same person. [...] You know, it may seem a bit strange but for me, it will be very hard if he isn't here anymore, and I may even miss all the stuff that I have got so used to, the ventilator, the bed, suctioning, etcetera.

The migration of advanced technology from the hospital to the home implies the migration of a (dreaded) form of dying to the home. In this form the body has lost all its capabilities and needs support for the most basic functions, but the *mind* lives on -synchronicity is lost. However, the wife in the quotation also says something quite different: as long as some form of communication between them remains possible, her husband's life remains worth living. As soon as that possibility disappears, her husband's life should be stopped by switching off the machine. This may be seen as a description of a good dying made possible by the technology: it makes it possible for the patient to die when the last reason to stay alive has gone.

A potential transformation in our ways of conceptualising the good death, provoked by this type of technology, may be that machinery such as the ventilator makes it possible to go on living as long as seems appropriate, even if it superficially conforms to an image of a bad death. This possibility of an appropriate or even beautiful death, even under these circumstances, can only be realised by the patients, the families, the caregivers and the technology in cooperation. It is not the technology that induces new forms of a good death all by itself; it is, as always, the technology plus the people, the other technologies and the infrastructure.

Another feared form of dying associated with medical technology is the increasing uncertainty or even disappearance of boundaries. Dying people who, until their last breath, are connected to machines by tubes, catheters, or infusion lines are often seen to have lost their borders. It is not clear anymore where they stop. This is the reason why in most cases, those who die at the ICU are detached from their machinery as much as possible. However, the migration of technology to the home turns the machinery into a more intimate part of the lives of people, comparable to their glasses and their clothes – they often live with this technology for several years. People enter their graves with clothes on, and sometimes with their glasses on, but usually not with their morphine pump or their nasal catheter. The following quote from a home care nurse about the death of one of her patients, referring to oxygen provision, shows how the continuation of such links to technical objects after death becomes at least conceivable:

> At the end of the day, his wife called me saying that she thought he had died. I went there and saw his oxygen tube still in place, with the cylinder switched off. He had a nasal oxygen tube which had become so much part of him that

it seemed natural, somehow, to leave it in place. But for his wife, it was clear that it had to be taken out, because she did not want to be reminded of his illness of the last few years. So I removed it, it was a strange feeling.

The idea that it could be 'natural' to leave a nasal tube in place runs counter to the idea that the connection to machines is what makes a dying process bad – unnatural, if you want. So again, the migration of advanced technology into the home could make new forms of dying acceptable, and even good. Contrary to what some sociologists argue (Walter 1994; Lawton 2000), dying may still be good even if the dying person or the deceased body remains technologically attached to the outside world.

Conclusion: caring machines

My aim was to try out an alternative to regarding technology as either a usurper of care or as a pure instrument, instead demonstrating that machines hold and perform various, sometimes conflicting and sometimes harmonious, concepts of good care. I think this attempt has shown a number of things. Firstly, taking seriously the idea of varieties of goodness creates a demand for empirical studies, not only studies of activities and opinions of the people involved, but also of the ways in which technological objects work within healthcare. Studying varieties of goodness in devices helps us understand the undeniable but always evasive normativity of technical objects.

Where new forms of care technology emerge, attention will have to be given to their normativity: into what kinds of care, homes, lives and deaths are they made to fit? How do they transform homes, care, lives and deaths to fit themselves? New forms of technology may be made to fit into existing forms of living (both in the sense of leading a life and being at home) and they may make new, good, bad, exciting, or dull homes and forms of caring and living possible. This becomes very concrete: parts of modern houses, for instance in houses for the elderly, will be built in ways that make the use of advanced home care technology possible. They will have the necessary outlets for fast Internet connection that enable monitoring at a distance, for instance for renal dialysis or artificial ventilation (obviously, care technology is not the only reason to provide houses with internet outlets).

I have tried to show that, among other things, advanced home care technology may be instrumental in the creation of new varieties of goodness, for instance new forms of good death, so that even forms of dying that many consider bad could become good or at least acceptable.

As announced in the introduction, this type of study would also have implications for empirical work in bioethics. I have worked with the idea that, in order to support the improvement of care, *varieties* of goodness, or versions of the good, need to be studied empirically. Again, why not just *the* good but versions of it? Because good care differs for different contexts, diseases, lives – it is not the same for the bed-ridden ALS patient as for the artificial oxygen-dependent COPD patient, for the friendly demented lady or for the child with a chronic disease. These differences require different versions of good care in the technology used in different situations.

This paper has shown a way in which the morality of the technical objects involved in healthcare can become an object of empirical studies. Even though we cannot interview them or have them fill out questionnaires, technical objects can be studied ethnographically by following them just as we follow human actors. Technological objects, obviously, do not deliberate about the good as humans (sometimes) do. It is through the way they work that they generate and maintain forms of good care and good living and dying (as humans also do). Healthcare technology performs good care; even though this may not make machines moral actors in the same way as humans, it does give them a place in the normative fabric of healthcare.

In this context of empirical ethics, it may be useful to raise a point about heuristics. Home care technologies for patients with breathing difficulties, both oxygen technology and artificial respiration, have served as cases in this paper because they have *migrated* from their original environment, the hospital, to the home and the streets. Migration appears to expose technology's 'built-in' normativities – it constitutes a sort of social experiment with technical objects. The migration and concomitant translation of machines to an environment that differs from the one they were originally designed for, puts a strain on their incorporated values and their varieties of goodness, making these more visible and – also – more vulnerable. So, if you want to study the normativity of technical objects, follow their migrations. Migration and translation may tell as much about the original version as about the translated technology (as much about hospital technology as about home technology). For the sake of focus, this paper has only discussed the home care part.

Not only the empirical study, but also the practice of doing bioethics may change when it takes the normativity of healthcare technology as its object. Some of bioethics' central metaphors, or exemplary situations, may prove too limited. The practical work of ethicists may need to move from balancing and giving weight to various values and normative principles to something closer to engineering: fitting, arranging and reshaping varieties of good care as performed in technological practices. Applied ethics in the original sense of plying or folding something to fit something else.

One could object that all I have been doing in this paper is discuss separate varieties of goodness, without paying attention to their interdependence. True. It is obviously necessary to investigate how the varieties of goodness I located in the technologies hang together and relate to each other. Or, better, are *brought* together, made to relate to each other in the everyday use of oxygen and of ventilators. Since part of the work of living with such technologies that most of my respondents had to do, lies in fitting and assembling the varieties of goodness they contain and express, empirical studies would need to describe and thereby support the way in which patients and their families succeed in doing just that: fitting, combining, relating forms of the good that are performed by different technologies.

References

Anonymous 1989. Recommendations for long term oxygen therapy (LTOT). European Society of Pneumology Task Group *Eur Respir* J, 2(2): 160-164.

Akrich, M. 1992. The de-scription of technical artefacts. In Bijker, W. E. & Law, J. (Eds.), *Shaping technology/building society*: 205-225. Cambridge, Mass.: MIT Press.

Arras, J. D. & Dubler, N. N. 1995. Introduction: ethical and social implications of high-tech home care. In Arras, J. D. & Dubler, N. N. (Eds.), *Bringing the hospital home. Ethical and social implications of high-tech home care*. Baltimore: Johns Hopkins University Press: 1-35.

Berg van den, J. H. 1969. *Medische macht en medische ethiek*. (Medical power and medical ethics) Nijkerk: Callenbach.

Callon, M. and Rahebarisoa, V. 1998. Reconfiguring the illness trajectory: the case of neuromuscular diseases. Unpublished Work.

Dufrenne, M. 1964. The aesthetic object and the technical object. *J Aesthetics Art Crit*, 23(1): 113-122.

Duwell, M. 1999. Aesthetic experience, medical practice, and moral judgement. Critical remarks on possibilities to understand a complex relationship. *Med Health Care Philos*, 2(2): 161-168.

Goldberg, A. I., Alba, A. A., Oppenheimer, E. A., & Roberts, E. 1990. Caring for mechanically ventilated patients at home. *Chest*, 98(6): 1543.

Kampelmacher, M. J., Rooyackers, J. M., & Lammers, J. W. 2001. CBO guideline 'Oxygen therapy at home'. *Ned.Tijdschr.Geneeskd.*, 145(41): 1975-1980.

Latour, B. & Akrich, M. 1994. A summary of a convenient vocabulary for the semiotics of technology. In Bijker, W. & Law, J. (Eds.), *Making technology/shaping society*. Cambridge, Mass: MIT Press.

Law, J. 1991. Introduction: monsters, machines and sociotechnical relations. In Law, J. (Ed.), *A sociology of monsters. Essays on power, technology and domination*. London: Routledge.

Lawton, J. 2000. The dying process. Patients' experiences of palliative care. London: Routledge.

Noddings, N. 1995. Moral obligations or moral support for high-tech home care? In Arras, J. D. & Dubler, N. N. (Eds.), *Bringing the hospital home. Ethical and social implications of high-tech home care*: 149-166. Baltimore: Johns Hopkins University Press.

NVALT (Nederlandse Vereniging van Artsen voor Longziekten en Tuberculose) 2001. Richtlijnen zuurstof thuis. (*Guidelines for oxygen treatment at home*) http://www.nvalt.nl/

Petty, T. L. 1996. Lungs at home. *Monaldi Arch Chest Dis*, 51(1): 60-63.

Petty, T. L. 2000. Historical highlights of long-term oxygen therapy. *Respir Care*, 45(1): 29-36.

Ruddick, W. 1995. Transforming homes and hospitals. In Arras, J. D. & Dubler, N. N. (Eds.), *Bringing the hospital home. Ethical and social implications of high-tech home care*. Baltimore: Johns Hopkins University Press: 166-180.

Seymour, J. E. 2000. Negotiating natural death in intensive care. *Soc.Sci.Med.*, 51(8): 1241-1252.

Simondon, G. 1985. *Du mode d'existence des objets techniques*. Paris: Aubier.

Von Wright, G. H. 1963. *Varieties of goodness*. New York: Humanities Press.

Walter, T. 1994. *The revival of death*. London/New York: Routledge.

Willems, D. 2000. Managing one's body using self-management techniques: practicing autonomy. *Theor.Med.Bioeth.*, 21(1): 23-38.

Willems, D. 2004. Geavanceerde tghuiszorgtechnologie: morele vragen bij een ethisch ideaal (Advanced home care technology: moral questions about an ethical ideal). In Gezondheidsraad (Ed.), *Signalering ethiek en gezondheid 2004*: Den Haag: Gezondheidsraad. http://www.ceg.nl/

Perhaps tears should not be counted but wiped away
On quality and improvement in dementia care

Ingunn Moser

There is a growing concern with the quality of practice in health care. But how to attend to the quality of practice, and of care practices in particular, in meaningful ways?

Increasingly, the question of quality in health care is becoming linked to a form of evaluation that works by proving and aims to convince outsiders (politicians, health administrators, insurances, publics) that something is efficient and worth paying for. As such it shifts the focus away from *improving* onto *proving* and accounting (Mol 2006).

This method of accounting was developed in a specific context, – that of the need for regulation and cost control of drug development.[1] Drug development involves markets, investments and profits. In this situation, public authorities need to know that their budgets are being well spent, and that people's health and safety is being protected. The question here is how to control such activities while leaving space for the actors to invest in research and development of new therapies. The solution that has emerged is to let pharmaceutical companies carry the burden of proof and publicly demonstrate that their new products are cost-efficient. Evidence in the form of statistically significant values on selected parameters of efficiency is collected in large, randomized, blind clinical trials (RCTs).

Many now doubt how well this method works for drugs.[2] One thing is sure, it certainly does not work for care practices. This does however not mean that in care everything is as it should be. The concern with quality and improvement of practice is legitimate and welcome. But it makes little sense to force the drug model, the RCT model, with its specific versions of evidence and knowledge, on other kinds of health care practices.

This was obvious at a recent meeting about the role of care, and particularly so-called 'environmental approaches' in dementia care in

Norway.[3] After presentations and discussion, a well known professor of geriatric psychiatry exclaimed in a mixture of despair and disillusionment: 'But what shall we do? Count tears?'

From the perspective of care, counting tears makes no sense. Tears ask to be wiped away, not counted. As the overoptimistic claims for a pharmaceutical cure to dementia are dwindling, and care approaches are increasingly recognized, the issue of their quality still remains. Should efforts be geared towards proving that they work in some external and accountable way? Or should it be invested in care practices' own capacities for improvement?

The argument I make here is that an RCT-type of accounting should not be forced on dementia care practices. First, there are no investors, markets, profits, or money. Neither is there an infrastructure for large, randomized clininal trials. Second, the method does not fit. It does not make sense to blind or randomize the prescription of comfort, music therapy, or the Marte Meo Method. It does not make sense to require that its effects be proved independent of (human, subjective) relations, when those relations are precisely what one acts on and through. It does not make sense to require that effects and efficiency should be measured against single and individualized parameters for the health of brains and bodies, when improvements are sought for situations, activities and daily life in wards involving not just single patients and their individual conditions, but fellow patients and carers, too. Dementia on a care ward is not mainly located in individual brains and bodies, but in interactions and daily life. This is also why the question as to whether the brains can be cured or repaired is not the first thing that is relevant. What is urgent in the context of daily care for people with dementia is rather how to make life bearable, and preferably even pleasant and good, here and now.

Instead of becoming obsessed with proving and accounting, I argue that we should trace and articulate ways of attending to quality that are already at work within care practices. Following others, I argue that it is possible to learn from and build on these (Mol 2006, 2008, Pols 2004, 2007, Thygesen 2009). If we turn to dementia care practices on their own terms, we learn that these have nothing to do with proving that they are good or cost-effective. Instead practice revolves around the double aim of finding ways of acting, and creatively *improving* this action and interaction in and as part of daily life, and thereby also improving the daily life and condition(s) of the patients. In order to make practices, relations and daily life conditions available to action and intervention, care approaches mobilize their own specific methods, instruments, analysis and knowledge. However, these are not made for outsiders, but for people who work there. They are not made to reveal, transport and circulate truths about the situation on the ward, but are geared instead towards the persistent improvement of care practices and care interactions.

I develop this argument by working through excerpts from fieldwork on care approaches in dementia care undertaken in two nursing homes in Norway.[4] These made use of a large repertoire of tools and approaches that also pass as 'environmental treatments', including sensory gardens, music therapy and the Marte Meo method. In this chapter I concentrate on the employment of the last of these. The Marte Meo method is a form of interaction and communication therapy that was originally developed in clinical psychology for improving communication between parents and infants. Over the last ten years it has become more widely used in care for people with dementia in Norway and the Nordic countries.[5] The method makes particular use of excerpts of video-recordings of interactions in supervision sessions.[6]

Improving, not proving

Please let me take you to the sheltered ward in nursing home B, where they use this method. What follows is from a Marte Meo supervision session. This means that the staff are working on a situation or activity that has been reported as problematic. The sessions take place in one of the living rooms on the ward. They are focussing on excerpts of videotaped carer-patient interactions. These have been recorded during the last few weeks before the supervision session and then analysed and prepared for presentation by the head nurse, who is trained as a Marte Meo therapist.

The example concerns Mr. Hansen brushing his teeth. Mr. Hansen is 66 and has been diagnosed with severe dementia. It is the very first supervision session in this case. With everyone gathered in a circle around the television, the head nurse presents the agenda. 'You all know Mr. Hansen', she starts, 'and that his ability to care for himself is dwindling, and that he suffers from hallucinations and delusions. Physical care, and particularly now, brushing his teeth, are situations in which Mr. Hansen feels threatened or invaded. So he resists care and exhibits what some of you experience as 'challenging behaviour'. There have been episodes when carers have been physically attacked and frightened. 'But Mr. Hansen does not know how to use his toothbrush nor how to proceed with the task himself. So what do we do? Research tells us that neglect of dental care in nursing homes often leads to toothache, problems with eating and undernourishment as well as 'challenging behaviour' because many patients cannot identify and express their irritation. Therefore doing nothing, skipping it or leaving it for the next shift are not options. It is our responsibility to find a solution and work out a shared way of going about it so that the situation becomes recognizable, predictable and safe for Mr. Hansen.

The head nurse turns on the video recorder. Everyone looks at the television. We see Mr. Hansen in his room with one of the carers. The camera zooms in and focuses on Mr. Hansen's face. The head nurse freezes the picture and comments: 'Look at his face and eyes: what do they express? How is Mr. Hansen doing? He is irritated or angry, isn't he? He is talking to himself'. She starts the film again. The picture zooms out and the head nurse comments: 'Look, he is focussing on the floor or on something we cannot see. He is not present in the situation with the carer. So how can she establish contact with him and call him back?' Then we see the carer coming out from the bathroom, approaching Mr. Hansen and calling him by his name. Mr. Hansen recognizes his name and looks up. She repeats it. The tone is mild and friendly. Mr. Hansen responds with a 'yes!', straightens up and comes towards her. She reaches out and lays her hand on his arm. He looks at her and she responds to him by smiling and holding his arm. She says: 'I will help you get your teeth brushed'. The head nurse stops the film again and points out how the carer uses both verbal and non-verbal means to get Mr. Hansen's attention. In addition to calling his name and naming the activity they are about to start, she uses her voice, eyes, facial expressions, gestures as well as physical contact to try to establish a friendly and safe relationship, and to make sure he knows she is there and sees him, and that he has relevance for her.

The film continues. The head nurse interprets and articulates what is happening: The carer guides Mr. Hansen to the bathroom with a supporting arm, eye contact, and naming and describing what they are doing. In front of the sink Mr. Hansen looks into the mirror, where he first sees himself and then her. The carer smiles and says: 'There you are, and here I am'. The carer resumes contact by looking at him in the mirror, and for a moment they look at and acknowledge each other. When she comes back with the toothbrush, he lets her brush his teeth. There is no problem. The carer keeps talking calmly while she is brushing his teeth. In this way she actively maintains the relationship and the contact. She carries him along by talk that recognizes and supports him. Mr. Hansen tries to say something and the carer acknowledges that it hurts and is uncomfortable. Perhaps his gums are sensitive. Just need to do it a little bit longer, and then they will be done. Mr. Hansen shifts, stirs, and turns his head away. The carer stops brushing to give him a break and the opportunity to speak. She waits a little and starts again. She gives more support and guidance: 'You are doing very well! Now you can just spit into the sink and rinse your mouth'. She hands him a glass of water. Even if Mr. Hansen no longer knows how to use a toothbrush or brushing his teeth, he seems to recognize what is happening, and can do the last part, rinsing his mouth, on his own. The carer praises him and concludes the activity: 'That was good, wasn't it, to have your teeth brushed! Now we are done'.

This story in which brushing Mr. Hansen's teeth is made into the object of video-recording and supervision illustrates what a care approach to dementia works *for*; it is about *improving* rather than *proving* the 'good' of care practice. However, *how* does it do this, precisely? In what follows I focus on this in detail, for the particularities, practicalities and even technicalities of care practices are all crucial. As is often the case, the devil is in the detail.

To start, I would like to draw attention to how the head nurse guides her colleagues by introducing, commenting and analysing the video. The exercise directs their attention and tells them what to look for and how. It also articulates the process by adding words to what is happening. It points out and articulates elements of the interaction around the brushing of Mr. Hansen's teeth that are usually enmeshed in hectic practical and bodily activities. It breaks the interaction down into its components, or at least a selection of them; emphasizes some of these; demonstrates how they interact and interfere with one another; articulates how they are mobilized; and suggests how one might build on and activate them in a better way, and for the better, in care interactions on the ward. In this way it makes care practice an object of collective reflection and improvement.

Next the story from the fieldwork reveals the importance of the video camera and recording. Video has become a commonly used instrument, not only in various clinical therapeutic approaches, but also as evidence in the court room, in nursing education, and in leadership training. It is important in this context because it mediates and renders the elements of interactions in dementia care, and of care skill in general, visible, present, and available in new ways. So what does this mean and how does it work?

First, the recordings literally bring the handiness, attitude and relational capacities that are all so important to care work, but which are difficult to pin down, yet alone articulate, out as distinct, embodied, material and practical skills. Thus if, as is often argued, human relations, are the most important tools in dementia care, it appears that these have to do with the positioning and disposition of bodies in relation to one another. With posture, gesture, physical touch and manual guidance, with the use of voice and pitch, eye contact and facial expression, and with pace, rhythm and turn-taking in communication and interaction. Likewise, attitudes are exhibited as very physical, embodied and concrete rather than as an ideal and abstract. Moreover capacities for caring that are usually seen to be innate and subjective are externalized and de-subjectivized. The film clippings thus foreground the embodied and choreographic aspects of care, that involve relating, coordination and synchronization, management of proximity and distance, and the creation of conditions for co-presence.

Second, the video camera allows the head nurse to focus on and trace minute details of interactions in relative isolation, that is to say, to disentangle them from the ongoing flux, the dynamics and the often chaotic life on a care ward. It becomes possible to freeze, slow down, rewind and review the interactions later – and if necessary over and over again. However, beyond that, the video technology also makes it possible to reintroduce the interactions to the carers involved in objectified form. It also allows them to take distance from behind the camera, and see and relate to the interactions from the outside, as objects for collective reflection and analysis. Moreove, the video recordings also work as a trigger for experimenting, and for rendering abstract things present and accessible. For instance, this happened later in the same meeting when toothbrushes were handed out and everyone was encouraged to assume the role of patient as well as carer to experience what it is like to have someone try to get into your mouth with a stick, and to experiment with ways of positioning and providing support when brushing someone else's teeth.

One more way in which the video camera and films make care relations and care skills visible and available deserves mention. Care relations and care skills are already available in theory. One can for instance read about them in books about interaction therapies in psychology, and in nursing theory. Using different styles, philosophers and ethnographers also articulate care practices and goals and help to make them available for reflection.[7] However, unlike psychology, nursing theory, philosophy and ethnography, which all use words and texts, the film and guided analysis make the contents of dry volumes on the topic of care available in a manner that can be easily accessed and shared in the middle of everyday care practices.

Improvements in and through interactions in daily life

This starts to show how a care approach involving the Marte Meo method and video-supported supervision works, and what it works *for*. However, what kind of improvement does this entail? What does it work *at*, and *through*? These are the issues I now address. To think about them I will introduce another story from the ward.

It is a morning shift, the nurses are busy helping people get up and get ready for breakfast, and I follow them around. We arrive at Mrs. Andersen's, whose morning care routine has been experienced by many carers as quite troublesome, if not 'challenging'. The problem is that Mrs. Andersen, who is about 80 years old, starts crying, screaming and becoming verbally aggressive with carers when they perform nursing activities such as washing, dressing, and moving her into her wheelchair. All the way through this she screams 'ow, ow, ow, ow...'. It is difficult to know the reason, and difficult to know what to do. It may be that moving her body, or parts of her body, after a night in bed, causes her pain or upsets her.[8] Pain relief has been tried, but does not help – on its own. Perhaps she is also afraid, either of pain or because she does not recognize the situation and understand what is about to happen. Or she might simply find it uncomfortable to be stripped of her warm duvet, washed all over, rolled over, washed again, rolled back, dressed, strapped in a lifting device, moved to the toilet, and then lifted over into a wheelchair. Mrs. Andersen screams and swears. The head nurse therefore contacted her relatives and asked for permission to make her morning care routine the subject of a series of video-recordings and Marte Meo supervision sessions. By the time I arrive to do fieldwork, they have already been working on it for a while and feel that they have made quite some progress.

When she enters Mrs. Andersen's dimly lit room, the nurse walks over to the bed, bends over, gets close to Mrs. Andersen's face and softly wishes her good morning. Mrs. Andersen opens her eyes, looks up at the carer, and responds by wishing the carer a good morning, too. 'Would you like us to let some light and sun into your room?', the carer asks, and Mrs. Andersen nods. The carer walks around the bed and draws the curtains back. Then she goes to the bathroom to prepare for the morning care routine. Looking around in Mrs. Andersen's room, I become aware of a few notes on the wall behind the head of her bed. Three in all, they include guidelines about physical care plus the lyrics of two old popular songs.

The guidelines say that Mrs. Andersen needs predictability, safety, and understanding. They urge everyone to follow the instructions carefully in order to build a shared and recognizable way of getting through the morning care routine and other nursing activities. The aim, it states, is to prevent unrest and anxiety in relation to physical care. The instructions are as follows: start with a form of 'relational warming up', for instance by saying her name and greeting her close up with a 'good face' and sustaining smile before proceeding. Make sure she has seen and heard you. Then make sure Mrs. Andersen knows what is about to happen. Describe what you are doing, and do not stray from the situation here and now. Do not ask questions, do not introduce other things from outside the here and now, and do not bring up too many things at once – one thing at a time. Give ample support and recognition during each action. In addition, use music and singing. Involve her in singing her favourite songs. If necessary, use one of the CDs on her coffee table.

The carer returns from the bathroom with Mrs. Andersen's teeth, bends over again and says: 'Here you have your teeth first. Push them up with your tongue... That's it... So, then, are you ready, Mrs. Andersen, for your morning wash?' Mrs. Andersen looks up into her face and says 'yes...' The carer starts to hum a song and brings some water and a towel to Mrs. Andersen's bedside. 'How does that song go again, about the girls from Bergen', she asks aloud. She starts with the first verse, and waits for Mrs. Andersen to join in and continue with the next. And Mrs. Andersen does, when the carer starts, she completes the verses. The carer brings out a facecloth and, in between the singing, says in passing that she will just wash her face a little. Mrs. Andersen starts crying 'ow, ow, ow, ow...' but when the carer starts singing she also gets caught up in singing again and completes the verse while the carer finishes the washing. The carer tells her that she is going to take off her vest. Mrs. Andersen starts moaning and screaming, but gets caught up in singing once again. The carer washes her upper body and gently raises her arms to wash underneath. She then tells her that she will have to turn her over to wash her back. '...turn over', repeats Mrs. Andersen. '- Are you ready?', asks the carer. 'Yes, to turn around', answers Mrs. Andersen. 'Can you sing me a song?', asks the carer, 'you are such a good singer, Mrs. Andersen'. Mrs. Andersen gets going again. The carer turns Mrs.

Andersen over towards her own body and holds her steady with one arm while washing her with the other. Mrs. Andersen gets turned over again, and then gets dressed. Getting clothes over her head and arms is difficult and it is probably also painful. Mrs. Andersen begins crying and at one point curses the carer. Getting up in the lift and over into the wheelchair is no better. The carer moves the lift closer, tells Mrs. Andersen to grasp hold of her, swings her legs down and her body up, supports her with one arm while putting the belt around her back with the other. Soon she is standing strapped up in the lift and is swung over into the wheelchair. All along she repeatedly gets caught up in singing the verses and chorus of one of the songs on the wall. 'Then we are almost don'e, says the carer, 'except for your hair, which needs brushing, and some perfume and lipstick!... So, now you look pretty! Lipstick and all!' Mrs. Andersen laughs and smiles and stretches out for the carer. 'You are a good one, well done, Mrs .Andersen', says the carer and returns the smile. 'We are all through now.'

The story from Mrs. Andersen's morning care routine shows more of how caring with the Marte Meo method works, and works a great deal. Things have improved. As the carers themselves put it, they have made considerable progress. However, how does it happen? What does it work at and through?

According to the traditional medical approach, there is nothing to be done about dementia. It cannot be cured. What I want to pick up on in the story above, however, is how in this care setting dementia is not primarily located and targeted in a deficient, individualized brain, but in interactions in daily life – and in care practices and interactions as part of daily life in particular.

This does not mean that dementia is not a reality that carers have to relate to, and an objective condition they are confronted with. The use of diagnostic labels such as 'challenging behaviour' and 'suffering from hallucinations and delusions' suggests that it is.[9] As with many conditions that people have to learn to live with these days, a cure or restored health are unattainable goals. Yet, in a dementia care setting, as with Mrs. Andersen, it is still not an option to let go and 'let nature take its course'. There are limits – but one cannot *not* act. In this situation, carers take upon themselves the challenge of making life with dementia *bearable*, and hopefully also *good* and pleasant, but at least *better* than if care were neglected. For this they invent ways of acting and improving in and through interactions in daily life. The Marte Meo method is one such way of acting – and a quite powerful one – in that it, as we have already seen, makes care relations and interactions available in new ways.

In this turn to daily life with dementia, the object of dementia care is framed in a different and much wider way than it is in the traditional, medical approach with its concern with cure. The relevant relations and interactions are no longer limited to intra-organic and neural processes, but are distributed in and across a broader daily life environment. Crucially, however, this does not exclude bodily, intra-organic or even neurological relations that can be targeted for instance through medication. In the case of Mrs. Andersen, pain killers were also introduced. Indeed, they were the first agents to be tested, and are still a part of Mrs. Andersen's morning care routine. They are present in the form of a sticking plaster that a nurse has gently, and more or less unnoticed by Mrs. Andersen, slipped on. Thus while attempts to make sense of care approaches often produce an opposition between 'medical' on the one hand, and 'care' or 'environmental' approaches on the other, or between 'pharmacological' and 'non-pharmacological' interventions, this is not necessarily the case in practice. Care approaches include, but do not restrict themselves to these so-called intra-organic relations.

Beyond this, the focus and object of dementia care approaches, and of the Marte Meo method in particular, not only include individual patients in their daily life environment. It includes carers, and sometimes other patients as well. Crucially, the focus is on the 'inter-action', that is, what is between, and either connects or disconnects, rather than on either one of the actors alone. The video-recordings are instrumental in this way of framing and refocusing, as well as letting relations appear as material and practical concrete instances rather than abstract concepts. What we learn from the cases of both Mrs. Andersen and Mr. Hansen is that critical elements in such interactions include verbal as well as non-verbal communication, exchanges, pace, rhythm and synchronization between actors and between the activities they are involved in. However, these interactions also involve elements and objects, other than the human actors, including facecloths, lifting devices, wheelchairs, medications, and procedures, that are mobilized along with voices, postures, and predictability. In addition, sometimes other elements, from the patient's history, such as music, are introduced.

The approach tries out and tests the qualities of each and every one of these elements in care interactions, but also the qualities of their interferences and interactions. Does music and singing, for instance, fit well with washing and morning care routines? Obviously, yes. Further, the approach not only tests them, it acts on, tinkers with, manipulates, works through and so *qualifies* any one of these individual elements in the interaction. For instance, the carers try a selection of facecloths with different textures until they find one that is softer and better. They introduce different forms of night clothing and jackets or blouses instead of pullovers. They employ different techniques and technologies for moving people. They experiment with different ways of positioning and establishing contact. They test different genres of music and ways of introducing, recorded or 'live'. In this way, step by step, meticulously and persistently, caring with Marte Meo works to lay down building blocks for a better and improved way of getting on, getting through difficult activities, and getting through the day.

Improving care practice(s), improving condition(s) for patients

The focus so far has been on the skills and capacities of the carers; how the use of the Marte Meo method make these visible and accessible in new ways; and how they are mobilized to improve care interactions, and thereby, daily life on the ward. However, improving the state of care practice also serves the further aim of improving the state and condition(s) of the individual patient. To see how the Marte Meo method mediates the patient and what possibilities this offers for engaging with the patient's condition, I return to my fieldwork and to Mr. Hansen and Mrs. Andersen.

When I reviewed the earlier video-recordings of Mrs. Andersen's morning care routine and discussed them with the head nurse, she explained that the idea is that it is the patient who provides the clues for the solution. What she looks for when analysing the videos is any sign or initiative by the patient or perhaps just a moment of contact they can pick up on.

In one of the recordings, a carer entered the picture and softly wished Mrs. Andersen, who was just waking up, good morning, and asked whether she would like to get up. Mrs. Andersen responded drowsily. However, when the carer came up to her with a facecloth in her hand and gently started washing her face, Mrs. Andersen immediately started crying and moaning: 'ow, ow, ow, ow...'. The carer tried to comfort her: 'Only a little. I will be careful. Only a little now...' Mrs. Andersen kept crying. Then the carer took Mrs. Andersen's hand: 'Hello, Mrs. Andersen!', got close to her face, laughed and smiled: 'Didn't you see me?' Mrs. Andersen was screaming throughout, but what the head nurse picked up on was the glimpse of contact when the carer took Mrs. Andersen's hand, got closer and realized she had not seen her or realized what was going on. The action just rolled over her. This was how they started working on what in the guideline for Mrs. Andersen's morning routine is called 'relational warming up'.

Similarly in the case of Mr. Hansen: When the head nurse began the video-taping of the first supervision session of tooth-brushing, the focus of attention was Mr. Hansen. The camera zoomed in as the head nurse was trying to capture his facial expressions, and not least, his eyes to determine how he was doing and how he was feeling, but also what he was doing and where his attention was focussed. The video showed his eyes and bodily attitude, tilted and directed at something on the floor, in a serious discussion with himself or some absent protagonist. The head nurse's interpretation was that he was not present in the situation with the carer, but involved in some other activity or perhaps visiting other spaces and realities in his mind. The question she posed to the collective of carers and colleagues was how to get in touch with him, draw him back or in some way create a shared reality in order to be able, and allowed, to perform necessary care activities. How does one build such a bridge? The excerpt from the video-recording shows one successful instance of a carer who, by verbal and non-verbal means, made contact, enticed Mr. Hansen into following her into a strange and possibly frightening activity, and carried him through it. However, perhaps other carers have other experiences they can build on?

Responding to the head nurse's invitation to share experiences, some carers relate that they have managed to get in touch with Mr. Hansen by talking about and engaging him in football. They know Mr. Hansen used to be a professional football referee. When he speaks to himself and addresses them in often unintelligible ways, he seems to be in a world of football and is probably reliving and performing his old professional role. In asking and talking about the local football team, they have tried to meet him in his own arena, and managed to connect through themes he takes a positive interest and engages in. Other carers bring in the experiences with the use of music and singing from Mrs. Andersen's morning care routine. Could this be of value in Mr. Hansen's case, too? Even if Mr. Hansen does not respond to or take part in music therapy sessions in the same way as Mrs. Andersen, he does respond when they hum or sing a verse from a local supporter's song.

What this shows is that in recording, analysis and supervision sessions, as much attention is paid to the patient, and her agency and her capacities, as to those of the carers. While the carers are indeed busy devising strategies for creating common ground and connections, they are not the only active ones. The practices they engage in not only offer patients positive identification, predictability and safety, and they not only entice and carry patients through unpleasant or frightening activities in more convenient ways. As if all agency resided with the professionals, whereas patients were only passively acted upon and led by the hand, exerting no other form of agency than resistance or 'challenging behaviour'. Instead I want to suggest that the method allows a different and more lively patient to emerge.

Again, the possibilities offered by the video-recordings are crucial: by disentangling interactions from the ongoing flux, dynamics and chaos of life on the ward; by making it possible to isolate and focus in on the individual patient; and by not granting privilege to the verbal over non-verbal, embodied and practical communication. The repeated recordings in combination with analysis and collective reflection in supervision sessions show patients acting, speaking and taking the initiative. Carers are enabled to see and hear and read their patients in ways they earlier could not.[10]

The case is parallel to what Nick Lee argues in an article on the use of videos in court cases with testimonies by children (2000). Here the role of video was to introduce the possibility for children to have a voice and agency rather than needing professionals to represent them and make their bodies speak. In our case the role of videos is to allow the possibility for patients with dementia to sign, speak and act rationally and meaningfully rather than having health professionals translate their bodily conditions for them into: severe dementia, hallucinating, displaying challenging behaviour.

What I want to add is that it is not only the patient with agency, voice and subjectivity who is mediated and made visible and present in new ways through the use of video, but it is also the conditions of possibility of this patient, and of agency, voice and subjectivity, too. The recordings show how conditions that used to enable, may turn out to disable people with dementia – as well as how a care approach to dementia may work to improve the *conditions for* and so the *condition* of individual patients.

What emerges from the video-recordings for instance is that the speed and pace at which most of the interaction in care occurs is a constant source of frustration (and the so-called 'challenging behaviour'). Things simply move too quickly; there is often no time for real exchange or dialogue, in which the patient is offered the possibility of responding in one way or another – whether verbally or nonverbally. By the time the patient reacts, the conversation and the carer have moved on. Or there are mismatches, problems with coordination and synchronization. There is a need to 'warm up', establish a link and shared reality, before moving on and proceeding with a task. Moreover, environments and activities that were once familiar become strange and opaque.

Yet the videos also show that creative, adaptive and tinkering strategies of care can work out successfully. Efforts to arrange for and build on the initiatives and capacities of the patient can and do manage to engage the patient. Local popular songs engage and carry Mrs. Andersen through her morning routine, and engaging Mr. Hansen with football talk and football songs offers him a position which he gladly adopts, and in which he happily takes part in any interaction. In such instances, he can become quite talkative and express his fear as well as gratitude without the usual 'word-salad'. Mr. Hansen's expressive 'thank you!!' following the tooth-brushing is memorable. Mrs. Andersen likewise reaches out to hold the carer's hands or face, smiles and makes jokes.

What happens here is that on the basis of the agencies, initiatives and communicative abilities of patients that become visible through Marte Meo recordings and supervision sessions, patients are invited and placed in positions of interaction in which they are acknowledged as actors and subjects (Moser 2009). This goes beyond offering positive identification, recognition, predictability and safety. What the carers are involved in here is the creation of, arrangements for, testing and establishing of conditions – and better and improved conditions – not only for necessary care activities, and for smooth and convenient life on the ward, but for sustaining patient capacities for agency, voice and subjectivity (Thygesen 2009).

The practice of the Marte Meo method in dementia care thus mediates and makes possible, not only a different and improved care practice, but different and improved conditions for the patient and life with a disease such as dementia. As the head nurse stated: 'We sometimes get a whole new patient'.

Knowledge is not about gathering facts and truths, but a tool in improving care

The stories and analyses have shown that a care approach makes use of method, analysis, knowledge and technology when attending to quality. However, they have also demonstrated that it does so within a logic and horizon of ongoing improvement of practice and daily life that differ in certain respects from that of the sciences and present-day requirements for evidence in medicine. The next question then is *how* it differs, but also what this makes of knowledge, and what the role of knowledge might be in this context and practice.

Here is a final story from the use of the Marte Meo method on the dementia care ward. When the head nurse had reached the conclusion that something had to be done about Mr. Hansen's tooth-brushing, and that they would try with the Marte Meo method, she first spent three rather frustrating weeks recording before she finally had (enough) material that they could start working on. As I have already suggested, the point of recording is not to document the situation on the ward, nor show how difficult it is, and how often things go wrong, but to illuminate the tiny bits and elements that do work, and then to use these as building blocks for better and improved patterns of interaction. It may only be a glimpse of positive contact, and an outsider would probably not even see it until it was pointed out. In the case of Mr. Hansen, it was a bit different: Suddenly, after three weeks of resistance or non-compliance, he gave his permission without any problem and gave the nurse access to his mouth. Suddenly brushing his teeth was ok, and not a problem. The question then was why, what happened, and how? Then the head nurse returned to the films again to study how this was built up. The edited excerpts she showed in the supervision meeting were a tiny and carefully chosen fraction of the tapes, those that focused on positive elements that might make the building blocks of a solution to the problem.

Further, the supervision meeting was not an isolated event, but an element in a process: meetings are repeated, there are three or four or more. The regular meetings drive the process onwards. Each identifies a set of issues that are brought up through the collective analysis and engagement with video-recordings. As we have seen in the case of brushing Mr. Hansen's teeth, the issues that came up during the first meeting concerned the establishment of contact and a shared space, a more supportive position during tooth-brushing, and better timing of the activity. Based on the discussion of each of these, the carers arrived at and agreed on a preliminary strategy for how to better facilitate brushing Mr. Hansen's teeth. These elements were then to be tested over a certain period of time until the next meeting. The aim, as we have seen, was to arrive at a shared way of proceeding and with provisional guidelines for everyone involved in care.

At the same time, and as part of this process, knowledge is gathered and fed into the process by way of different instruments, logs and records. These include standardized tests of mental status, depression and wellbeing; the patient/nursing record, the cardex; and often extra research into the history of the patient as well. In addition, a 24-hour deviation log is introduced a week or two before the Marte Meo process is started. This procedure logs and codes various forms of unrest, aggression or other 'challenging' or 'deviant' behaviour on an hourly basis. It produces a collection of maps of behavioural patterns, and changes in patterns, for instance of sleep and activity, unrest and agitation, based on colour codes. It gives an easy and powerful overview, both of the actual current situation and development over time – indeed, over weeks and months.

In the case of Mr. Hansen, the head nurse also introduced an extra log for registering results during tooth-brushing. This was posted on the inside of the cupboard in the patients' bathroom. Every day, morning and evening the responsible carer was required to tick off whether the action has been carried out, and whether the result is good, partial, or unsuccessful. If unsuccessful, a reason has to be stated as well as how many times the action has been attempted, and at what times.

For the next meeting, then, there is data, and there are new recordings. The recurring recordings again focus on and explore moments of positive contact and interaction. In the next supervision meeting on tooth-brushing, for instance, the excerpts of the recording show a nursing student drawing on her background as a dentist's assistant and gently leading Mr. Hansen into a chair, positioning herself behind him, letting him rest his head in her arm and maintaining eye contact and a comfortable overview of things while she brushes his teeth. Mr. Hansen is all sunshine. In this way the film clippings, the recurring recordings, also demonstrate changes, progress, and improvement. They may not *document* this in a way that is scientifically recognized, but they *demonstrate* for the carers that acting on and through interaction in daily life works.[11]

Similarly, in commenting on the significance of the logs and the collection of data, the head nurse first mentions that the rationale is to know whether the actions suggested in supervision meetings are having the desired effects, or if they have to try something else. However, then she quickly adds: 'But also so that we can all *see* the progress demonstrated before our very eyes. It is very motivating to see the changes, and to learn that if we work systematically to seek solutions with the patient and in interactions, and lay down a shared way of going about it, we sometimes get a whole new patient'.

The argument I develop here then is that the engagement in the Marte Meo method, and the use of video-recordings and gathering the data that it entails, is not primarily about providing documentation or evidence in the narrow sense. For this reason the supervision meeting differs from the academic seminar or practice of collective autoethnography that is reminiscent of; collecting data and documentation differs from academic research and truth-driven medicine; and the use of video deliberately omits most of the data. They are not designed to produce the same result over and over again, not meant to establish the truth about a given and definite reality, but to change and improve it. As a part of this, all the data produced and collected are fed directly into the process again rather than circulated and processed elsewhere, be it in laboratories or in research networks.

As such dementia care, and the Marte Meo method in particular, do not differ significantly from other clinical practices in which doctor and patient with long-term or chronic conditions by way of a tinkering process arrive at specific measures. Along the way various data are collected and collated. Interventions are tried out and either rejected or followed up. Annemarie Mol has described this as the process of 'doctoring' (2008). In this process, what counts is what works, and works for the better, and so makes an improvement in the specific everyday relations in which the patient is placed. Since the conditions of patients, in a broad sense which includes, but is not limited to bodily conditions, are subject to changes, what works often also changes over time. Working to improve care is therefore necessarily an ongoing effort, requiring a persistent, meticulous, tinkering process of care. It does not make much sense to fix the truth (at one point or another) in this endeavour.

Therefore what does this make of knowledge? The answer is that knowledge is not about facts or truths that are gathered and fixed, but rather a tool or instrument in improving care. Using this line of logic, many things can make relevant and useful knowledge. This is perhaps one reason why it is difficult from the outside to pinpoint what knowledge in care practice is, or for that matter, to define what the knowledge basis of care is. It includes many different traditions, as care is constantly gathering new ideas from various fields – trying them out, rejecting or incorporating them, revising and transforming them. This is certainly the case with the Marte Meo method: In seeking ways to help and improve the life of patients with dementia, carers picked up and tried out a method originally developed in other contexts. In incorporating this tool in and for dementia care, they also tinkered with and transformed the method itself. From being a psychologist's method in therapeutic work with her individual patients, it has now been lifted out of this bilateral relation and become a collective method and tool with a therapist as facilitator and other carers performing a form of reflexive auto-ethnography in their professional practice. Incorporated into a tradition of nursing and dementia care, the Marte Meo method has been turned into a tool and structure for methodical and systematic improvement of care practice. In a parallel way, music therapy on this ward is not only applied and prescribed individually, by a specialized therapist in relation to his patients, but also incorporated into this process of collective tinkering and collective appropriation and improvement of care skills and competence.

Conclusion

In this article I have traced and articulated one way of attending to quality in dementia care. I have shown how carers mobilize an approach called the Marte Meo method, which employs video-recordings of care interactions and supervision sessions to find ways of acting, and improving the ways of acting, in care for people with dementia. The aim is to improve daily life, thereby making the condition and life bearable, better, and preferably also good, for individual patients. Dementia in these care settings is not so much a matter of individual minds/brains that cannot be repaired as of interactions in and as part of daily life on a ward. The act of caring for people with dementia is therefore a matter of inter-acting and relating. It is a matter of acting on and through the things that connect or disconnect, and which include, but are not restricted to, humans and human relations.

The role and contribution of the video-recordings is to mediate the elements of care skills and care interactions in new ways, and thus to make them visible, present and accessible in new ways. They bring out and foreground the embodied, material, practical and choreographed aspects of care. They externalize and de-subjectivize them, and make them objects of collective reflection and improvement. However, the video-recordings also mediate the patients in new ways. They show patients with dementia acting, speaking and taking initiatives – and enable carers not only to see and hear and read their patients in new ways, but also to find ways of persistently and creatively improving the conditions for – and so the conditions of – individual patients. In so doing, the method, with the technologies, instruments, analyses and knowledge it sets in motion, transforms not only the care practice, but the object of the practice – the disease and the patient living with the disease.

However, this means that the trajectory of a life with dementia is no longer simply given and determined. Instead, people live – and die – with dementia in better or worse ways, and are treated and cared for in better or worse ways. In its better forms, dementia care practice persistently strives to create conditions for and enable better interaction, and also to afford people with dementia positions in which they can act and exert valued forms of subjectivity. In these approaches, a patient as well as a life with dementia emerges in ways that are less determined. This means she is less determined by the disease, she is not gone, lost, sailed away, or beyond reach, but acting and speaking in meaningful ways. Care approaches make the assumed one-way downward trajectory of, and life with, dementia available, and to a certain extent, even capable of being shaped. By tinkering, testing, trying out and qualifying every element that makes a part of and goes into the interactions of daily life, they demonstrate that care matters. There is no need to resign and let nature take its course. Moreover, there is no need to push RCT types of evaluating and accounting in dementia care practice either. Directing efforts into accounting and proving efficiency redirects attention away from sustaining capacities for improvement. Instead, as this article argues, we should rather relate to and build on what is already there, in care, and cultivate and articulate practices of improvement. We should foster reflection that is not just critical, but also creative.

Acknowledgements

I would like to express my gratitude towards the nursing homes that gave me access to conduct fieldwork for studying care approaches to dementia, as well as the staff and patients who gave me access to their daily life and worlds. Further I am indebted to the Norwegian Research Council for the post-doctoral grant that made this research possible and to my colleagues in the larger collaborative project 'Nature in Science, Politics and Everyday Practices' at the Centre for Technology, Innovation and Culture, University of Oslo; and John Law and Kristin Asdal for sustained academic collaboration and friendship. Finally I am also grateful to Bettina Sandgathe Husebø, Stein Husebø, Audun Myskja, Raj Gupta, Frode Aas Kristoffersen and Tone K. Sæther Kvamme for discussions of care approaches and nursing home medicine.

Notes

1. Trudy Dehue (1997, 2001) argues in a parallel way that the research design of RCTs is not a matter of timeless logic but developed in the context of expanding bureaucratic management needs, with research serving administrative knowledge making and decision making.

2. See for instance Trudy Dehue (2002, 2004), but also the special issue of Social Studies of Science devoted to the issue, 34 (2) 2004.

3. Environmental therapies or treatments is a term for care approaches to dementia that work on the assumption that dementia is not primarily located in individualized and bounded brains and bodies, but in a wider ecology or network of relations and interactions in daily life. They may for instance take physical environments into account or mobilize sensory gardens, music, food, and physical activity as elements in care. Sometimes these care approaches are designated 'non-pharmacological' or even 'non-medical' interventions, in order to separate them from traditional, curative approaches in medicine. This is however quite misleading, as environmental approaches usually include but do not limit themselves to pharmaceutical interventions.

4. The data were collected in relation with a research project on 'Alzheimer's Disease in Science, Politics and Everyday Care Practices', funded by a post-doctoral grant by the Norwegian Research Council. The project investigated the different and changing versions of Alzheimer's Disease in biomedicine, politics and care, and was based on fieldwork (with participatory observation as well as interviews, informal conversations and document analysis) in sheltered wards in two different nursing homes in Norway in a period of 7 months in 2006-2007. The project was approved by the Norwegian regional research ethical committees (REK-SOR) and the Norwegian Social Science Data Services (NSD). For reasons of anonymity, all names and identifications are fictitious.

5. Marte Meo is a method developed by Maria Aarts in the Netherlands about 25 years ago. Today it is used not only in parent-infant communication, but in many other areas too, including care for people with dementia. See Munch (2005) and Hyldmo (2002).

6. The supervision aims at supporting carers in identifying children's or patients' initiatives, agency and capacities in interactions with them, and to start from and support these when seeking solutions to problems in care. Hence the name Marte Meo: of one's own strength, or mars martis. However, and as will become clearer throughout, what in parent/infant therapy is and remains a tool in the professional's bilateral relation with a client, in dementia care has been taken further and turned into a collective tool for reflection on the professionals' practice.

7. This is a growing body of work, but the work of Mol (2006, 2008) and Pols (2004, 2007) needs mention. On dementia care in particular, see Chatterij 1998, 2006, Harbers, Mol and Stollmeyer 2002, Kontos 2003, 2006, Thygesen 2009.

8. On the issue of pain in patients with dementia, see the work of Bettina Sandgathe Husebø (2008).

9. It should be noted that these labels and ways of speaking contribute to produce a very particular version of the dementia disease, locating the problems in individualized brains and bodies again. This points to the different versions and the coexisting logics simultaneously at work in care practice, and the tensions between them. See Moser (2008).

10 Carers in interview note that the Marte Meo Method have helped them recognise the initiatives and signals of patients with dementia, and put it this way: 'But even if a person has dementia, this does not mean it is empty in there. You just have to find her language'. See Moser (2008).

11 If it does not work every time and with everyone, neither do the pills. Care approaches at least work a great deal.

References

Chatterij, Roma (2006) 'Normality and Difference. Institutional Classification and the Constitution of Subjectivity in a Dutch Nursing Home' in Leibing, Anne and Cohen, Lawrence (eds.) *Thinking about Dementia. Culture, Loss, and the Anthropology of Senility*, New Brunswick: Rutgers University Press.

Chatterij, Roma (1998) 'An Ethnography of Dementia. A Case Study of an Alzheimer's Disease Patient in the Netherlands', *Culture, Medicine and Psychiatry*, Vol. 22, No. 3, pp. 355-384.

Dehue, Trudy (2004) 'Historiography Taking Issue: Analyzing and Experiment with Heroin Abusers', *Journal of the History of the Behavioural Sciences*, Vol.40, No.3, pp. 247-264.

Dehue, Trudy (2002) 'A Dutch Treat: Randomized Controlled Experimentation and the Case of Heroin-Maintenance in the Netherlands', *History of the Human Sciences*, Vol.15, No.2, pp. 75-98.

Dehue, Trudy (2001) 'Establishing the Experimenting Society: The Historical Origin of Social Experimentation According to the Randomized Controlled Design', American Journal of Psychology, Vol. 114, No.2, pp. 283-302.

Dehue, Trudy (1997) 'Deception, Efficiency, and Random Groups. Psychology and the Gradual Origination of the Random Group Design', Isis, Vol. 88, pp. 653-673.

Harbers, Hans, Mol, Annemarie, Stollmeyer, Alice (2002) 'Food matters. Arguments for an Ethnography of Daily Care', *Theory, Culture and Society*, Vol. 19, No. 5/6, pp. 207-226.

Husebø, Bettina Sandgathe (2008) *Assessment of Pain in Patients with Dementia*, PhD Dissertation, Department of Public Health and Primary Health Care, University of Bergen.

Hyldmo, Ida (2002) 'Samspill i focus. Marte Meo metoden i arbeid med personer med demens', *Aldring og Livsløp*, Vol .19, No. 4, pp. 0-11. [Interaction in focus. The Marte Meo method in care for people with dementia' in *Aging and the Course of Life*].

Kontos, Pia (2006) 'Embodied Selfhood. An ethnographic Exploration of Alzheimer's Disease' in Leibing, Anne and Cohen, Lawrence (eds.) *Thinking about Dementia. Culture, Loss, and the Anthropology of Senility*, New Brunswick: Rutgers University Press.

Kontos, Pia (2003) ''The painterly hand': Embodied Consciousness and Alzheimer's Disease'', *Journal of Aging Studies*, Vol. 17, pp. 151-170.

Lee, Nick (2000) 'Faith in the Body? Childhood, Subjecthood and Sociological Enquiry' in Prout, Alan (ed.) *The Body, Childhood and Society*, London: Macmillan.

Mol, Annemarie (2008) *The Logic of Caring*. London: Routledge.

Mol, Annemarie (2006) 'Proving or Improving: On Health Care Research as a Form of Self-Reflection', *Qualitative Health Research*, Vol.16, No.3, pp. 405-414.

Mol, Annemarie (2002) *The Body Multiple. An Ontology of Medical Practice*. Durham: Duke University Press.

Moser, Ingunn (2008) 'Making Alzheimer's Disease Matter: Enacting, Interfering and Doing Politics of Nature', *Geoforum*, Vol. 39, No.1, pp.98-110.

Moser, Ingunn (2005) On Becoming Disabled and Articulating Alternatives: The Multiple Modes of Ordering Disability and their Interferences. *Cultural Studies*, 19, pp.667-700.

Munch, Marianne (2005) 'Marte Meo film-councelling, a supportive communication approach towards elderly with poor communication skills', *Mundo da Saude*, 29 (4).

Pols, Jeanette (2007) Which Empirical Research, Whose Ethics? Articulating Ideals in Long-term Mental Health Care. In Widdershoven, G. et al (eds.) *Empirical Ethics in psychiatry*. Oxford: Oxford University Press.

Pols, Jeanette (2004) *Good Care. Enacting a Complex Ideal in Long-Term Psychiatry*. PhD-thesis, Utrecht: Trimbos Instituut.

Thygesen, Hilde (2009) *Technology and Good Dementia Care: A Study of Technology and Ethics in Everyday Care Practice*. Oslo: Unipub.

The syndrome we care for

XPERIMENT! Bernd Kraeftner, Judith Kroell, Isabel Warner

Introduction

The following article describes the transformation of a research project and its protagonists. The project started five years ago when we (the authors and members of the 'Research Centre for Shared Incompetence') had a brief encounter with a syndrome. Or better, we briefly encountered two experts who spoke of their first hand experience with patients suffering from that syndrome. The meeting sparked our interest in the practices that emerge during the care of those patients.

At the time we were exploring how we might describe science and technology projects to a larger public. For some time we had been playing with the idea of working on decision making and informed consent in health care. (We were having doubts about the political and theoretical soundness of the idea of the 'public understanding of science'.) Informed consent was appealing because it looked as if it might a suitable place to explore the interdependence of 'science' and 'society'. So we met with these two experts, and we were impressed by their anecdotes even though we had not met any of their patients. In particular, we were struck by the fact that the patients suffering from this syndrome could not talk, move and were apparently unconscious for months, and in some cases, years on end. They were legally incompetent persons/bodies who lived in specialized wards supported by various professionals, family members (sometimes), and/or (just occasionally) friends. When we heard about this we immediately wondered: how are decisions made under such circumstances? How is consent achieved between comatose persons and carers?

This may sound rather paradoxical. How can people in coma decide? How can they express consent or dissent? As you may have suspected we are talking here of a syndrome called vegetative state. The term is applied to people who have undergone severe brain injury and subsequently remain in a state of prolonged coma. These are patients who are by definition considered to be devoid of consciousness and awareness. However, during our first encounter with the experts

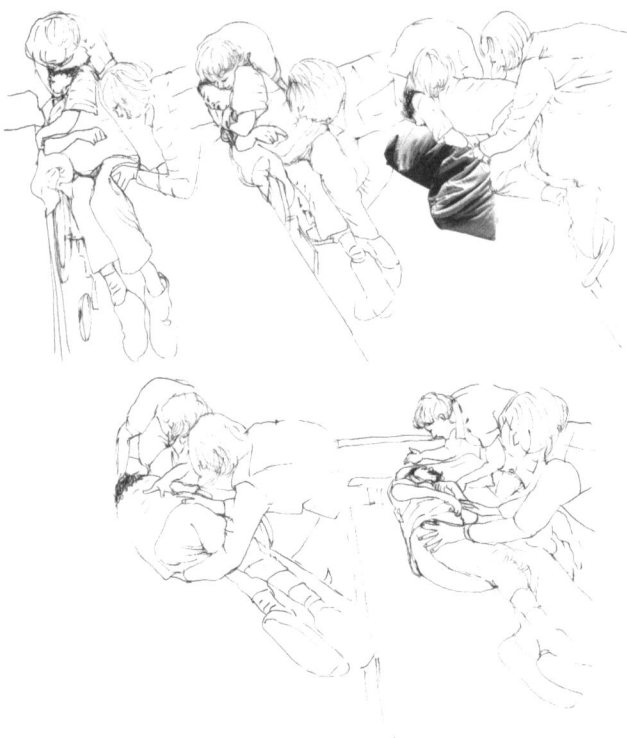

Figure 1: Two nurses 'rolling' a patient from wheelchair into bed.

we also learned that it is not entirely absurd to ask whether those patients are able to take an active part in clinical decision-making.

This is partly because the ambiguities of clinical assessment have led to the (fuzzy) demarcation of an additional syndrome. Called 'minimal conscious state', this reflects the fact that some patients show reproducible but inconsistent evidence of perception, communicative ability or, purposeful motor activity. It is also because care givers who look after 'their' patients daily (and often for years) tend to describe bodily, 'vegetative' symptoms as a kind of deliberate expressive behaviour. They talk, for instance, of sweating, mucus production, muscle spasticity, or the frequency of startle responses in this way. This is how we were introduced to a 'syndrome' that seemed to fit our research agenda.

Why do we talk about the transformation of our research project? To answer this, we want to relate to a dynamic which we became part of when we started our field work. For we started by 'gazing' at patients and their carers, and by making the results of this gaze public. But after a while we found ourselves asking about our motives for entering the field. We wondered about the circumstances in which we would prefer to stay alive rather than to 'vegetate'. We found ourselves immersed in the practical world(s) of the syndrome. And we found ourselves thinking about our relations with patients, carers and the syndrome itself. As a result a new question emerged. We started to wonder about how we could contribute to the 'care of a syndrome'.

In the beginning, of course, we were not concerned with the dynamics of this change, or indeed with 'our' care of the syndrome. Instead we were confronted with patients in need of meticulous care 24 hours a day. So this is how we started: by watching practices of care. And this is where we start now, by focusing on the care for persons and bodies: on *care with moving*.

Moving and being moved.
Imagine a hospital or a nursing home ward. You enter a long corridor with doors to the left and right. Some doors are open, some are closed. None of the staff are around. Walking along the corridor you look into a room and see four to six beds with prominent bed rails. It is quiet and you go in. You step closer to a bed and you recognize a patient almost entirely hidden beneath blankets and support cushions. She lies motionless and silent. You realize that you have started to behave very carefully. You say 'good morning' quietly and unassertively, but you get no answer. You look at her face but there is no reaction. You turn round. Some of the patients are staring at the ceiling. Others seem to be looking at you. But when you look again you can see that there is no eye contact. You turn round again. There is no reaction. It is almost as if you were invisible. How to proceed? You start to think about your own reactions and responses. Should I start to talk or stay quiet? Should I touch her and move her passive limbs? Should I sit down and read her a short story? Should I start to move her out of bed or leave her alone and let her rest? How to handle the situation and these bodies/persons?

We've already said that patients cannot move their bodies. They spend most of their days and nights on their back or on their side, lying on the two square meters of a hospital mattress. The decision to move those bodies/persons, to transfer them from bed to a wheelchair, to train, touch or guide them depends entirely on others. But what are the signs, symptoms or cues that tell the carer that someone needs to be moved? The answer depends on whether the syndrome is tought

CHAPTER 14

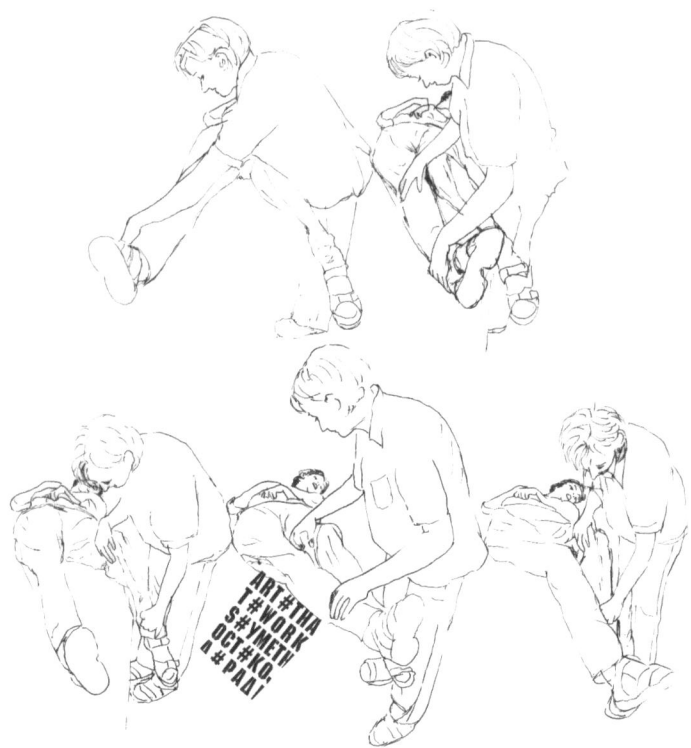

Figure 2: Nurse moving patient to the edge of the bed.

to be in transition, or permanent, and then on whether rehabilitation efforts are considered beneficial, or futile – even harmful. In the first case, of course, the aim is to provide a better 'quality of life': can something be done to improve the condition of the patient or at least prevent deterioration? Whereas in the second case it is a matter of allowing the patient to die in peace: can measures be avoided that might prolong suffering or undermine his or her dignity?

In what follows we describe some scenarios that show that motion or (passive) motor activities of patients are considered to be important and beneficial for patients with the syndrome. Neurologists say that the only neuro-rehabilitative principles with verified effects so far are 'repetition, constraint-induced therapies and endurance'. Nevertheless, please keep in mind that this is not as obvious as it sounds. The behaviour and responses of patients is often minimal and ambivalent. Your own actions tend to erase the cues that might help in reaching mutual 'informed consent', and the latter is an idea that informs how you rather than the patient act. There is certainly no clear-cut plan or 'algorithm' that prescribes how to handle bodies or 'care for moving'.

Scenario 1

'When I enter the room, Patient Green and Patient White are lying on a mat on the floor, and Patient Singer is being moved by the cycling ergometer. Mara, the physiotherapist, is about to move Patient Green through his ranges of motion. However, she does not get very far because she constantly has to come to the aid of Mrs. Green, the wife of Mr. Green; and Mrs. White, the mother of Patient White. Patient White is being leaned headfirst over a big ball. Three persons and six hands try to lift the distorted body and arrange it in a balanced position. Mara has to help everywhere. Transfers from the bed to the

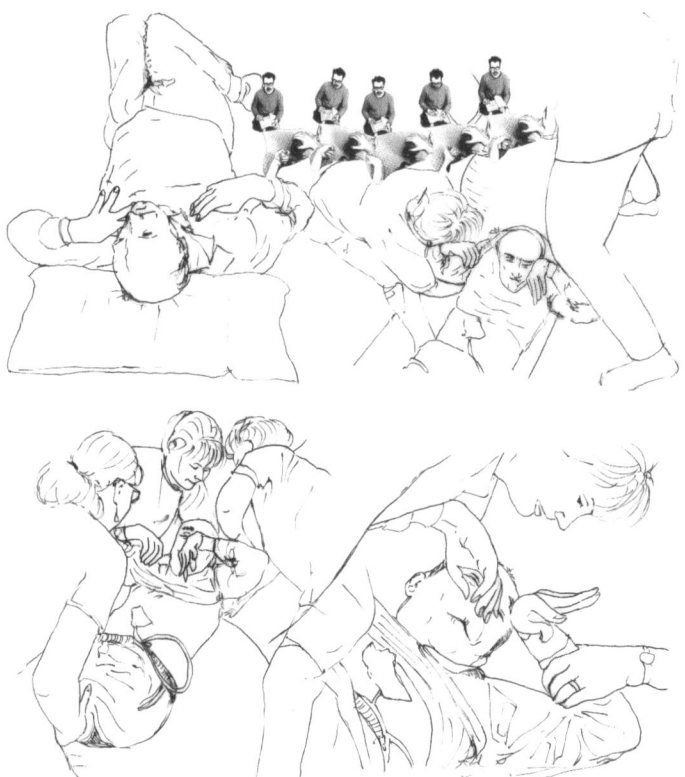

Figure 3: Three family members, with the help of a physiotherapist, exercising transfer techniques

wheelchair, from the bed to the mat on the floor repeatedly take place. Resolute handling, withdrawal reactions, grimaces and ridden up T-shirts. But practice makes perfect and there is a positive spirit in the room.' (field note, 25.11.2004).

Following the advice of the experts, some family members think of 'movement' as therapeutic. However, the physiotherapists are so short of time that they sometimes give priority to patients who lack support from family members or friends. This can cause friction, and relatives may, as Mrs. Green puts it in a leaflet, treat it as a reason for 'taking advantage of the available human resources (physiotherapists) with the help of the relatives'. By advising two or three family members, one physiotherapist can exploit her or his expertise more effectively and work with three to four patients at the same time.

In our conversations with family members, we encounter a range of motives for taking part. These include: the rejection of therapeutic nihilism; the wish to draw on any remaining potential in the patient; the desire to stimulate training and learning; curiosity about experimenting with new techniques and devices; impatience or anger about what goes on in the ward; guilt about missing any chance to help and the experience of solidarity and sociability.

If you were to ask Mara whether any of this was state of the art physiotherapy, in all likelihood she would say no. She would probably say that proper treatment demands skill and experience. All the tugging, pulling, pushing, distorting, and painful gripping needs to be avoided. As well as any incautious handling that works against the resistance of developing muscular spasticity and body tensions. She would probably mention, the danger of occupational illness caused by improper handling. Then she would most likely add that she underestimated the difficulty of all this, and that though she wants to support the relatives, professionals sometimes need to take corrective action, because being active as an end in itself does not always achieve the therapeutic goal. Thus, from the point of view of 'a professional' (here the physiotherapist), how these patients are handled could be called 'non-state-of the-art-practice' or even 'bad care'. This is never made formally clear: accounts, feedback and comments are all unofficial. But here is the question. Could it be that in these circumstances any physical interaction is better than correct handling – the 'good' care – of bodies?

Scenario 2

The nurse bends the body of the young man forward; then she moves his legs and feet out of the bed, pivoting him on his buttocks; finally, she sits down beside the 27 year-old and positions the lower part of his pelvis on her right thigh. She carries him along the edge of the bed to the wheelchair. To move him into the chair, she tries to use the distribution of body mass and tension to minimize her effort. Nevertheless this is an intensive and intimate movement. It takes a lot of effort, and it is best done jointly. The two have known each other for almost 8 years.

The patient cannot move his body by himself. Along with his other symptoms, he suffers from quadriplegia. Both his legs and arms are paralysed, with either increased or decreased muscle tone. It is not clear whether he is aware of his environment. He shows no reactions

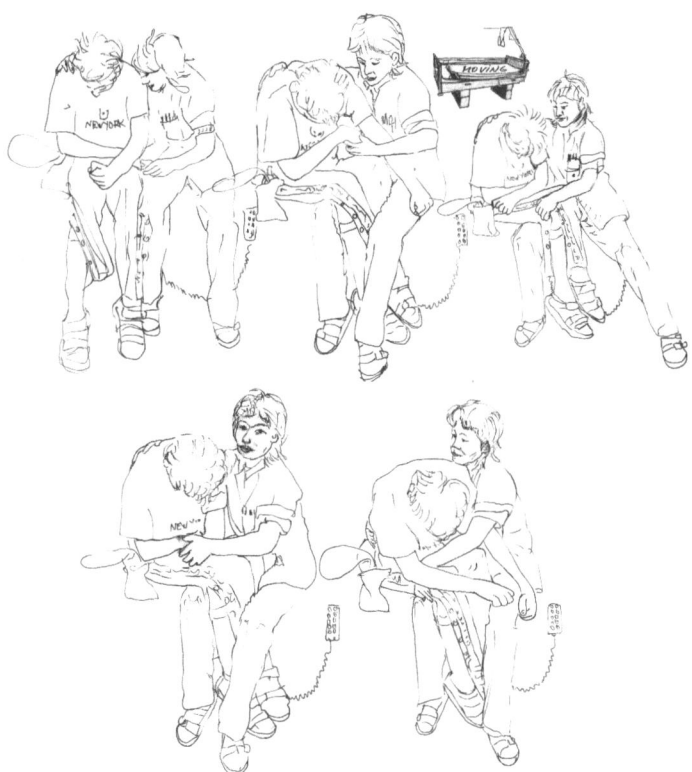

Figure 4: Nurse transferring a patient from bed to wheelchair. part 1

CHAPTER 14

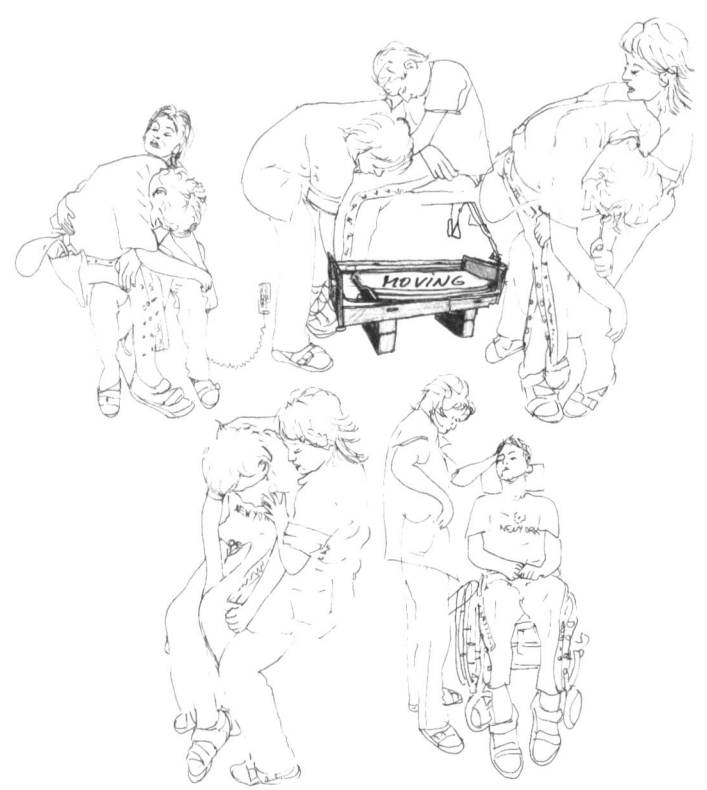

Figure 5: Nurse transferring a patient from bed to wheelchair. part 2

to the presence of various visual, auditory, tactile, olfactory, or gustatory stimuli. But even if he were aware of his environment what would he perceive lying in his bed all day? The assumption that the complete loss of any motor function may lead to or worsen sensory deprivation is a reason for acting for the nursing staff. When his general condition is stable he is moved daily to the wheelchair for up to four hours. He is taken to other places on the ward: to the lounge, to the television outside the room, or, sometimes, to the park for a walk.

Most of the nurses consider human movement to be fundamental to perception, learning and improvement in health. And stimulatory choreography, this skilled touching and moving, guiding and adapting, is taught on costly training courses.

These techniques form an important part of the therapeutic nursing approach developed by the nursing staff over a number of years. Yet, although they are essential to 'professional handling' of these bodies/persons, these practices also lead to contradiction. Sometimes this is explicit. It might take the form of an anonymous letter to the local authority. If this happens it leads to an official investigation. Here is an example:

> (...) In the nursing home P., five patients have suffered severe (bone) fractures since the middle of 2003. (...) These incidents seem to have occurred through inappropriate mobilization techniques. These are vegetative patients, who are unable to move by themselves. They have severe alterations of their joints, muscles and bones. At the ward, they do not approve of lifting devices. Even small and not particularly muscular nurses from the staff have to take patients out of bed, without the aid of lifting devices. (...). But our vegetative patients are not able to help! (...) If one comments and asks if this method is appropriate for these kind of patients, the answer is: 'You can't make an omelette without breaking eggs'. They (...) apply kinaesthetic practices, but nobody asks if these methods are appropriate for this group of patients. (...) At the end of the day, who can be called to account for this?

The letter appears to be written in good faith. The author asks the authorities to attend to a deplorable state of affairs so that further 'side-effect fractures' might be prevented. It is not clear whether the author of the anonymous letter is part of the so-called multidisciplinary team, or a member of a patient's family. For her or him, these incidents show the need to act on behalf of the patients. Here, then, the contradiction is made explicit. Often it is expressed implicitly. For instance by members of the nursing staff who may refuse to use their own bodies (together with those of the patients) as a lifting device, for reasons of health and safety. (Of course, some colleagues in turn disapprove of the way those nurses use mechanical lifting devices.)

In scenario 2 we see it again. Good care may be turned into bad care, depending on who is caring, and whether the syndrome is considered to be a state in transition, or permanent.

Scenario 3

For weeks, Dr. Lippschitz, the ward doctor, has been trying to secure preoperative clearance for reconstructive contracture surgery of Mr. Richards' distorted ankle. A contracture is the stiffening of a joint that prevents it from being moved through its normal range. It can be caused by lack of continuous physiotherapy – for instance the continuous (passive) movement of the ankle and the spastic lower limbs of Mr. Richards. Mr. Richards is legally incompetent, so Mrs. Lippschitz has had to collect statements from the neurologist, the internist and the physiotherapist. These statements have been forwarded by the legal guardian of the patient to the district court. The court has sought expert advice from a surgeon.

Dr. Lippschitz is sitting in the small office of the ward and talking to this surgeon on the phone. After a short conversation, she puts down the receiver. She is angry. She says that his comments imply that the nursing team wants the operation to try to make its life easier; that it has less to do with improving the quality of life of the patient than that of the nursing staff who are, says the surgeon, probably positioning the patient wrongly or not working with him enough.

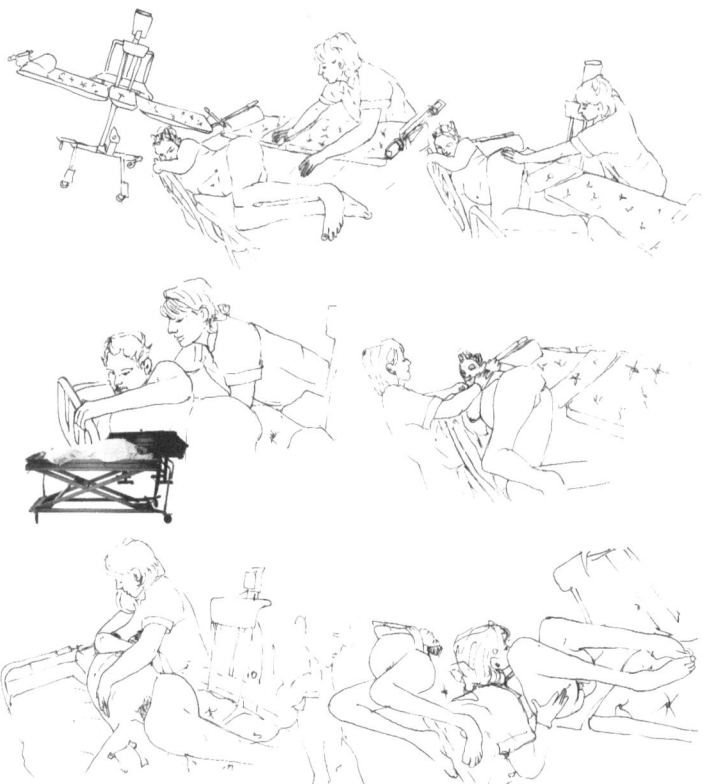

Figure 6: Patient being transferred to a lifting device

Dr. Lippschitz is disappointed. The surgeon is not going to recommend the operation to the court.

Here's how the medical experts voted:

Internal view (ward doctors):

- *Neurologist*: 'Yes' ('the operation will have no negative effects on the neurological status')
- *Internist (Dr. Lippschitz herself)*: 'Yes' ('there are no objections to the planned medical intervention from the perspective of the internal specialists'.)
- *Physiotherapy specialist*: 'No, but' ('conservative measures not promising – except for optimal and optimized positioning. Notable perioperational risk, however, this has to be evaluated by the surgeon')

External view (consultation):

- *Surgeon*: 'No'

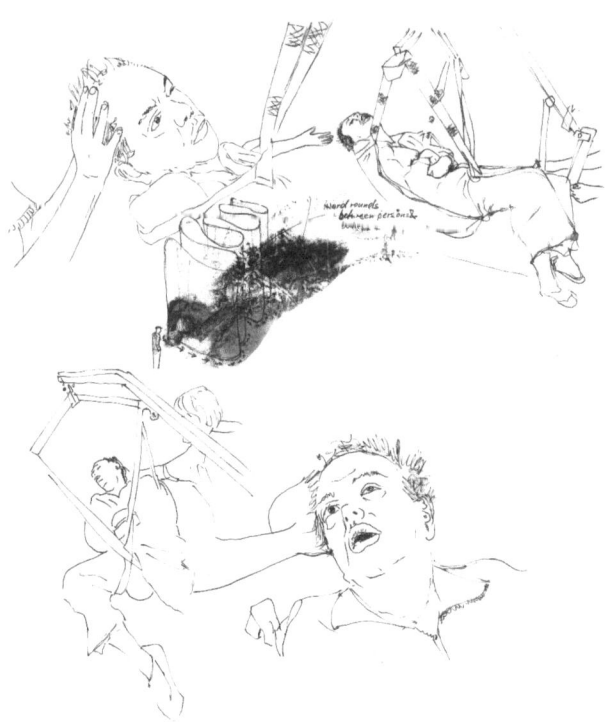

Figure 7: Patient being transferred by means of a lifter

But it is more complicated. The ward doctors are not seeking the operation because of the distorted ankle. The initiative has come from the nursing staff. Dr. Lippschitz knows that the nurses are closest to the patients, so she follows their advice. But obtaining informed consent is complicated. Mr. Richards cannot say 'yes' or 'no'. If he were able to do so then no-one would interfere, even if the operation were risky. But since he can't, everyone involved is worried since no-one wants to be accused of negligence. Indeed the ward doctor worried that this would happen. Knowing that 'recurrent ulceration' is not a strong indication for an operation, she wrote instead: 'Danger of infection due to recurrent ulcerations'.

But the surgeon has disagreed. The implication is that the ward doctor's willingness to listen to the nursing staff reflects bad care. Nurses have no authority to participate in the decision-making process. Qualified medical professionals make such decisions. None of this is officially stated. Instead, it is turned informally into 'negligence' on the part of the nurses that has led to recurrent ulceration. It is a consequence of the actions of the nurses. Distorted logics and ankles. Does bad nursing causes ulceration? Or is it that a bad ankle causes ulcerations that cannot be prevented even by good (nursing) care?

Transition zone

Care of moving – that is what we have been describing. But if you watch how these patients are cared for there are many other forms of care too: of cleaning, loving, or treating, writing, or excreting; care of communicating, or temporalizing, defining, or individualizing, and, of course, care of eating and feeding.

This is what we did: from each of these care procedures, we created a visual arrangement of more or less controversial practices that we intertwined to create a configuration. For some this was an artistic installation. We called this 'A Topography of the Possible. What is a Body/a Person?' For us this was a method for displaying the syndrome that textbooks call 'vegetative state' as a dynamic configuration. (In German textbooks it is referred to as 'Apallic Syndrome' or 'Coma Vigil'.) We were not trying to depict 'bad care'. We were not seeking to criticize the scientific disciplines or professionals from the outside. Instead we were trying to sensitize people to the relationships between practices and meanings, and show how the latter might change with the frame of reference. One could categorize our endeavour as something like a visual ethnography. This did not sim-

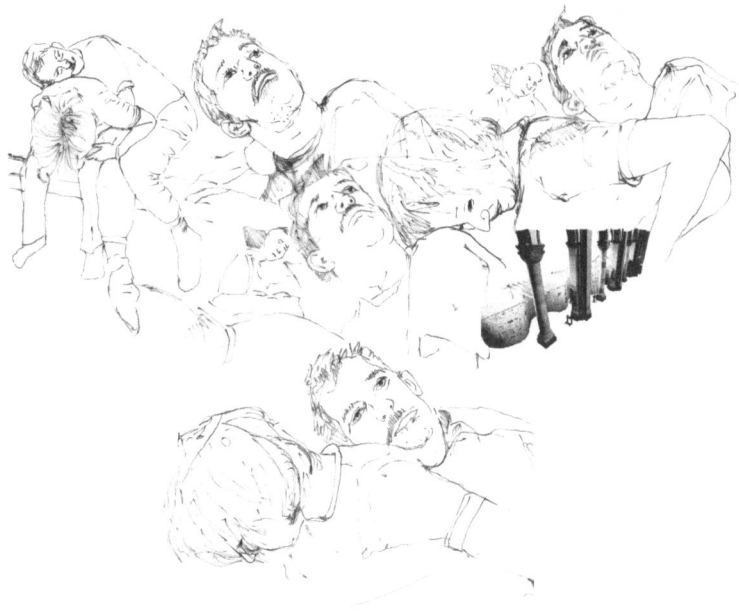

Figure 8: Nurse establishing 'body communication'

ply rely on text, photographs or video. It also used painting and techniques of montage to visually juxtapose, articulate, and relate practices that are usually difficult to take in at a single glance.

We showed this installation in various exhibitions. Often we found that it provoked debates about 'big' ethical questions, rather than discussions about the complex and mundane relations of sometimes cumbersome care procedures. It seemed as if the syndrome and the taken-for-granted moral dimensions of the topic attracted more interest than the 'praxiography' itself.

You will probably know the big questions: they centre around our conceptualizations of life, and whether it is worthwhile living in a 'vegetative' state. Bereft of perception, intelligence, reason and the capacity for voluntary movement, such patients are only capable of visceral functions: digestion, circulation, body temperature, breathing. Does it make sense to keep them alive and at what cost? Are there remnants of consciousness, or the soul? Do patients feel pain? Will they wake up in the end, or inevitably remain in a coma for the rest of their lives? And, of course, there is the question as to whether 'we' should withdraw nutrition and let 'them' die? Please keep in mind that we are talking of severely disabled people with a heterogeneous clinical picture. Even experts do not know how to categorize them 'properly'. The same experts frequently feel the need to avoid generalized predictions about outcomes or treatment. So there are no clear-cut answers to any of these questions. Rather, there are issues to do with quality, with the level of cumbersome care, and case management. And this is what we were trying to visualise for the public. So we were caught in wild oscillations between different reductionist, holistic, philosophical and spiritual arguments. Yet this wasn't just how audiences far removed from concrete experience of the syndrome reacted. It also showed up in our own reasoning and, interestingly, among staff and family members (an additional group of experts) when they visited our installation. It was as if they were looking at something strange and exotic that had little to do with them, and they seemed to feel obliged to classify what they were doing on a daily basis morally, or to rank this. Whereas in practice these big questions rarely played a dominant role. But then, how to get back to the questions of care?

Transformation

We would like to come back to the transformation we referred to at the beginning of our account. This transformation has to do with who we are (as members of a research/art group), the way in which we work, with our long-standing presence (in the field), and how this is related to a topic that obviously has much to do with care. Furthermore, perhaps it also has to do with the altered meaning we started to give to the word 'care'. We started to use it in the sense of the German word *kümmern*. This has several meanings but has no direct relation to nursing care. When translated into English, a rather superficial glance at the dictionary includes the following: to pay attention, to worry about, to tend, to attend to, to care about, /for/; to look after/to, to see about/to, to take care, etc. And we think this has something to do with the problem that we started to explore. We came to see our work as a kind of care/*kümmern* for the syndrome. A form of care that we have rarely made explicit to ourselves or others – until now.

Well you will probably say – how can that be? All this visual stuff you are producing – the exhibitions, how can you say that you are not making something explicit? Well, yes, we did this in a very standard way. We did this in the way it is done in journalism, TV-documentaries and sometimes in social science and the arts. This is a moment when people start to observe, to gaze, to describe, to use 'something' (a topic, a problem, etc.). They run away with it and then they start to work with it. What happens next? The answer is that they move, displace themselves, and travel on to the next 'something'. Leaving behind good or bad descriptions, analyses, reflections, disclosures, and all the rest. This is a mode of care that seeks to make 'something' explicit, and most of the time our work is read in this way. But we are increasingly struggling with a feeling of unease about this. This is because our understanding of caring for 'something' (a topic, problem, event) has started to change.

In our 'care for moving' section we tried to show some mundane moments in careful care, and a little about the people interested in the well-being of marginalized patients. You may have been surprised that alongside these taken-for-granted everyday practices we also included an anonymous letter, a debate about the authority to decide on an operation, or discussion of professional ethics about what it means to handle bodies with care. But we included these because we wanted to show how intricate 'care for moving' can be, or better, how intricate it can be to make explicit whether 'something' is to count as good care or not.

Good care or bad care?

We have tried to show that it is sometimes difficult to decide this question. Who should judge whether something is 'bad care'? As we have mentioned, instead of mainly seeing 'bad care' we repeatedly witnessed care that was unequivocally good. We witnessed it in situations with doctors, nurses, family members, and therapists.

Frequently, especially in nursing care, we encountered a form of care, that is not made explicit, that is not talked about or explained. This was not only to be found at the bedside, but also in situations where straightforward nursing knowledge is being made explicit. Take, for instance, the working group of ward nurses undertaking a research project on the effectiveness of specific nursing concepts. In its meetings, we found inarticulate, bodily, 'fleshy' or visceral forms of knowledge and practical experience that lay beyond big, strategic intentions, plans or programs. Here, we realized that the vegetative patient becomes a set of embodied categories including: weight; body or muscle tension; changes in the body that might be abrupt, continuous, or show signs of decrease or increase; smells; breathing rhythms; skin colour and temperature; facial expressions; minimal involuntary movements; vocalizations; and utterances.

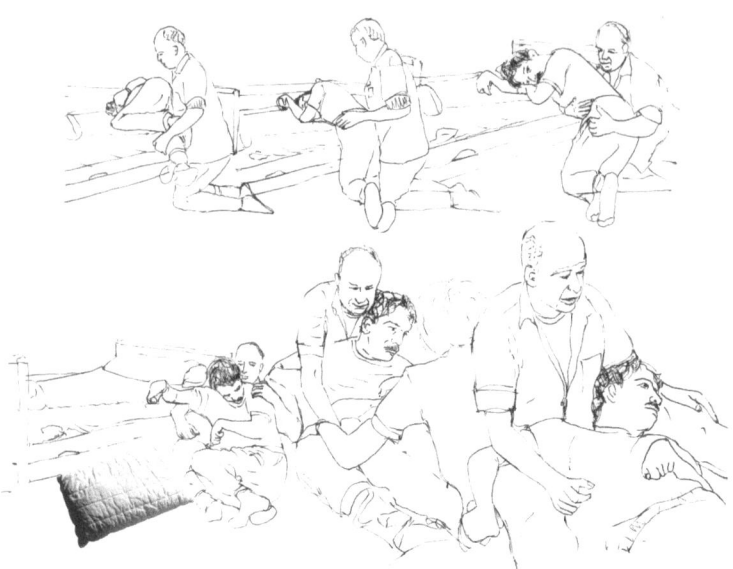

Figure 9: Physiotherapist transferring patient from bed to the floor

Yet, it was interesting to see how reluctant the caregivers were to provide explicit categories for what they described as 'gut-feelings'. Everybody agreed that it is important to gather, write down and talk about signs and symptoms. This would allow implicit knowledge to be communicated with other disciplines.

Nevertheless some worried that making care explicit for research purposes was in tension with taking care of patients themselves. And this had nothing to do with laziness or shortage of time. It was rather that while it might be beguiling to make care explicit this also missed the point. To do so was to put care at risk by intruding into a quiet realm, by disrupting concentration, or by undermining its skills by making these explicit.

Nevertheless, our account also shows that (disciplinary) practices of care may be made explicit when it is necessary to make different versions of care commensurable. How do you move bodies and persons? How do you relate versions of careful care, make them commensurable, without knowing in advance whether this or that form of care is good or bad? How do you contribute to what one might think of as evolution or drift in shared knowledge or ideas to do (for instance) with moving, when these forms of practice may not previously have existed in that form?

Today we ask ourselves: What was it that actually happened there in the field with us? For a book about care, why not simply attempt to describe, sketch, show, the care that we saw? Perhaps the answer is this. That we are quite similar to the nurses, and have become reluctant to demonstrate our gaze at or on 'something'. Instead, we have apparently become interested in, paid attention to, worried about, attended to, and cared for the version(s) of the syndrome that we enacted in the course of our stay in the field. So what does care, then, mean for us?

Presence and 'Inarticulateness'

We think that it has something to do with our continuous presence (in the field). We are simply there. What would they say if you were to ask the nurses, therapists, family members, the chief physician, administrators, the head nurse, even the patients (some of them demonstrate awareness of their environment): who are these people who regularly spend time at the ward doing various more or less strange things? They would probably hesitate and search for words. Yes, some would remember that this group has a funny name – something like 'The Research Centre for Shared Incompetence'. They would smile and say that they think that it has something to do with art (they know our exhibition work), or journalism or maybe sociology (we asked them for contributions to a book).

Perhaps, they would add, it also has a medical background (we are working at the bedside with some patients). Or possibly it is a kind of research (we conduct 'pillow research' and are part of the nursing research team). Or film making (we provided several short films for events organized by the Austrian Coma Vigil Association). Or perhaps we are there for private reasons, or as volunteers workers (we were involved in the administration of the estate of a patient who died, and did other kinds of 'social work')?

Four years ago we had a clear aim. Inspired and motivated by the book *The Body Multiple*, various other texts and previous experiences, we intended to do a kind of visual ethnography. This provided legitimacy for us and for those we wanted to observe, and allowed us to enter and stay in the field. But during the last two to three years our attitude changed. Along with our attempt to look at, listen to, understand, and describe 'something', we also began to do 'something' *together with* the carers. We stayed at the site and hung around without far-reaching plans, strategies, programs or any mission to help, to advise, or perhaps to criticize or reveal something discreditable like

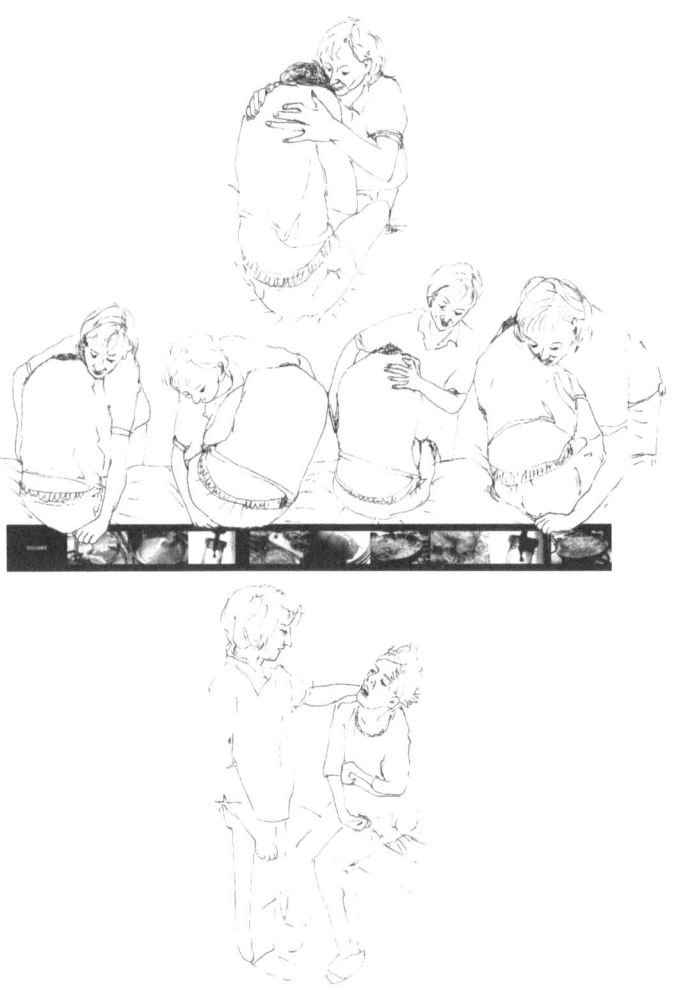

Figure 10: Nurse moving a patient in sitting position alongside the edge of the bed

inequality, discrimination, or bad care. We worked in a way similar to the 'found footage' approach in film-making, in which people work with – sometimes literally - film fragments they have found, without shooting new footage. So we waited (and we still wait) for situations, opportunities, coincidences in which to share our (in)competences and develop our work (or care?) for the syndrome.

Our presence and the work that we do seems to be appreciated (so far, nobody has chased us away). Yet, people do not talk about it much. Yes, we think that our presence and some of our work has had some impact on the understanding of care of the vegetative and minimally conscious patients in the ward, but we have never made this explicit. Like the nurses, we rarely classify or categorize the activities that have followed from our comparatively undirected interest. People consider us to be part of the 'care for the syndrome', and we come and go, involved in practicalities, quite like the family members who spend a lot of time with their next of kin. These people care for 'their' patient, they develop their own styles and logics of care and some of them also engage with more public dimensions of the syndrome.

We entangled ourselves in the care for the syndrome without having a working contract, and without having filled out forms for the ethical committees that decide about research. We developed the sentiment that we have a right to do so since we provide care for the syndrome because we are involved. This is *kümmern*: we attend to it, pay attention it, worry about it, and all the rest.

'Explicitness' in the form of (art)work(s) and artefacts

From time to time we feel the need to make something of our work explicit: when we feel the necessity of making our realities, our 'care practices', commensurable with protagonists in the field. Instead of showing our work, the images, the photographs, the 'visual ethnography', to an external audience (though we have done this too), we have shown it to an internal audience and tried to test it with those who may be directly affected by our suggestions.

At such moments we have tried to make our care explicit in the form of (art)works and artefacts and/or initiatives or performances that might perhaps create moments of translation. These are moments of problematisation that might elicit concern and interest and so enrol patients and non-patients, including ourselves and inserting them (and us) into new and surprising roles. (Yes, here we are alluding to a sociology of translation, but less as a tool for description than as a guide for construction or enactment). So here are the questions. Could the care for 'something' (in this case for a syndrome) also be applicable as a method of work in the arts or the social sciences? Might it be made to belong to those who are doing the careful and or careless mundane work of care that tries to help patients and/or to enrich the syndrome by their respective practices? In the context vegetative state might it be possible, for us, to forget or leave undetermined for a moment the 'big' and centring questions about life and death? So that this care at least temporarily implies a kind of decentring of the patient. And that it defers decisions that follow from an outside 'gaze': whether this is blunt, humanist, cold or empathic, loving, hating or dissecting, holistic or reductionist. Instead it attempts to create some mutually shared experiences of care in the field. Here are three examples to illustrate what this might mean.

- We conduct what we call 'pillow research'. Pillows are ubiquitous. They form part of the everyday handling and positioning of patients. They are almost part of them. They embody situated knowledge in, but not just in, the clinical routine. Pillows are also part of the worlds of doctors, nurses, family members, administrators, researchers and artists. They are part of our memories and they have a history. Pillow research explores the construction of pillows in a very broad sense of the word. It is an attempt to experiment with forms and functions of sculptural medico-technical artefacts in the context of the routines of clinical nursing. Thus the notion of what a pillow is, or what it can do, should be the result of a collaborative procedure in the ward. Our experimental work with pillows in the clinical context may touch (in the best case 'translate') issues that are part of the syndrome including diagnosis, consciousness or 'knowing' bodies.

- We took part in the research working group of the nursing staff mentioned above. This tries to explore and test the effects of innovative nursing concepts. After two years of watching, we decided to become active, and initiated and helped to implement a new assessment technique. Suddenly we found ourselves in the middle of a turbulent collective experience involving the medical staff and family members that might alter and improve some aspects of the daily lives of patients. This experience also helped us to think through our ideas about the 'big' holism/reductionism dualism because it brought 'holistic' and 'embodied' care concepts together with a reductionist, neuro-cognitive stimulus-response paradigm for assessment.

- Finally, we experimented with the question: how does it feel to become a family member of a person/body who is suffering from the syndrome? This was driven by a feeling of responsibility for a patient who no longer has any relations with the outside world. But how does this relate to our care for (a version of) the syndrome? A photographic novelette might illustrate this. These workings and works make matters explicit in a way that goes beyond text or words. It gives us the opportunity to articulate our standpoints, relations and realities. It is the (sometimes risky) attempt to make them commensurable. It is work that continues.

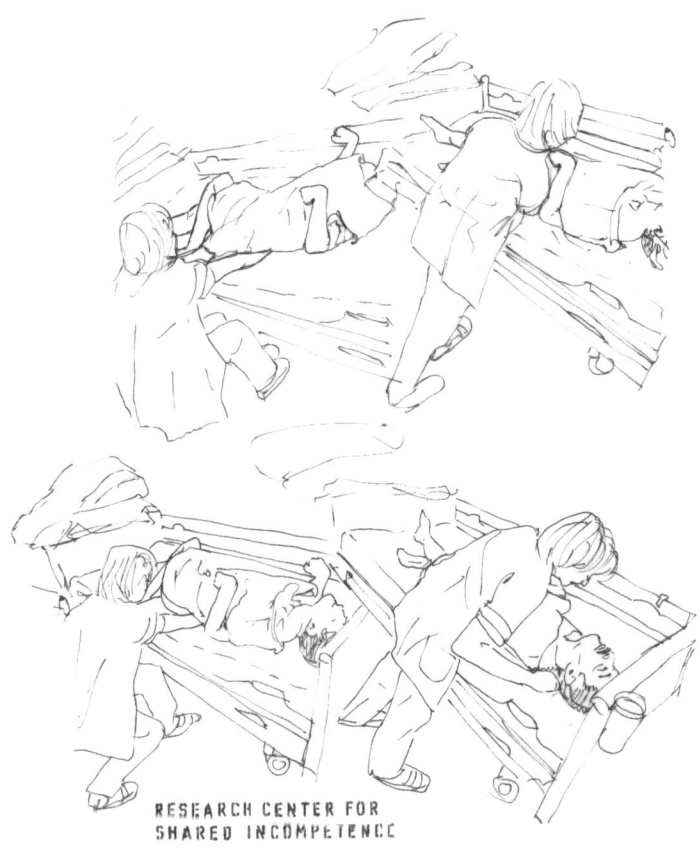

Figure 11: Nurse pulling the pelvis of the patient towards the edge of the bed

As a result of our quest for the creation of moments of commensurability, our work(s) change. It is elusive, open ended, and fragmentary. It drifts. These moments are important pointers or markers that help us to refine our version(s) of the syndrome. Of course, the creation of these gatherings of things (strange objects, initiatives, procedures, artworks) is an act of translation and transformation, that brings disruption, disturbance, loss or abandonment. In this it is like the experience of the nurses when they try to make their embodied categories explicit. These shifts between the inarticulate and the explicit create constraints that have become a prerequisite of our work as it has developed over the past few years. They are the result of our entanglement in the care for a syndrome that transformed us and that we wanted to describe – to make explicit – in this article.

Acknowledgements

The project 'Performing Shared Incompetence - A Topography of the Possible. What is a Body/a Person?' has been realized within the transdisciplinary research programm 'TRAFO' of the Austrian Ministry of Sciene and is further developed as 'Pillow Research' within the 'Translational Research Programm' of the Austrian Science Fundation (FWF). Further we want to thank John Law for correcting the English.

List of authors

Blanca Callén is a researcher in the Social Psychology, Department at the Autonomous University of Barcelona (UAB) and consultant professor at the Faculty of Psychology at the Catalonia Open University (UOC). Email: blanca.callen@uab.cat

Miquel Domènech is Senior Lecturer in Social Psychology at the Universitat Autònoma de Barcelona. His research interests centre broadly on the field of science and technology studies (STS), with a special focus on the relationship between technical innovation and power relationships. At the Universitat Autònoma de Barcelona he leads GESCIT (Grup d'Estudis Socials de la Ciència i la Tecnologia) a group of researchers on Science and Technology Studies. Email: Miquel.Domenech@uab.cat

Hans Harbers, farmer's son and trained as a sociologist, is Associate Professor in Philosophy of Science, Technology & Society at the Department of Philosophy, University of Groningen, Netherlands. Email: j.a.harbers@rug.nl

Henriette Langstrup is assistant professor at the Department of Health Service Research, University of Copenhagen. Her current research is concerned with 'the home' in the political, clinical and everyday management of chronic illness. Email: helan@sund.ku.dk

John Law is Professor of Sociology at the Open University in the UK, and a director of the ESRC Centre for Research on Socio-Cultural Change. He writes on non-coherent methods; people technologies and animals; biosecurity; agriculture and disaster; and alternative knowledge spaces. His personal web page is at www.heterogeneities.net

Daniel López is lecturer in Social Psychology at Universitat Oberta de Catalunya. He is currently working on the implementation of new technologies in care settings, specifically Home Telecare, and the technoscientific controversies of the new care policies in Spain. Email: dlopezgo@uoc.edu

LIST OF AUTHORS

Annemarie Mol is Socrates Professor of *Social Theory, Humanism & Materialities* at the University of Amsterdam. As a member of the Department of Sociology & Anthropology she just started a long-term joint research project on *The eating body in Western practice and theory*. Email: a.mol@uva.nl

Tiago Moreira is Lecturer in Sociology at Durham University (UK). He has published on the collective production of health care standards and regimes of therapeutic development and evaluation. His current research focuses on health care priority setting, the governance of ageing research and the role of patient organisations in the knowledge society. Email: tiago.moreira@durham.ac.uk

Ingunn Moser is professor and dean in the Department of Nursing and Health Care, Diakonhjemmet University College, Oslo, and also professor of sociology in Bodø University College. She has published extensively on disability, subjectivity and embodiment in relation to new technologies. Her most recent research deals with the different and changing understandings of dementia, and with care approaches to dementia in particular. Email: moser@diakonhjemmet.no

Jeannette Pols Works as a postdoc researcher at the department of General Practice, section Medical Ethics, Academic Medical Centre (AMC), University of Amsterdam. Her research interests are normativities in care, medical technology at home and knowledge of chronic patients. Email: a.j.pols@amc.uva.nl

Vicky Singleton is Senior Lecturer in the Centre for Science Studies and the Centre for Gender and Women's Studies, Department of Sociology, Lancaster University, UK. She practiced as a Registered General Nurse prior to academia and her key research interests are in health policy and practices as well as in farming. Email: d.singleton@lancaster.ac.uk

Janelle S. Taylor is Associate Professor of Anthropology at the University of Washington, in Seattle. She is currently pursuing research on medical education as well as on dementia. Email: jstaylor@uw.edu

Francisco Tirado is Senior Lecturer in the Social Psychology Department of the Universitat Autònoma de Barcelona and full member of the Group for Social Studies of Science and Technology (GESCIT). His main research interests are: a) power relations and political action in socio-technical contexts and b) biopolitics and technology. Email: franciscojavier.tirado@uab.es

Dick Willems studied medicine and philosophy at the Universities of Groningen (Netherlands) and Paris-IV. Having worked for 15 years as a general practitioner, he is now a professor of medical ethics at the University of Amsterdam. Email: d.l.willems@amc.uva.nl

Myriam Winance has a research position at the INSERM (National Institute for Medical research). As a member of the CERMES (Research Centre on Medicine, Science and Society), she works on disability. Email: winance@vjf.cnrs.fr

Brit Ross Winthereik is Associate Professor at the IT University of Copenhagen. Her current research centers on the role of instruments and formalized objects for knowledge production in development aid partnerships and within the academy. Email: brwi@itu.dk

XPERIMENT!/SHARED INC.
The working group XPERIMENT! (Bernd Kraeftner, Judith Kroell, Isabell Warner) operates the Research Centre for Shared Incompetence as a research strategy that employs and transforms methods from the sciences and the arts. The transdisciplinary group explores the messy and heterogeneous interfaces between science and society and for this purpose conducted research projects funded by the Austrian Ministry of Science, the WellcomeFoundation/SciArt, London; the ZKM, Karlsruhe, the Humboldt University, Berlin etc. Currently (2008-2010), the group (together with L. Peschta and G. Ramsebner) works on the research/art project 'Pillow Research: multiple diagnoses and hidden talents", sponsored within the 'Translational-Research-Program' of the Austrian Science Foundation. The group (together with M. Guggenheim) recently started with a long-term project that focuses on provision and care in the event of anticipated emergencies within the 'Arts & Science Call 2009' of The Vienna Science and Technology Fund (WWTF). Email: collective@xperiment.at

Lay out and typography
Rob Kreuger works as scientific illustrator and graphic designer at the Academic Medical Centre (AMC/University of Amsterdam. Webpage: www.medischeillustraties.nl